S.T.A.B.L.E.® – Cardiac Module

Recognition and Stabilization of Neonates with Severe CHD

Second Edition

Kristine A. Karlsen, PhD, APRN, NNP-BC, FAAN

The S.T.A.B.L.E. Program Author/Founder

Park City, Utah

Clinical affiliation

Neonatal Nurse Practitioner

Neonatal Intensive Care Unit

Intermountain® Primary Children's Hospital

Salt Lake City, Utah

Collin G. Cowley, MD, FAAP, FACC, FAHA

Medical Director, Pediatric Cardiology

PEDIATRIX Specialty Care of Utah

Former Professor of Pediatrics

Division of Pediatric Cardiology

University of Utah

Salt Lake City, Utah

S.T.A.B.L.E.® – Cardiac Module
Recognition and Stabilization of Neonates with Severe CHD

SECOND EDITION ISBN: 978-1-937967-17-8

John S. Gibb, MA
Medical Illustrator/Animator

Kristin Bernhisel Osborn, MFA
Graphic Designer

Notice

This educational program provides general guidelines for the assessment and stabilization of sick infants with suspected congenital heart disease. Because of rapid advances in nursing and medicine, independent verification of diagnoses, stabilization recommendations, and drug utilization and doses, should always be made by the healthcare professional. Medical decisions should not be made based solely upon the content herein. Changes in nursing and medicine may impact the patient care recommendations contained in this book. It is the responsibility of the reader to verify their care practices are current with any new evidence that arises. To the fullest extent of the law, no responsibility is assumed by and no damages may be assessed against the authors, the content reviewers, the publisher, or S.T.A.B.L.E., Inc., for any injury and/or damage to persons as a matter of negligence, or otherwise, or from any use of the instructions, guidelines, or recommendations contained in the content herein. While caring for infants, healthcare professionals may encounter situations, conditions, and illnesses not described in this book. It is strongly recommended that additional nursing and medical education materials and consultation with neonatal and cardiology experts are utilized when necessary. Use of this book implies your acceptance of this notice.

Cardiothoracic Surgery and Cardiology

American Academy of Pediatrics Section on Cardiology and Cardiac Surgery

Michael Carr, MD, FAAP, FACC
Pediatric Cardiology
Ann & Robert H. Lurie Children's Hospital of Chicago
Program Director, Cardiology Fellowship
Associate Professor
Northwestern Feinberg School of Medicine
Chicago, Illinois

Aaron "Rusty" Eckhauser, MD, MS
Associate Professor
Pediatric Cardiothoracic Surgery
Division of Cardiothoracic Surgery
Salt Lake City, Utah

Lloyd Y. Tani, MD, FAAP, FAHA, FACC, FASE
Professor of Pediatrics
Division of Pediatric Cardiology
University of Utah/Primary Children's Hospital
Salt Lake City, Utah

Neonatology

Diane E. Lorant, MD, FAAP
Project Chief – Neonatology Reviewers
Associate Professor of Clinical Pediatrics
Division of Neonatal-Perinatal Medicine,
Department of Pediatrics
Riley Hospital for Children
Indianapolis, Indiana

American Academy of Pediatrics Committee on Fetus and Newborn

American Academy of Pediatrics Section on Neonatal-Perinatal Medicine

Ryan McAdams, MD
Neonatology Division Chief
Division of Global Pediatrics
Department of Pediatrics
University of Wisconsin School of Medicine and Public Health
Madison, Wisconsin

Mary L. Puchalski, DNP, APRN, CNS, NNP-BC
Ann & Robert H. Lurie Children's Hospital of Chicago
University of Illinois at Chicago
Chicago, Illinois

Elizabeth Rex, RN, MSN, NNP
UCSF Benioff Children's Hospital
Intensive Care Nursery and Emergency Transport
Oakland, California

Elizabeth Sharpe, DNP, APRN, NNP-BC, VA-BC, FAANP, FAAN
Associate Professor Clinical Nursing
NNP Specialty Track Director
The Ohio State University
Columbus, Ohio

Howard Stein, MD, FAAP
Director of Neonatology
Ebeid Children's Hospital
Professor of Pediatrics
University of Toledo College of Medicine and Life Sciences
Toledo, Ohio

Genetics

Sabrina Malone Jenkins, MD
Assistant Professor of Pediatrics
Department of Pediatrics Neonatology
University of Utah
Salt Lake City

Laila Andoni, MS, CGC
Licensed Certified Genetic Counselor
Primary Children's Hospital
Salt Lake City, Utah

Lindsay Meyers, MS, LCGC
Certified Genetic Counselor
Sr. Manager, Cardiology and Pediatric Genetic Services
Genome Medical Services
S. San Francisco, California

This book is dedicated to all of the little heart warriors who fight to survive

and to all the healthcare professionals who work tirelessly to save their lives and

improve their outcomes. And to my family – Torbjorn, Annika, and Solveig,

whose support throughout these years has allowed me to work, learn, and write.

— Kris A Karlsen

I want to express my gratitude to Kris Karlsen for her vision and tireless efforts

in guiding this project and for allowing me the opportunity to participate.

I'd like to dedicate my efforts to the spirit of collaboration among all healthcare

providers and institutions that make real progress possible.

— Collin G. Cowley

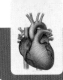

Acronyms Used in this Book . . . . Inside front cover

Introduction 1

Part 1 History and Patient Assessment **3**

Incidence of Congenital Heart Disease (CHD) 3

History and Patient Presentation 4

Neonatal History 4

Pregnancy, Labor, and Delivery History 4

Maternal Medical History. 5

Recurrence Risk. 5

Patient Assessment

Neurologic Status 8

Physical Appearance – Size and Features. 9

Infant of the Diabetic Mother (IDM) 10

Small for Gestational Age (SGA) Infants 12

Syndromes and Chromosomal Abnormalities Associated with CHD 13

Trisomy 21 (Down Syndrome) 13

Trisomy 18 (Edwards Syndrome) 16

Trisomy 13 (Patau Syndrome) 17

What does it mean? Let's talk about a persistent Patent Ductus Arteriosus (PDA). 18

Monosomy X (Turner Syndrome – XO chromosome). 19

CHARGE Syndrome 20

VACTERL Association. 22

22q11.2 Deletion Syndrome (22q11.2DS) 22

What does it mean? Conotruncal. 24

Color 25

Oxygen Saturation 26

Vital Signs – Respiratory Rate and Effort 29

Vital Signs – Heart Rate and Rhythm 30

Treatment of Supraventricular Tachycardia (SVT) 34

Adenosine 36

Vital Signs – Blood Pressure (BP) 38

Shock 43

Bruit 44

Pulses 45

Skin Perfusion and Appearance. 46

Precordial Activity 48

Heart Sounds. 49

Table of Contents

Heart Murmur 52

Liver Size and Location. 57

What does it mean? Situs solitus, situs inversus, and heterotaxy. 58

Diagnostic Tests 62

Differential Diagnosis 64

Part 2 Clinical Presentation and Stabilization of Neonates with Severe CHD 67

What does it mean? Let's talk about CHD that is ductal dependent. 68

Pharmacology – Prostaglandin E1 (PGE, Alprostadil, Prostin) 70

Left-Sided Obstructive Lesions, Ductal Dependent for Systemic Blood Flow 72

Underlying Concepts 72

Coarctation of the Aorta 74

Interrupted Aortic Arch 76

Aortic Valve Stenosis 78

Hypoplastic Left Heart Syndrome 80

Left-sided Obstructive Lesions – Clinical Presentation 82

Left-Sided Obstructive Lesions – Chest X-Ray 82

Left-sided Obstructive Lesions – Initial Stabilization 84

Case Study: 1-Day old infant with HLHS 85

Cyanotic Congenital Heart Disease, Not Ductal Dependent for Pulmonary Blood Flow 86

Underlying Concepts and Stabilizing the Cyanotic Neonate with Suspected CHD . . . 86

Tetralogy of Fallot 88

Tetralogy of Fallot – Clinical Presentation 90

Tetralogy of Fallot – Chest X-Ray 91

Tetralogy of Fallot – Initial Stabilization 92

What does it mean? Let's talk about hypercyanotic/tet spells. 93

Hypercyanotic/Tet Spell – Treatment Principles. 95

What does it mean? Let's talk about Double Outlet Right Ventricle (DORV). . . 98

Tricuspid Atresia 102

Tricuspid Atresia – Clinical Presentation 104

Tricuspid Atresia – Chest X-Ray 106

Tricuspid Atresia – Initial Stabilization 107

Truncus Arteriosus 108

Truncus Arteriosus – Clinical Presentation 110

Truncus Arteriosus – Chest X-Ray 110

Truncus Arteriosus – Initial Stabilization 111

Total Anomalous Pulmonary Venous Connection 112

Supracardiac TAPVC 114

Cardiac TAPVC 116

Table of Contents

Infracardiac TAPVC (also called infradiaphragmatic). .117

Total Anomalous Pulmonary Venous Connection – Clinical Presentation 118

Total Anomalous Pulmonary Venous Connection – Chest X-Ray 118

Total Anomalous Pulmonary Venous Connection – Initial Stabilization 119

Ebstein Anomaly 120

Ebstein Anomaly – Clinical Presentation 122

Ebstein Anomaly – Chest X-Ray 122

Ebstein Anomaly – Initial Stabilization 123

Cyanotic Congenital Heart Disease, Ductal Dependent for Pulmonary Blood Flow 124

Underlying Concepts 124

Stabilizing the Cyanotic Neonate with Ductal Dependent Pulmonary Blood Flow. 125

Pulmonary Atresia with Intact Ventricular Septum (PA-IVS). 126

Pulmonary Atresia with Intact Ventricular Septum (PA-IVS) – Clinical Presentation 128

Pulmonary Atresia with Intact Ventricular Septum (PA-IVS) – Chest X-Ray 128

Pulmonary Atresia with Intact Ventricular Septum (PA-IVS) – Initial Stabilization 129

What does it mean? Let's talk about PA-IVS and Ventriculocoronary Connections.. 130

Pulmonary Atresia and Ventricular Septal Defect (PA-VSD). 132

Pulmonary Atresia and Ventricular Septal Defect (PA-VSD) – Clinical Presentation 134

Pulmonary Atresia and Ventricular Septal Defect (PA-VSD) – Chest X-Ray 135

Pulmonary Atresia and Ventricular Septal Defect (PA-VSD) – Initial Stabilization 135

Transposition of the Great Arteries (TGA) 136

Transposition of the Great Arteries – Clinical Presentation 138

Transposition of the Great Arteries – Chest X-Ray 140

Transposition of the Great Arteries – Initial Stabilization .141

What does it mean? What is the difference between D-TGA and L-TGA? 144

Part 3 S.T.A.B.L.E. – Cardiac Module 147

Introduction 147

Sugar and Safe Care Module 147

Glucose Production and Utilization Rate 148

Initial IV Fluid Rate and Target Glucose Levels 148

IV Access and Central Lines 149

Umbilical Vein Catheter (UVC) 150

Umbilical Artery Catheter (UAC) and Peripheral Arterial Line (PAL) 152

Umbilical Catheter Safety. 154

Peripherally Inserted Central Catheter (PICC).. 155

Temperature Module 158

Table of Contents

Airway Module 159

O₂ Saturation, Hemoglobin, and CHD 160

O₂ Content 160

What does it mean? What is Regional Oximetry Monitoring – Near Infrared Reflective Spectroscopy (NIRS) Monitoring? . . 161

Pulse Oximetry Screening (POS) for Critical Congenital Heart Disease (CCHD) 162

Blood Pressure Module 166

Methods for Measuring BP 166

Oscillometric Measurement – How Does it Work? 167

Lab Work Module 168

Blood Sugar 168

Blood Gas 168

Lactic Acid/Lactate 168

Electrolytes and Renal Function Tests 169

Ionized Calcium 170

Magnesium 170

Liver Function Tests 171

Complete Blood Count with Differential 172

Cardiac Enzymes: B-Type Natriuretic Peptide (BNP) and Troponin . . . 173

What does it mean? Let's talk about Genetic Testing. 174

Emotional Support Module 176

Appendix – Palliative and Surgical Repair Options 179

References 216

Index 227

Cardiac Module *2nd edition*

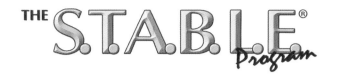

Sugar, Temperature, Airway, Blood Pressure, Lab Work, and Emotional Support

Introduction

The S.T.A.B.L.E. Program is an educational program designed for all maternal/child healthcare professionals (nurses, physicians, respiratory therapists, and prehospital providers) to address the pretransport stabilization and postresuscitation care of sick neonates. All information in The S.T.A.B.L.E. Program applies to neonates with cardiac conditions. This resource includes additional guidelines for neonates with severe congenital heart disease (CHD).

Part 1 will focus on the history and physical examination of neonates with suspected CHD; Part 2 will focus on the presentation and stabilization of infants with severe structural heart disease; and Part 3 will discuss The S.T.A.B.L.E. Program postresuscitation stabilization modules — Sugar, Temperature, Airway, Blood pressure, Lab work, and Emotional support — and adaptations that may be necessary when caring for neonates with CHD. An Appendix is included to explain the palliative and surgical options to address the cardiac defects described in this book.

Incidence of Congenital Heart Disease (CHD)

Worldwide, approximately 8 babies per 1,000 live births, or just under 1% of all babies born, will have some form of CHD.[1-3] Globally, this rate equates to 1.35 million babies born each year with CHD.[3] In the United States, with an annual birth rate just under 4 million,[4] 39,000 infants will have CHD and approximately 25% will have the most severe forms, that are known as critical congenital heart defects (CCHDs).[5,6] These infants will require care by neonatal and cardiac experts in the first days to weeks of life. Prompt, effective care of neonates with CHD can reduce secondary organ damage, improve short- and long-term outcomes, and reduce mortality.[7]

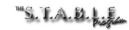

Cardiac Module
2nd Edition – Part 1

Incidence of Congenital Heart Disease

› Worldwide just under 1% of newborns will have CHD
  ▪ Not all will be severe forms
› Each year approximately 39,000 infants born in the U.S. will have CHD (annual U.S. birth rate ~ 3.9 million)
  ▪ 10,000 (1/4) will be critically ill at birth or soon after birth as a result of their CHD

U.S., Annual Rate of CHD

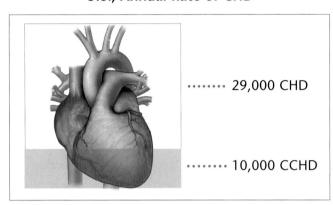

········ 29,000 CHD

········ 10,000 CCHD

39,000 infants will have CHD and approximately 25% will have the most severe critical congenital heart defects (CCHDs).

Infants Born with CHD Per Year

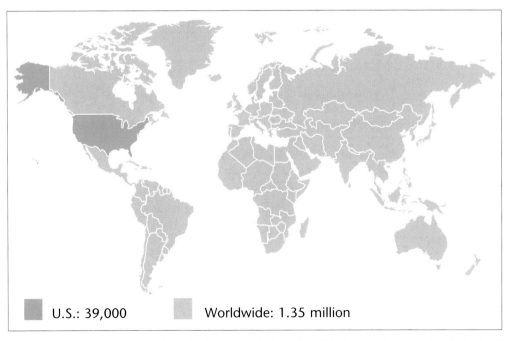

U.S.: 39,000   Worldwide: 1.35 million

Worldwide, approximately 8 babies per 1,000 live births, or just under 1% of all babies born, will have some form of CHD.

History and Patient Presentation

When a neonate presents with cyanosis, respiratory distress, and/or shock, the process of determining whether signs and symptoms are due to pulmonary, cardiac, infectious, neurologic, or other causes begins.[2] Information valuable to differential diagnosis includes evaluation of the presenting signs and timing of presentation, as well as family, pregnancy, and maternal medical history.

Neonatal History[2,8]

A baby who presents with severe cyanosis, congestive heart failure (CHF), and/or cardiovascular collapse within the first hours, days, or weeks of life must be evaluated for CHD. The timing and history of symptom onset are very important. A term infant who has been well the first few days of life, but who becomes tachypneic, feeds poorly, sleeps more than normal, and/or displays signs of shock should prompt consideration of left-sided obstructive CHD with a closing ductus arteriosus. The infant with early onset respiratory distress following a difficult birth or born to a group B streptococcus positive mother is more likely suffering from pulmonary disease or the effects of sepsis. A preterm infant is more likely to have pulmonary causes of respiratory distress, although cardiac disease does occur in both preterm and term infants.

Pregnancy, Labor, and Delivery History

Pregnancy, labor, and delivery complications should be carefully evaluated for risk factors that could affect the cardiovascular system or conditions that mimic CHD.[2] For example, intrauterine and perinatal hypoxia are risk factors for development of myocardial dysfunction, as well as persistent pulmonary hypertension of the newborn (PPHN). Risk factors for sepsis should be identified, as septic

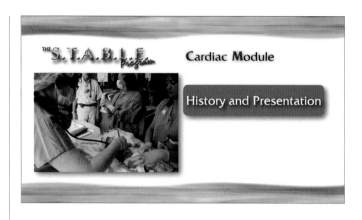

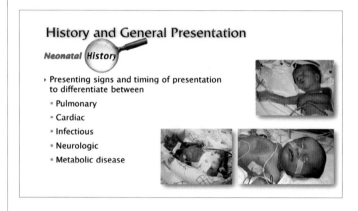

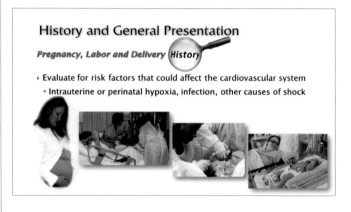

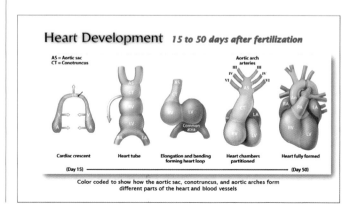

neonates may present in shock similar to those with left heart obstructive lesions. Other causes of shock, including maternal/fetal hemorrhage, should be identified and treated.

Maternal Medical History[1,9-24]

The heart develops very early in pregnancy. Between the 15th and 50th day after fertilization, the four-chamber heart has formed. After that, the heart continues to grow and mature.[25] Exposure to teratogens early in pregnancy, including alcohol, drugs of abuse, viruses, certain medications, and even elevated glucose levels, increases the risk for CHD. Maternal illnesses that may result in fetal anomalies including congenital heart defects, include diabetes, obesity, connective tissue disorders, and phenylketonuria (PKU). However, in the case of diabetes and PKU, it should be noted that strict preconception and intrapartum metabolic control can decrease or even eliminate risk to the developing fetus. Table 1.1 on page 6 summarizes maternal exposures, conditions, and illnesses that increase risk for CHD.

Recurrence Risk[18,26-32]

When a sibling or parent has a congenital heart defect, the question of recurrence risk arises. Family counseling involves consideration of many factors, including the type of CHD, other family members with CHD, and presence of genetic syndromes or other congenital anomalies.[33] Generally speaking, when one sibling has a congenital heart defect, the recurrence risk for other siblings ranges between 2% and approximately 4%. However, there is some evidence that left heart obstructive lesions, such as coarctation of the aorta, hypoplastic left heart syndrome, and aortic stenosis or atresia, are associated with an even higher risk of recurrence than other forms of CHD. Although not clearly understood why, when the mother has a congenital heart defect, the recurrence risk for CHD is higher in her offspring than when the father has CHD.

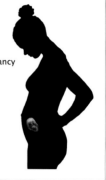
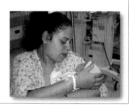
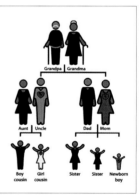
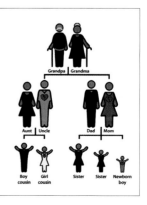

Exposures That Increase Risk for Congenital Heart Defects	
Drugs of Abuse	
Alcohol	VSD, ASD, PDA, TOF
Amphetamines	VSD, ASD, PDA, TGA
Medications	
Retinoic acid	Conotruncal defects
Antiepileptic agents Phenytoin, Trimethadione, Valproic acid, Hydantoin, Carbamazepine, Lamotrigine	Various CHDs associated: PAtr, PS, AS, COA, ASD, VSD, TGA, TOF, HLHS
Angiotensin-converting enzyme (ACE) inhibitors taken during 1st trimester	ASD, VSD, PDA, PS
Lithium	Ebstein anomaly and other CHDs
Hormones: Progesterone, Estrogen	VSD, TGA, TOF
Viral Infection	
Rubella[a]	PDA, branch PA stenosis, TOF, VSD, ASD, myocarditis, hydrops
Coxsackievirus B and cytomegalovirus (CMV)	Various CHDs if infection in early pregnancy Viral myocarditis if infection later in pregnancy
Zika[b]	ASD, VSD, PDA
Medical Conditions	
Pre-gestational type 1 and type 2 diabetes (preexisting diabetes during fetal cardiogenesis) **Gestational diabetes mellitus (GDM)**	TOF, TGA, Truncus, TA, VSD, COA, AV septal defects, cardiomyopathy
Obesity[c]	Various heart defects, including conotruncal, LVOT, and RVOTO defects
Systemic lupus erythematosus and connective tissue disorders	Complete heart block and cardiomyopathy
Maternal phenylketonuria[d]	COA, HLHS, TOF, ASD, VSD

a. The last major rubella epidemic in the U.S. was in 1965; however, rubella continues to affect immigrants.[21]

b. In one study,[34] 40% of infants with ZIKA viral exposure had cardiac defects but none was critical.

c. Positive associations are reported with higher categories of body mass index (BMI).

d. Strict preconception metabolic control can eliminate the risk.

VSD (ventricular septal defect), ASD (atrial septal defect), TOF (tetralogy of Fallot), PDA (patent ductus arteriosus), TGA (transposition of the great arteries), PAtr (pulmonary atresia), PS (pulmonary stenosis), AS (aortic stenosis), COA (coarctation of the aorta), HLHS (hypoplastic left heart syndrome), PA (pulmonary artery), Truncus (truncus arteriosus), TA (tricuspid atresia), LVOT (left ventricular outflow tract), RVOTO (right ventricular outflow tract obstruction)

Table 1.1. Exposures that Increase Risk for Congenital Heart Defects.[1,9-24,34]

The importance of performing a thorough physical exam cannot be emphasized enough, as exam findings often overlap among conditions. Diagnostic tests helpful in generating a differential diagnosis, as well as definitive diagnosis, include a chest x-ray, blood gas, lactate, other labs, echocardiogram, and electrocardiogram.

This patient assessment review will be organized in the following order:

- Neurological status
- Physical appearance – size and features
- Color and oxygen saturation
- Vital signs
- Bruit
- Pulses
- Skin perfusion

- Precordial activity
- Heart sounds
- Heart murmurs
- Liver size and location
- Diagnostic tests
- Differential diagnosis

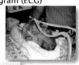

Differential Diagnosis for CHD

Physical Exam
› Exam findings often overlap between conditions
› Be alert for clues that indicate CHD

Diagnostic Tests
› Chest x-ray
› Blood gas, lactate, other labs
› Echocardiogram
› Electrocardiogram (ECG)

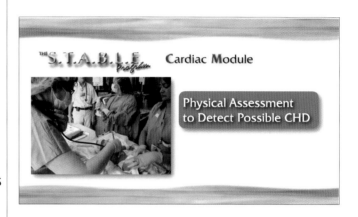

THE S.T.A.B.L.E. Program   Cardiac Module

Physical Assessment to Detect Possible CHD

Physical Assessment for CHD

› Neurological status
› Physical appearance
  ▪ Size and features
› Color and oxygen saturation
› Vital signs
  ▪ Respiratory rate and effort
  ▪ Heart rate and rhythm
  ▪ Blood pressure

› Bruit
› Pulses
› Skin perfusion
› Precordial activity
› Heart sounds
› Heart murmur
› Liver size and location
› Diagnostic tests
› Differential diagnosis

Patient Assessment

Neurologic Status

Infants with severe forms of CHD may be in significant distress with severe cyanosis, respiratory distress, and an advanced state of shock.[35] Therefore, it is important to perform a rapid assessment to determine whether the infant needs immediate resuscitation. Assess level of consciousness, tone, and response to touch. If the infant is unresponsive or appears in significant distress, provide immediate support to establish oxygenation, ventilation, and circulation.[36]

Normal

No signs of "distress" are observed.

The infant is active and alert and has good tone, a strong cry, and a normal feeding pattern.

Abnormal

Early signs of deterioration include a poor feeding pattern, weak suck, disinterest in feedings, and a change in level of consciousness, including increased sleepiness or difficulty in awakening the infant.

If in shock, the infant may display a range of symptoms including "distressed" facies, irritability, weak cry, lethargy, poor or flaccid tone. If shock is advanced, the infant may be unresponsive.

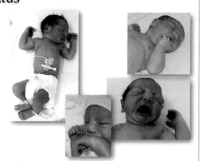

Neurological Status

Normal
- No signs of "distress"
- Active
- Alert
- Good tone
- Strong cry
- Normal feeding pattern

Neurological Status

Normal
- No signs of "distress"
- Active
- Alert
- Good tone
- Strong cry
- Normal feeding pattern

Abnormal
- Early signs of deterioration → poor feeding / weak suck, disinterest in feeding
- Change in level of consciousness
  - Increased sleepiness, difficulty awakening infant
- Signs of shock
  - Irritability
  - Weak cry
  - Lethargy, poor tone
  - Unresponsive / comatose

Patient Assessment

Physical Appearance – Size and Features

Normal

The size of the infant's head, body length, and weight is within normal limits or appropriate for gestational age (AGA).

The infant appears well-nourished, and there are no visible anomalies or malformations.

Abnormal

Large for Gestational Age (LGA)

LGA infants are defined as those with a birth weight greater than the 90th percentile for their gestational age.[37,38] Infants may be LGA because of ethnic[39] or genetic factors[40] or, in the case of male infants, because of a higher percentage of lean body mass.[41] However, infants may also be LGA because of the effects of elevated maternal glucose levels during pregnancy.[38] Therefore, when an infant is born LGA the underlying cause should be investigated. This includes the possibility that the mother was not recognized as being diabetic or that she developed gestational diabetes mellitus (GDM).

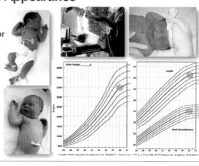

Infant Size and Appearance

Normal
- Appropriate growth for gestational age (AGA)
  - Weight
  - Length
  - Head circumference
- Well-nourished
- No visible anomalies

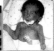

Infant Size and Appearance

Normal
- Appropriate growth for gestational age (AGA)
  - Weight
  - Length
  - Head circumference
- Well-nourished
- No visible anomalies

Abnormal
- Large for gestational age (LGA)
  - Assess for maternal diabetes risk
- Small for gestational age (SGA)
  - Assess for dysmorphic features which may be secondary to a chromosomal abnormality or syndrome

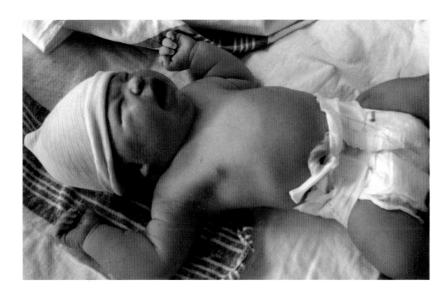

Term, 4.5 kg, LGA infant.

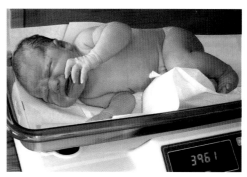

37-week gestation, 3.96 kg, LGA female infant.

Infant of the Diabetic Mother (IDM)[1,3,19,21-24,32,42-53]

Pregestational type 1 and type 2 diabetic women give birth to infants with congenital malformations, including CHD, at rates higher than nondiabetic women. The incidence of cardiac malformations in IDM patients is estimated between 3 and 6%. The etiology is multifactorial, but the leading cause appears to be maternal hyperglycemia that is teratogenic in the early stages of fetal development. Strict glycemic control prior to the onset of, and during pregnancy decreases the frequency and severity of adverse outcomes in the offspring. Thus, it is very important that women with pregestational type 1 and type 2 diabetes seek assistance from experts to receive education, counseling, and sometimes treatment to achieve glycemic control before becoming pregnant.

Gestational Diabetes and Obesity[54-59]

Worldwide, the incidence of GDM is increasing and is likely related to increasing rates of maternal obesity. As many as one-third of reproductive-aged women are obese, which has major implications for this worldwide public health issue. In addition to maternal obesity, other risk factors for developing GDM include past history of GDM or delivering a LGA infant, glycosuria, a maternal family history of type 2

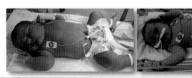

Infant of Diabetic Mother (IDM)

‣ Type 1 or 2 diabetes at onset of pregnancy
  ▪ Structural CHD (3 – 6% incidence)
‣ *Leading cause* → hyperglycemia is teratogenic in early organogenesis
‣ Gestational diabetes mellitus (GDM) → ↑ risk for CHD
  ▪ May have hyperglycemia secondary to undiagnosed type 2 diabetes

diabetes, and women with certain ethnicities that are associated with a higher incidence of diabetes (Latina, African American, Asian American, Native American, and Pacific Islander).

Women with GDM also have an increased risk for CHD in their offspring. It is postulated that some women with GDM may actually have undiagnosed type 2 diabetes with the fetus exposed to the adverse effects of hyperglycemia in early pregnancy. An elevated prepregnancy body mass index (BMI) is also associated with an increased risk for delivering an infant with CHD. The higher the BMI, the higher the risk for CHD and other malformations. One theory for this risk is that obese women are more likely to have higher blood glucose concentrations during early fetal heart development.

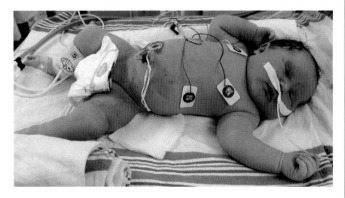

39-week gestation, 5.1 kg, infant of a diabetic mother.

Hypertrophic Cardiomyopathy (HCM)

In the second and third trimesters, the IDM fetus may develop a complication called HCM, which is an increase in thickness of the interventricular septum and the right and left ventricular free walls. In some cases, the septum is disproportionately affected (asymmetric septal hypertrophy). The exact mechanism is not known, but it is postulated that poor control of maternal diabetes leads to fetal hyperinsulinemia that, in turn, results in cardiac visceromegaly. The increased myocardial fiber size and number cause thickening of the ventricular walls that may impact ventricular filling. Impaired cardiac output may present with signs of CHF, including tachypnea, cyanosis, tachycardia, and cardiomegaly. In severe cases, HCM may be associated with obstruction to blood flow out of the left ventricle. The incidence of HCM is estimated at approximately 33% of diabetic pregnancies, but not all cases of HCM result in clinical decompensation. The infant's heart usually returns spontaneously to its normal size over the first few months of life.[49]

Congenital Heart Disease (CHD)

In pregestational type 1 and type 2 diabetic women, there is a 3 to 6% incidence of CHD in the IDM,[49] especially if glucose control was suboptimal prior to and in the very early stages of pregnancy.

Infant of Diabetic Mother (IDM)

LGA Infant

Hypertrophic Cardiomyopathy
- Develops during 2nd and 3rd trimester
- Hyperinsulinemia leads to visceromegaly → ↑ myocardial fiber size and number → septal hypertrophy
- Can cause cardiomegaly, congestive heart failure, left outflow tract obstruction

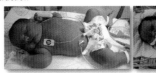
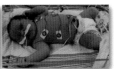

Infant of Diabetic Mother (IDM)

LGA infant

Structural CHD (3 – 6% incidence)
Most common lesions reported:
- Ventricular septal defect
- Atrial septal defect
- Transposition of the great arteries
- Truncus arteriosus
- Tricuspid atresia
- Tetralogy of Fallot
- Coarctation of the aorta
- Hypoplastic left heart syndrome

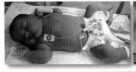
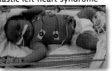

The most common cardiac defects include:
- ▶ **Ventricular septal defect (VSD)***
- ▶ **Atrial septal defect (ASD)***
- ▶ **Transposition of the great arteries (TGA)**
- ▶ **Truncus arteriosus (Truncus)**
- ▶ **Tricuspid atresia (TA)**
- ▶ **Tetralogy of Fallot (TOF)**
- ▶ **Coarctation of the aorta (COA)**
- ▶ **Hypoplastic left heart syndrome (HLHS)**

* See Figures 1.2 and 1.3 on page 15 for illustrations of VSD and ASD.

Small for Gestational Age (SGA) Infants

SGA infants are usually defined as those with a birth weight below the 10th percentile for their gestational age. Growth in utero is influenced by genetics, the ability of the placenta to deliver oxygen (O_2) and nutrients to the fetus, and intrauterine growth factors and hormones.[60] In a study comparing infants without CHD to those with prenatally diagnosed minor (VSD, ASD, rhabdomyoma) to major CHD*, birth weight less than the 10th percentile was statistically more frequent in infants with major forms of CHD. This conclusion was reported in consideration of factors that were controlled for: exposure to tobacco, African American race, chronic hypertension, and single umbilical artery. These findings support the importance of monitoring inutero growth and fetal well-being once major forms of CHD are diagnosed.[61]

Additional fetal factors that may be associated with growth restriction and SGA size include chromosomal abnormalities such as trisomy 21, 18, and 13, monosomy X, and microdeletions as well as single gene conditions such as found with CHARGE syndrome. CHD is commonly associated with all of these genetic disorders.[19,62]

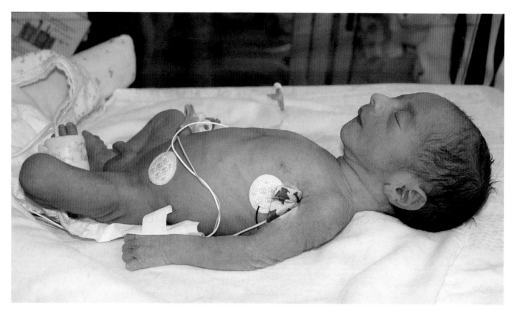

34-week gestation, intrauterine growth restricted (IUGR) infant.

---

* Major types of CHD included hypoplastic left heart, atrioventricular canal defect, hypoplastic right heart, transposition of the great arteries, tetralogy of Fallot, and mixed/complex cardiac defects.

Syndromes and Chromosomal Abnormalities Associated with CHD

Trisomy 21 (Down Syndrome)[19,33,63-67]

The incidence of Down syndrome is 1:700 live births, with increasing incidence as maternal age increases. Cardiac malformations are found in 40 to 50% of children with trisomy 21. The infant should also be assessed for duodenal atresia and umbilical hernia.

The most common cardiac defects include:

▶ **Atrioventricular septal defect** (also known as endocardial cushion defect or atrioventricular canal defect) occurs in 2% of all forms of CHD and accounts for approximately 50 to 60% of cardiac defects affecting infants with Down syndrome (see Figure 1.1, page 14).

▶ **Ventricular septal defect (VSD)**

▶ **Atrial septal defect (ASD)**

▶ **Patent ductus arteriosus (PDA)***

▶ **Tetralogy of Fallot (TOF)**

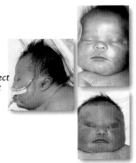

Chromosomal Conditions

Trisomy 21 – Down Syndrome
› 40 – 50% incidence CHD
▪ 50 – 60% have atrioventricular septal defect (AVSD)
  ▪ Also called *endocardial cushion defect* or *atrioventricular (AV) canal defect*
▪ Ventricular septal defect
▪ Atrial septal defect
▪ Patent ductus arteriosus
▪ Tetralogy of Fallot

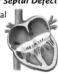
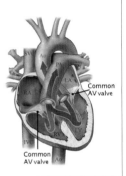

Chromosomal Conditions

Endocardial Cushion Defect
› Incidence: 2% of all forms of CHD
› May have partial or complete defect

Complete Atrioventricular Septal Defect
› Atrial and ventricular septal defect and common atrioventricular (AV) valve → mitral and tricuspid valve bridging leaflets

Common AV valve

Definitive Physical Features

▪ Small size, low birth weight

▪ Short round head with a flat facial profile

▪ Epicanthal folds, upslanting palpebral fissures

▪ Short nose, flat nasal bridge

▪ Small oral cavity with protruding tongue and an open mouth

▪ Small ears, overfolding of angulated upper helix

▪ Short neck, excess nuchal skin

▪ Short fingers, square hands, clinodactyly (curving of the fifth finger inward), single transverse palmar crease

▪ Wide gap between the first and second toes

▪ Hypotonia, hyperextensibility of the joints

▪ Broadened iliac bones

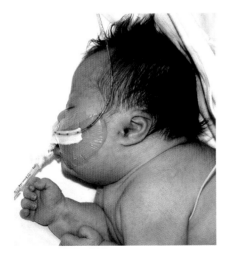

Term, 3 kg infant with Trisomy 21, ASD, and VSD.

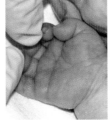

Single transverse palmar crease.

---

* Refers to persistent patency of the ductus arteriosus (DA) after the first month of life when the DA should be completely closed. See **What does it mean? Let's talk about a *persistent* patent ductus arteriosus (PDA) on page 18.**

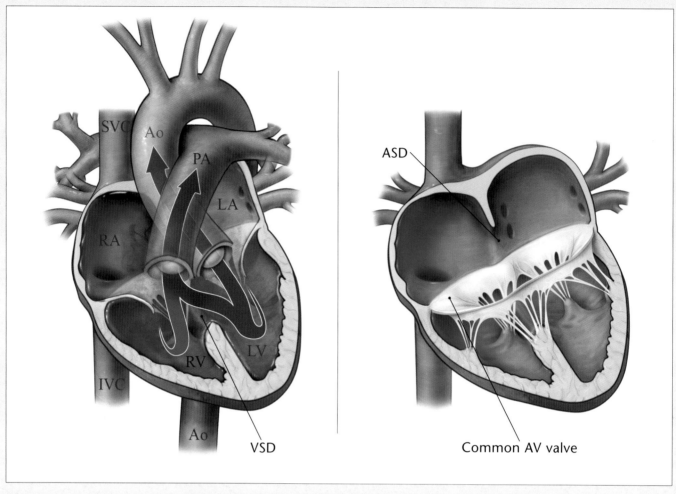

Figure 1.1. Complete atrioventricular septal defect (AVSD).[68-70]

The normal heart has four chambers (right and left atria and right and left ventricles) that are separated by two walls of tissue (atrial septum and ventricular septum). In complete AVSD, endocardial cushion tissue that forms the atrial and ventricular septum failed to close, leaving an ASD (primum type that is lower down in the atrial septal area), a VSD, and failure to form separate tricuspid and mitral valves. Instead, there is a common atrioventricular (AV) valve that spans the entire septal defect (hence, the alternate name – AV canal).

Five leaflets attach the common AV valve to the ventricular tissue. AVSD is classified as balanced or unbalanced. This illustration demonstrates a balanced AVSD where the atrioventricular tissue is fairly equally committed to each ventricle and the ventricles are equal in size.

In an unbalanced AVSD, one ventricle is hypoplastic with associated unequal commitment of the AV valve tissue. The status of balanced versus unbalanced AVSD may have significant implications for stability in the neonatal and early infant period, as well as the available repair options in later infancy.

NORMAL CARDIAC PHYSIOLOGY – TRANSITION FROM FETAL TO NEONATAL

Index
1. Introduction ....
2. Ductus Arteriosis ....
3. Ductus Venosus ....
4. Umbilical Vein ....
5. Foramen Ovale ....
6. Umbilical Artery ....
7. Placenta...
8. Lungs ....
9. Right Ventricle..
10.Left Ventricle   3

1. Introduction

Oxygen delivery to the tissues for a fetus in utero is a much different task than for the neonate, and the fetus has many unique mechanisms designed to maximize the efficiency of circulation. Once a baby is born however, it must begin to function with a circulatory system that resembles that of an adult. During the first 10 minutes after birth, the average heart rate is between 120-200 beats per minute (bpm). Thereafter, the average is approximately 120-130 bpm. Tachycardia may result from volume depletion, cardiorespiratory disease, drug withdrawal and hyperthyroidism (link tachycardia section). Bradycardia often results from apnea and is often seen with hypoxia (link bradycardia section). Given that the contractile strength of the neonatal heart has not had a chance to adjust to the new pulmonary and systemic circuitry and pressures, the neonate is highly dependent on heart rate for maintenance of cardiac output and blood pressure. Furthermore, the vasoconstrictive response of the neonate to hemorrhage or volume depletion is less that that of an adult. Following is a summary of the changes that occur in the cardiovascular system soon after birth.

2. Ductus Arteriosis

Ductus Arteriosis is a shunt from the descending aorta to the left pulmonary artery near the bifurcation of the pulmonary trunk. It stays open in the fetus because low PaO_2 and circulating prostaglandins (PGE_2) are vasodilatory on the ductus. In the neonate, when pulmonary oxygen saturation increases, there is less circulating PGE_2 and the ductus closes off. This usually occurs within the first day of life in the term infant. Permanent closure due to fibrosis takes 4-6 weeks, and the remnant is referred to as the ligamentum arteriosum.

3. Ductus Venosus

Ductus Venosus is a shunt of oxygenated blood from umbilical vein to IVC, bypassing the liver. The crista dividens in the right atrium deflects 1/3 of this blood through the foramen ovale, to the left atrium. The ductus venosus closes physiologically as soon as the umbilical vein is obstructed with the clamping of the cord, but with time it closes anatomically, and becomes the ligamentum venosus.

4. Umbilical Vein

The Umbilical Vein carries oxygenated blood from the placenta to the fetus in intra-uterine life. It flows into 1) the Ductus Venosus and 2) the IVC before it enters the liver. With the clamping of the umbilical cord, the umbilical vein closes physiologically, and after a few days anatomically. The remnant of this structure is called the round ligament of the liver (or ligamentum teres), and is clinically significant as it may be responsible for spreading tumors from the peritoneum to the umbilicus later in life.

5. Foramen Ovale

Foramen ovale is a flap valve in the atrial septum that shunts highly oxygenated blood from the IVC to the left ventricle. From the left atrium oxygenated blood is pumped through the aorta to the coronary circulation and the great vessels of the head and neck. The foramen ovale functionally closes at birth when the pressure in the left atrium (increased systemic resistance because loss of the placental parallel circuit) exceeds the pressure in the right atrium (decreased pulmonary resistance because of expanded lung vasculature with breathing), forcing the flap valve closed. It takes several months however for the atrial septum to fibrose, giving permanent closure to the foramen ovale, and leaving behind only the fossa ovalis.

6. Umbilical Artery

Two umbilical arteries carry deoxygenated blood from the internal ileac arteries of the fetus to the placenta. Delayed clamping of the cord in an infant held at a level higher than the placenta with delivery may decrease total blood volume as the blood is displaced to the placenta through the umbilical artery.

7. Placenta

Clamping of the umbilical cord removes the low resistance systemic diversion to the placenta, thereby forcing more blood to the lower limbs. This also increases systemic resistance, directing a larger proportion of blood through the pulmonary circulation.

8. Lungs

The cause-effect relationship of the onset of breathing and pulmonary vascular resistance is not completely understood. However, increased PaO_2 in the breathing neonate compared to the fetus lowers pulmonary vascular resistance and allows more blood to flow to the pulmonary circulation. The closing ductus arteriosus contributes to a higher blood flow to the lungs as less blood is diverted from the pulmonary trunk to the aorta. PO2 rises from 20-30 mmHg in the fetus arterial blood to 60 mmHg at approximately 1 hour of life to 80-90 mmHg at 24 hours of life.

9. Right Ventricle

The right ventricle is the dominant ventricle in utero. It pumps 65% of the total cardiac output. In the neonate, a decreased pulmonary vascular resistance and closed ductus arteriosus requires less force from the right side of the heart.

10. Left Ventricle

The left ventricle is relatively quiescent in utero because of the parallel structure of the circulatory system, but as the ductus arteriosus closes, the left ventricle becomes responsible for the increasing cardiac output to the body. In the neonate, the systemic vascular resistance increases much more than the size of the fetus does, exerting much force onto the left ventricle, thereby causing hypertrophy of the left ventricle.

References

1. Smyth, JA. Fetal-neonatal Transition. Growth & Development: Week 2 lecture notes. 2005.
2. Behrman, RE. and Kliegman, RM. Nelson Essentials of Pediatrics. W.B. Saunders Company. Philadelphia, USA: 2002.

Acknowledgements
Writer: Brook Glanville

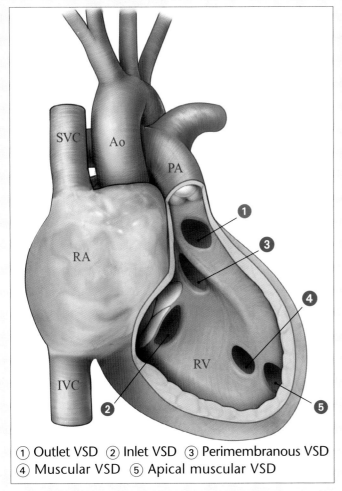

① Outlet VSD ② Inlet VSD ③ Perimembranous VSD
④ Muscular VSD ⑤ Apical muscular VSD

Figure 1.2. Ventricular septal defect (VSD) – incidence and locations.[65,71-73]

VSDs occur in the septum between the right and left ventricles. After bicuspid aortic valve (BAV), which occurs in 0.5 to 2% of the population, VSD is the most common form of CHD (40% of cases of CHD). Like ASD, VSD may be an isolated defect or occur in association with other CHD lesions. More than one VSD may be present. A VSD may be adjacent to the aortic and pulmonary valves (① outlet VSD), just inferior to the tricuspid and mitral valves (② inlet VSD), in the part of the septum adjacent to the tricuspid and aortic valves (③ perimembranous VSD), or in the septal muscle (④ muscular VSD). Small muscular VSDs are commonly seen in the neonatal period and frequently close spontaneously without intervention.

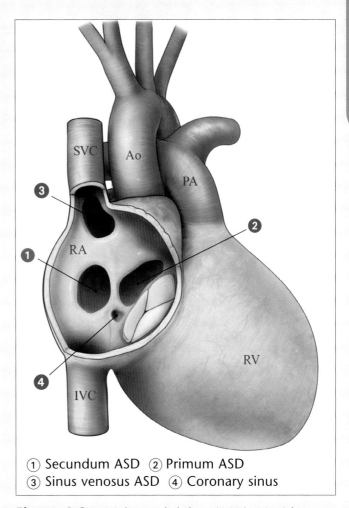

① Secundum ASD ② Primum ASD
③ Sinus venosus ASD ④ Coronary sinus

Figure 1.3. Atrial septal defect (ASD) – incidence and locations.[65,71,74]

ASDs occur in the septum between the right and left atria. An ASD is a common finding in approximately 30 to 50% of all forms of CHD and is an isolated finding in 5 to 10% of cases of CHD. The most common location for an ASD is in the atrial septum in the region of the fossa ovalis and is called a secundum ASD (75% of ASDs). The fetal structure, foramen ovale is also located in the midatrial septal region of the fossa ovalis. Because of the location, on echocardiography it may be challenging at times to determine whether the defect is a ① secundum ASD or a patent foramen ovale (PFO). The second most common type of ASD occurs in the ostium primum area near the tricuspid valve (② primum ASD; approximately 20% of ASDs; and part of the spectrum of AVSD). An ASD located near the superior vena cava is called a ③ sinus venosus ASD (approximately 5% of all ASDs; and is often associated with partial anomalous pulmonary venous drainage). At times, there may be an ASD at the ④ coronary sinus, but this ASD is rare.

Trisomy 18 (Edwards Syndrome)[33,63,67,75-81]

The incidence of Edwards syndrome is approximately 1:8000 live births;[75] affected infants are three times more likely to be female than male.[67] Pulmonary hypertension often complicates the clinical management of babies with trisomy 18. Cardiac malformations are found in 90% of children with trisomy 18.

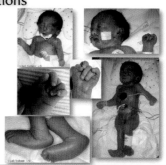

Chromosomal Conditions

Trisomy 18
› 90% incidence CHD
  - Ventricular septal defect
  - Atrial septal defect
  - Patent ductus arteriosus
  - Pulmonary stenosis
  - Tetralogy of Fallot
  - Double-outlet right ventricle
  - Polyvalvular disease

The most common cardiac defects include:

▶ **Ventricular septal defect (VSD)**

▶ **Atrial septal defect (ASD)**

▶ **Patent ductus arteriosus (PDA)***

▶ **Pulmonary stenosis (PS)**

▶ **Tetralogy of Fallot (TOF)**

▶ **Double-outlet right ventricle (DORV)**

▶ **Polyvalvular disease (2 or more valve leaflets are dysplastic)**

Definitive Physical Features

- Small size, low birth weight
- Prominent occiput, narrow bifrontal diameter
- Short palpebral fissures, ptosis of one or both eyelids
- Pinched appearance of the nose
- Low-set malformed ears
- Micrognathia, small oral opening
- Short sternum
- Hands held in a clenched position with overlapping of the flexed third and fourth fingers by the second and fifth fingers, hypoplasia of nails
- Rocker bottom feet with prominent calcaneus
- Single umbilical artery, genitourinary defects
- Inguinal or umbilical hernia
- Cutis marmorata

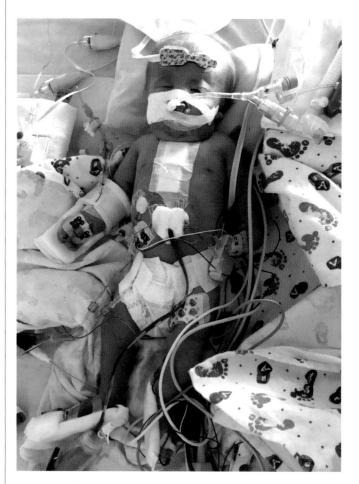

Infant with Trisomy 18 and a double outlet right ventricle (DORV) cardiac defect; post-operative following VSD repair. For more information about DORV, see page 98.

---

*Refers to persistent patency of the ductus arteriosus (DA) after the first month of life when the DA should be completely closed. See **What does it mean? Let's talk about a *persistent* patent ductus arteriosus (PDA)** on page 18.

Trisomy 13 (Patau Syndrome)[33,63,67,75,77,79,81]

The incidence of Patau syndrome is approximately 1:10,000 to 1:20,000 live births.[75] As with trisomy 18, pulmonary hypertension often influences the clinical picture and management of children with trisomy 13. Cardiac malformations are found in 80 to 90% of children with trisomy 13.

The most common cardiac defects include:

▶ **Ventricular septal defect (VSD)**

▶ **Atrial septal defect (ASD)**

▶ **Patent ductus arteriosus (PDA)***

▶ **Polyvalvular disease**

▶ **Dextrocardia**

See footnote on page 16.

Definitive Physical Features

■ Small size, low birth weight

■ Microcephaly, central nervous system (CNS) malformations including holoprosencephaly and scalp defects

■ Central facial anomalies, midface hypoplasia-dysplasia, cleft lip and/or cleft palate

■ Sloping forehead, broad bulbous nose, low-set malformed ears, loose nuchal skin

■ Microphthalmia, anophthalmia, hypotelorism, coloboma of the iris, cataracts

■ Polydactyly, single transverse crease, flexion deformities of the hands, fingers, and wrists

■ Rocker bottom feet

■ Urogenital abnormalities, polycystic kidneys, single umbilical artery

■ Omphalocele, umbilical or inguinal hernia

■ Hypoplastic or absent ribs

■ Hypoplastic pelvis

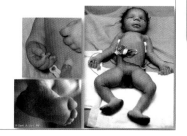

Chromosomal Conditions

Trisomy 13

› 80 – 90% incidence CHD
▪ Ventricular septal defect
▪ Atrial septal defect
▪ Patent ductus arteriosus
▪ Polyvalvular disease
▪ Dextrocardia

It is important to acknowledge that because approximately 50% of infants with trisomy 18 or 13 will survive longer than a week and about 6 – 12% of infants will live past 1 year, the still widely used terms of "lethal abnormality" and "incompatible with life" are inappropriate and misleading. Families of children with these disorders assert quite eloquently their objection about the use of "lethal" in these settings (p. 943).

The trend in neonatal intensive care in the last three decades has been to place significant weight on parental decision-making, usually in the context of the "best interest of the child." Parents appreciate partnership in decision-making. Overly simplified and value-laden terms such as "lethal," "vegetative," and "hopeless" not only are inaccurate, but also convey an implicit message from the outset. Initial counseling of the family should be realistic and accurate and not unnecessarily grim and bleak (p. 944).

Dr. John Carey. Management of Genetic Syndromes, 4th ed., 2021.

What does it mean?
Let's talk about a *persistent* Patent Ductus Arteriosus (PDA)[82-84]

In utero, prostaglandin E_2 (PGE_2) helps maintain ductal patency because of its relaxant effect on smooth muscle contained within the ductus arteriosus (DA). PGE_2 is produced primarily in the placenta. When the infant separates from the placenta at birth, circulating levels of fetal PGE_2 drop precipitously. At the same time, the arterial PO_2 rises, causing constriction of the smooth muscle contained within the DA. In normal term infants, functional closure of the DA begins shortly after birth with complete anatomic closure by 4 days of age. However, in progressively younger gestational ages the PDA closes at a slower rate. This may be due in part, to the immaturity of the DA both structurally and functionally in terms of being able to respond to the normal signals that induce closure.

The impact of a persistently patent ductus arteriosus is the potential for developing pulmonary overcirculation. As pulmonary vascular resistance drops in the days and weeks after birth, blood will shunt readily from the aorta through the DA to the pulmonary artery and to the lungs. This left-to-right shunting through the PDA leads to pulmonary overcirculation with increased blood returning to the left side of the heart, increasing left heart workload. The consequences of long-term, increased left heart workload include atrial and ventricular enlargement and, eventually, a risk of myocardial dysfunction. In addition, especially in preterm infants, the organs and tissues perfused by the aorta may receive less blood flow because of the shunting of blood from the aorta to the pulmonary artery. The aortic diastolic pressure drops and may result in decreased perfusion pressure, increasing the risk for end-organ ischemia.

Signs that the PDA is hemodynamically significant include tachypnea, increased work of breathing, bounding pulses and a widening pulse pressure as the diastolic blood pressure declines, a hyperactive precordium, cardiomegaly with increased pulmonary vascularity on chest x-ray, and a rising B-type natriuretic peptide (BNP).* Clinicians refer to this phenomenon of increased pulmonary blood flow at the risk of systemic blood flow as an "aortic run-off lesion." Options for closing the PDA include pharmacologic, percutaneous transcatheter occlusion, or surgical intervention.

---

*BNP is explained in the Lab work module on page 173.

Monosomy X (Turner Syndrome — XO Chromosomes)[33,66,67,85]

The incidence of Turner syndrome is 1:2000 liveborn female infants. Ninety-five percent of affected fetuses are miscarried by 28 weeks gestation. Thirty percent of children with Turner syndrome have cardiac malformations. Unless other genetic testing is indicated, consider obtaining a karyotype on a female infant with COA.

The most common cardiac defects include:

▶ **Coarctation of the aorta (COA)**

▶ **Bicuspid aortic valve with or without aortic stenosis**

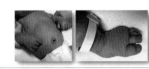
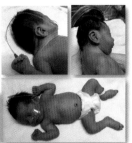

Chromosomal Conditions

Turner Syndrome (XO chromosomes)
› 30% incidence CHD
  ▪ Coarctation of the aorta
  ▪ Bicuspid aortic valve
    ▪ With or without aortic stenosis

Definitive Physical Features

- Short stature
- Downslanted palpebral fissures, epicanthal folds and ptosis
- Low-set, posteriorly rotated ears
- Micrognathia
- Short, webbed neck or redundant skin on the back of the neck
- Low posterior hairline
- Broad chest with widely spaced hypoplastic nipples
- Lymphedema of the dorsum of the hands and feet
- Hypoplastic convex nails
- Inguinal hernia

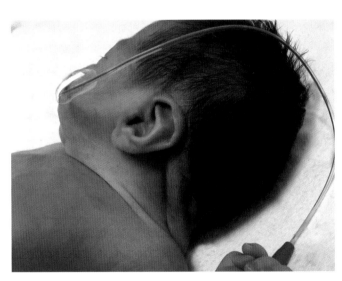

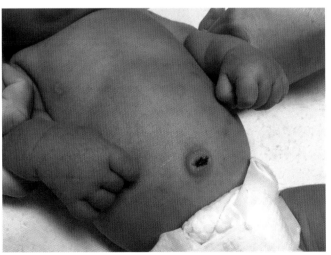

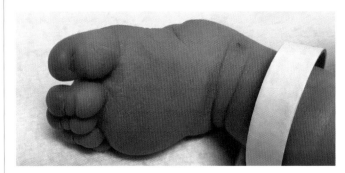

Late preterm infant with Turner Syndrome. Note the low posterior hairline, short neck, excess nuchal skin, wide-spaced nipples, and lymphedema of the hands and feet.

CHARGE Syndrome[86-93]

This is a multiple congenital anomaly syndrome that is most commonly caused by mutations in a single gene (*CHD7*) located on chromosome 8. The incidence of CHARGE is estimated between 1:8,500 to 1:17,000 births, depending on the case series. Table 1.2 summarizes the clinical characteristics of the CHARGE acronym.[90]

Diagnosing CHARGE Syndrome

With the advent of advanced genetic testing, a criteria to establish a diagnosis of CHARGE now also includes presence of pathogenic *CHD7* variants, plus one other major characteristic (see Table 1.3). However, not all infants with suspected CHARGE will have advanced genetic testing done. Therefore, most diagnostic criteria overlap to include establishment of a clinical diagnosis of CHARGE if there are either of the following:

- 3 major characteristics (Table 1.3), or;
- 2 major and 3 minor characteristics.[93]

The minor characteristics of CHARGE syndrome include the following:[93]

- **Developmental delay**
- **Heart or esophagus abnormalities**
- **Feeding difficulties or dysphagia**
- **Structural brain abnormalities**
- **Gonadotropin or growth hormone deficiency and genital anomalies**
- **Renal anomalies**
- **Skeletal/limb anomalies**
- **Facial features (square face)**

Cranial nerve dysfunction or anomalies are one of the major diagnostic characteristics (Table 1.3), yet this item is not included in the CHARGE acronym. Cranial nerve anomalies

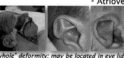
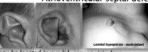

CHARGE Syndrome

| Mutation in CHD7 gene on chromosome 8 |

- Coloboma
- Heart defects
- Atresia of the choanae
- Restricted growth and development
- Genital abnormalities
- Ear anomalies or deafness

- 75 – 90% incidence CHD
  - Aortic arch abnormalities
  - Tetralogy of Fallot
  - Truncus arteriosus
  - Double outlet right ventricle
  - Transposition of great arteries
  - Atrioventricular septal defects

Coloboma: cleft, "keyhole" deformity; may be located in eye lid, cornea, iris, lens, ciliary body, retina, choroid, optic disk → request ophthalmology evaluation

may lead to major problems with feeding and gastrointestinal dysfunction, thus contributing to an increased risk for morbidity and mortality in children with CHARGE syndrome.

The *CHD7* gene is actively involved in the very early development of the heart. Therefore, mutations in this gene can alter how the heart forms. Seventy-five to 90% of children with CHARGE syndrome have cardiac malformations.

The most common cardiac defects include:

- **Left-side obstructive lesions including interrupted aortic arch type B (IAA, type B)**
- **Aortic arch abnormalities**
- **Tetralogy of Fallot (TOF)**
- **Truncus arteriosus (Truncus)**
- **Double outlet right ventricle (DORV)**
- **Transposition of the great arteries (TGA)**
- **Persistent patent ductus arteriosus (PDA)**
- **Septal defects:**
  - **Atrioventricular septal defects (AVSD)**
  - **Ventricular septal defect (VSD)**
  - **Atrial septal defect (ASD)**

Clinical Characteristics of the CHARGE Acronym	Percent with Characteristic
Coloboma – unilateral or bilateral (may involve the iris, retina, or optic disk)	75-90
Heart defects	75–90
Atresia of the choanae (or choanal atresia – unilateral or bilateral)	35-60
Retardation of growth and developmental delay (developmental delay in 75-100% of patients)	35-70
Genital abnormalities (genital hypoplasia) (males: micropenis, cryptorchidism; females: hypoplastic labia)	60-70
Ear abnormalities or deafness	90-100

Table 1.2. Clinical characteristics of CHARGE syndrome and percentage of patients with each characteristic.[93]

Major Diagnostic Characteristics of CHARGE Syndrome		Frequency
Coloboma – unilateral or bilateral	Implications for visual impairment	75-90%
Atresia of choanae (or choanal atresia – unilateral or bilateral; or stenosis), or orofacial clefting	Uncoordinated sucking and breathing	35-60%
Cranial nerve (CN) dysfunction or anomaly	CN I (olfactory) Absent or decreased sense of smell	86-95%
	CN V (trigeminal) Dysfunctional muscles of mastication; decreased facial sensation	
	CN VII (facial): Facial palsy, abnormal taste, abnormal esophageal sphincter, abnormal hyoid and laryngeal movement	
	CN VIII (vestibulocochlear): Hypoplasia of auditory nerve	
	CN IX (glossopharyngeal): Abnormal taste and sensation, impaired tongue movement	
	CN X (vagus): Abnormal swallowing and peristalsis, gastroesophageal reflux and aspiration	
	CN XII (hypoglossal): Impaired tongue movement	
Ear anomalies or deafness	Outer ear – short, wide ear with little or no lobe, often protruding and usually asymmetric	80-95%
	Middle ear: ossicular malformationss	
	Mondini defect of cochlea	
	Temporal bone abnormalities; absent or hypoplastic semicircular canals	
Pathogenic *CHD7* variants		

Table 1.3. The major diagnostic characteristics of CHARGE syndrome and frequency of each characteristic.[86,92,93]

VACTERL Association[94-99] (expanded VATER acronym)

Vertebral anomalies

Anal atresia

Cardiac defects

Tracheoesophageal fistula (TEF)

Esophageal atresia (EA)

Renal anomalies

Limb/radial anomalies (including limb-length discrepancy, limb hypoplasia, radial anomalies, radial hypoplasia, isolated thumb anomalies, polydactyly, and digit hypoplasia)

This is a nonrandom association of congenital malformations that occur together more commonly than would be expected by chance alone. At this time, no specific common etiology has been identified. Two additional features, cardiac and limb/radial, are added to the VATER acronym. Although there is no specific combination of features that confirms the diagnosis, a common approach is to consider the association when three of the features are present. Especially in infants who present with TEF/EA or anorectal malformation, investigation for other features of VACTERL should be undertaken. Since neurocognitive impairment is not associated with VATER/ VACTERL, the prognosis is positive, provided there is optimal surgical correction of any severe malformations (cardiac defects, TEF/ EA, and anal atresia). The incidence of VATER/ VACTERL is reported as 1:10,000 to 1:40,000 live births. There is an increased frequency of occurrence in infants of diabetic mothers. A single umbilical artery is observed in 70% of cases; therefore, this finding should prompt

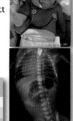

VACTERL Association

VACTERL	40 – 80% incidence CHD
› Vertebral anomalies	› Ventricular septal defect
› Anal atresia	› Tetralogy of Fallot
› Cardiac defects	› Double outlet right ventricle
› Tracheoesophageal fistula	
› Esophageal atresia	
› Renal defects	
› Limb anomalies	

# of Systems Affected	Percentage of Cases
3	75%
4	25%
5	uncommon

careful evaluation for any other features of VATER/VACTERL. Cardiac anomalies are present in 40 to 80% of affected individuals.

The most common cardiac defects include:

▶ **Ventricular septal defect (VSD)**

▶ **Tetralogy of Fallot (TOF)**

▶ **Double outlet right ventricle (DORV)**

22q11.2 Deletion Syndrome (22q11.2DS)[33,52,62,100-104]

As shown in Figure 1.4, a microdeletion located in the critical region of the long arm of chromosome 22 causes 22q11.2DS, which is also referred to as **DiGeorge syndrome** or velo-cardio-facial syndrome. One in 64 infants with CHD have this microdeletion. 22q11.2DS affects both males and females and occurs in approximately 1:4000 to 1:6000 live births. The neurocognitive impact in affected children is variable. Motor delays, often related to hypotonia, as well as speech and language deficits are common. Intellectual levels may be impacted and psychiatric disorders, including attention deficit hyperactivity disorder, autism, anxiety, and mood disorders; and psychotic disorders, including schizophrenia, may occur.

22q11.2DS (Continued)

Seventy-five to 85% of children with 22q11.2DS have cardiac malformations and infants with conotruncal and/or aortic arch abnormalities are more likely to have 22q11.2DS. See page 24, *What does it mean? Conotruncal*, for more information.

The most common cardiac defects include:

▶ **Tetralogy of Fallot (TOF)**

▶ **Interrupted aortic arch (IAA)**

▶ **VSD with aortic arch anomalies, including COA and right aortic arch**

▶ **Truncus arteriosus (Truncus)**

▶ **Pulmonary atresia with VSD (PA-VSD)**

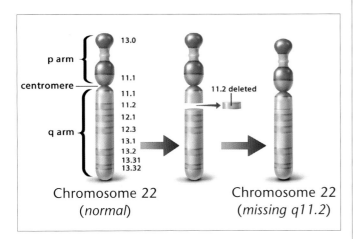

Figure 1.4. Microdeletion on the long arm of chromosome 22 seen in DiGeorge syndrome.

Physical Features

- Hooding of eyelids, downslanting eyes, narrow palpebral fissures, hypertelorism

- Prominent nose with squared nasal root, short philtrum

- Cleft of secondary palate

- Micrognathia, "fish mouth" appearance

- Low-set posteriorly rotated ears

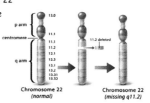

Chromosome 22q11.2 Deletion Syndrome

- Missing small part of chromosome 22
- Also known as *DiGeorge syndrome* and *velo-cardio-facial syndrome*

Manifestations

- Facial malformations
- Varying degrees of parathyroid and thymic hypoplasia
  - Evaluate for hypocalcemia
- Cardiac defects
- Variable neurocognitive impact

Deletion detected by Fluorescent In Situ Hybridization (FISH) chromosome analysis or Single Nucleotide Polymorphism (SNP) microarray testing

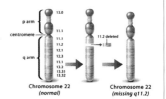

Chromosome 22q11.2 Deletion Syndrome

- 75 – 85% incidence CHD
- Tetralogy of Fallot
- Interrupted aortic arch
- VSD with aortic arch anomalies – coarctation of aorta and right aortic arch
- Truncus arteriosus
- Pulmonary atresia with VSD

Deletion detected by Fluorescent In Situ Hybridization (FISH) chromosome analysis or Single Nucleotide Polymorphism (SNP) microarray testing

Multisystem Derangements

- Velopharyngeal incompetence, which has implications for feeding and speech difficulties.

- The palate is commonly affected and may complicate feeding and speech.

- Metabolic, including hypocalcemia secondary to hypoparathyroidism.

- Immunologic, including absent or hypoplastic thymus, which has implications for chronic and problematic infections.

What does it mean? Conotruncal[62,105,106]

In the very early weeks of gestation, the heart is the first organ to develop. The "conotruncal" area refers to the region that gives rise to the outflow tract (aorta and pulmonary artery) and interventricular septum. Disturbance of formation results in the following 'conotruncal' heart malformations: tetralogy of Fallot, pulmonary atresia with ventricular septal defect, double-outlet right ventricle, truncus arteriosus, transposition of the great arteries, and interrupted aortic arch type B. Closely related to development of the conotruncus is the concurrent development of the face, eyes, ears, thyroid and parathyroid glands and thymus. Thus, disruption during this very early stage of fetal development can result not only in cardiac abnormalities, but also in craniofacial malformations and glandular dysfunction.

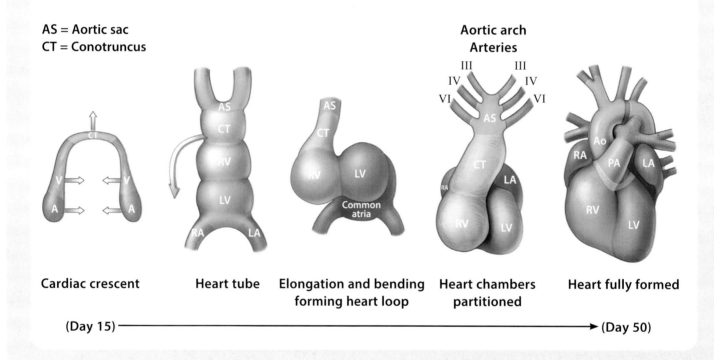

AS = Aortic sac
CT = Conotruncus

Aortic arch Arteries

Cardiac crescent
(Day 15)

Heart tube

Elongation and bending forming heart loop

Heart chambers partitioned

Heart fully formed
(Day 50)

Color coded to show how the aortic sac, conotruncus, and aortic arches form different parts of the heart and blood vessels.

Patient Assessment[2,107-110]

Color

Normal

Pink skin and mucous membranes.

In darker skinned neonates, the mucous membranes should be evaluated for pink color.

Abnormal

Central cyanosis: Bluish discoloration of the tongue and mucous membranes caused by desaturation of arterial blood indicate cardiac and/or respiratory dysfunction.

Cyanosis

The color of **reduced hemoglobin** (Hb) or Hb that is not bound to O_2 is **purple**. It takes at least 3 to 5 grams per deciliter (dL) of reduced Hb for cyanosis to be apparent.

To apply this principle, consider the infant with a Hb of 20 gm per dL. Even though O_2 content is sufficient, desaturation of 3 to 5 grams (15 to 25% of the Hb means that cyanosis will be apparent when the O_2 saturation is 75 to 85%. In addition, a Hb > 20 gm per dL increases the risk for hyperviscosity that can impair O_2 delivery to the tissues. Signs of hyperviscosity include cyanosis, tachycardia, tachypnea, hypotonia, poor feeding, tremors, hypoglycemia, hypocalcemia, and jaundice.

Color

Normal

▸ Pink color

▸ Assess mucous membranes in darker skinned neonates

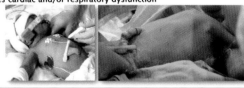

Color

Abnormal

▸ **Central cyanosis** – bluish discoloration of tongue, mucous membranes, and skin
  ▪ Caused by desaturation of arterial blood
  ▪ Indicates cardiac and/or respiratory dysfunction

If the infant's Hb is 15 gm per dL, then cyanosis will be visible when the O_2 saturation is 67 to 80%. When the Hb is 10 gm per dL, cyanosis will be visible when the O_2 saturation is 50 to 70%. At this point, the infant will also be significantly hypoxemic. *Therefore, it is important to interpret saturation values and cyanosis in the context of the infant's Hb level.* Figure 1.5 illustrates these concepts.

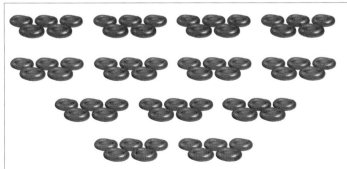

	Hb 20 gm/dL — O_2 saturation 100%; pink color, no cyanosis is apparent
	Hb 20 gm/dL — O_2 saturation 75 to 85% and **cyanosis may be apparent**
	Hb 15 gm/dL — O_2 saturation 67 to 80% and **cyanosis is apparent**
	Hb 10 gm/dL — O_2 saturation 50 to 70% and **cyanosis is apparent**

Figure 1.5. Hemoglobin (Hb) level, O_2 saturation with 3 to 5 gm per dL of reduced Hb, and when cyanosis may be apparent. (Each RBC represents 1 gram of Hb).

Patient Assessment

Oxygen Saturation*

Oxygen (O_2) is transported to the tissues bound to Hb. O_2 saturation is the percentage of Hb bound to O_2. When infants are cyanotic, oxygen is given to improve arterial O_2 saturation.

Cyanotic CHD should be suspected when there is a minimal increase in O_2 saturation or arterial PO_2 when the infant breathes 100% O_2.

Infants presenting with shock should be assessed for presence of a **left heart obstructive lesion** such as critical COA. In these infants, the cardiac defect is severe despite the responsiveness of the O_2 saturation and PaO_2 to O_2 administration.

Figure 1.6. Illustration of a right-to-left shunt through the PDA secondary to increased PVR and vasoconstricted pulmonary arterioles. Because of increased PVR, blood shunts via the pathway of least resistance, R to L through the PDA, into the aorta. Typically, significant R to L ductal shunting leads to a saturation in the right hand at least 5 to 10% higher than saturation in either foot. If shunting is primarily R to L at the patent foramen ovale (PFO), then there may be no appreciable difference in preductal and postductal O_2 saturations.

Preductal and Postductal O_2 Saturation

At times, it is of diagnostic value to evaluate both the preductal and postductal O_2 saturation to determine whether there may be a right-to-left shunt at the DA, as may occur when there is a noncardiac clinical problem called persistent pulmonary hypertension of the newborn (PPHN; see Figure 1.6). Characterized by persistently elevated pulmonary vascular resistance (PVR), the pathophysiology of PPHN usually falls into one of three categories, although overlap between categories is possible:

1) Pulmonary arteriolar vasoconstriction in association with lung parenchymal disease such as meconium aspiration syndrome, pneumonia, respiratory distress syndrome, or bronchopulmonary dysplasia;

2) Reduced pulmonary vascular bed with lung hypoplasia, such as seen with congenital diaphragmatic hernia; or,

3) When the lung parenchyma is normal, but there is remodeled, muscularized pulmonary vasculature (also called idiopathic).

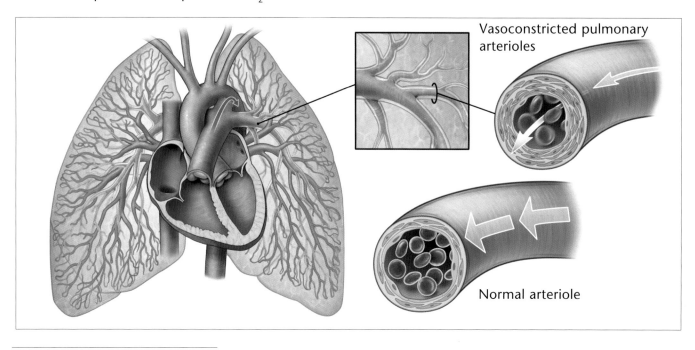

* See the S.T.A.B.L.E. – Cardiac Module PowerPoint presentation for a video on O_2 saturation and normal heart anatomy.

To monitor preductal and postductal saturation, attach a pulse oximeter probe to the right hand and to either foot. Allow the reading to stabilize and then record your findings.

In addition to monitoring preductal and postductal O_2 saturations in ill-appearing infants, pulse oximetry screening to detect critical congenital heart defects (CCHDs) is being performed in many hospitals worldwide.[111-116] Otherwise healthy appearing infants are screened before discharge to home with the purpose of detecting *lower than normal O_2 saturation values* secondary to previously undiagnosed CCHDs. For information specific to CCHD screening, see page 162.

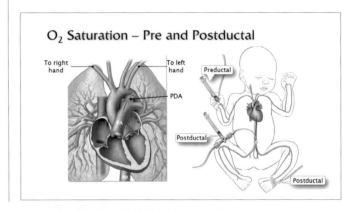

Oxygen (O_2) Saturation

Preductal and Postductal O_2 Saturation
- Right hand → preductal
- Foot → postductal
- Useful to evaluate for **R**-to-**L** shunt at ductus arteriosus
  - Right hand (preductal) saturation *greater* than foot (postductal) saturation indicates shunting through the ductus arteriosus
  - May indicate persistent pulmonary hypertension, coarctation of the aorta, or interrupted aortic arch

O_2 Saturation – Pre and Postductal

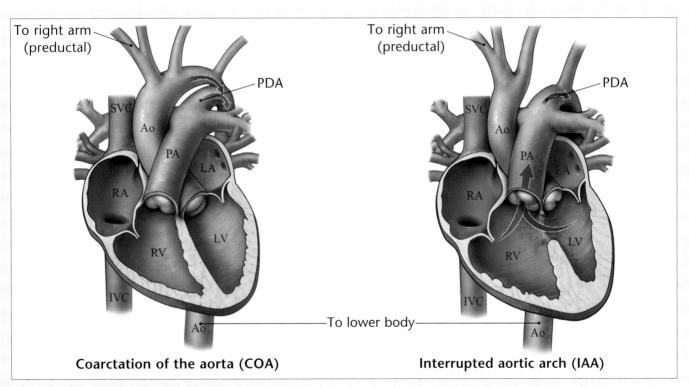

Coarctation of the aorta (COA)

Interrupted aortic arch (IAA)

Figure 1.7. Differential cyanosis (higher O_2 saturation in the right hand, lower O_2 saturation in the foot), that may be observed with COA and IAA. While the PDA is open, desaturated blue blood can shunt from the pulmonary artery, through the PDA, and into the aorta. Pulse oximetry screening may detect a difference between the right hand (preductal) and the foot saturation (postductal).

Reverse Differential Cyanosis

A higher O_2 saturation in the right hand compared to either foot indicates a right-to-left ductal shunt as just described. *Reverse differential cyanosis*, where there is a lower O_2 saturation in the right hand compared to the foot, suggests transposition of the great arteries (TGA) with pulmonary hypertension (see Figure 1.8), or TGA with critical COA/IAA. In TGA, the aorta originates from the right ventricle and the pulmonary artery originates from the left ventricle. When infants have TGA, continuous assessment of preductal O_2 saturation is critically

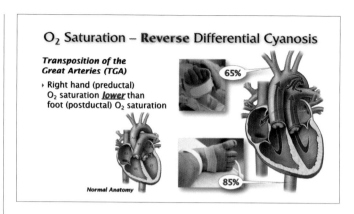

important because the O_2 saturation in the right hand is the same O_2 saturation of the blood perfusing the brain.

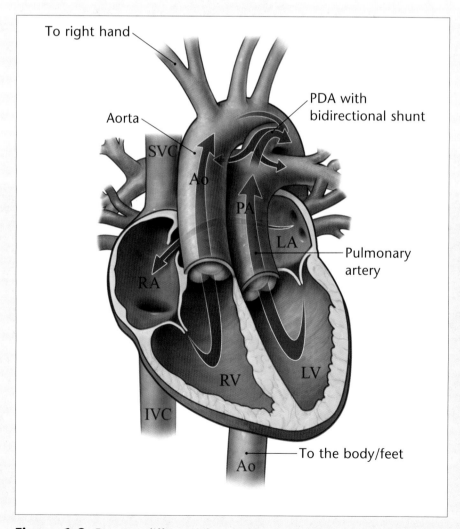

Figure 1.8. Reverse differential cyanosis secondary to Transposition of the Great Arteries (TGA).

The pathway of blood flow in this illustration is as follows: Blue, deoxygenated blood returning to the right side of the heart is pumped from the right ventricle into the aorta, to the brachiocephalic artery that branches into the right subclavian artery (to the right hand) and the right carotid artery (to the brain). Red, oxygenated blood returning from the lungs to the left side of the heart is pumped from the left ventricle into the pulmonary artery, through the PDA and into the aorta (to the body). In the presence of pulmonary hypertension, which is not uncommon in TGA, blood is preferentially shunted through the PDA into the aorta. Thus, the color of the blood in the right hand is more desaturated than the color of the blood in the distal aorta (i.e., reverse differential cyanosis). Infants with TGA may also have critical COA or IAA (not shown), which has the same effect on blood flow as pulmonary hypertension.

Patient Assessment

Vital Signs – Respiratory Rate and Effort*

Normal

The respiratory rate is 30 to 60 breaths per minute.

Breathing is not labored.

Symmetric breath sounds are heard.

Abnormal

Tachypnea

A respiratory rate > 60 breaths per minute, without signs of respiratory distress (comfortably tachypneic), may be one of the first signs of cardiac disease.

Respiratory Signs of CHF[118] may include:

► **Increased work of breathing**

► **Tachypnea**

► **Retractions**

► **Grunting**

► **Nasal flaring**

► **Abnormal blood gas (respiratory acidosis or mixed respiratory and metabolic acidosis)**

Respiratory Rate < 30 (Bradypnea)

A slow respiratory rate, in association with labored breathing and a declining neurologic status may signal that the infant is becoming exhausted. Bradypnea (respiratory rate < 30 per minute) may also represent a decrease in central respiratory drive because of hypoxic ischemic encephalopathy, prematurity, medications that depress respiratory drive (e.g. opioids), or other illnesses.

Respiratory Rate and Effort

Normal
› Respiratory rate 30 – 60 per minute
› Easy breathing effort
› Symmetric breath sounds

Abnormal
› Respiratory rate > 60
  ▪ "Comfortable tachypnea" → May have normal or lower O_2 saturation
    · May be an early sign of CHD

Let's explore "why" …

Respiratory Rate and Effort

Respiratory Signs of Congestive Heart Failure
› Increased work of breathing
› Tachypnea
› Retractions
› Grunting
› Nasal flaring
› Abnormal blood gas
  ▪ Respiratory or mixed respiratory and metabolic acidosis

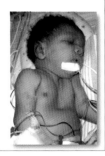

Gasping is an ominous sign of impending cardiorespiratory arrest. This extremely critical state should be treated the same as though the infant is apneic. Immediately provide positive pressure ventilation. If the infant's heart rate is low and not rising, establish an advanced airway via tracheal intubation or insertion of a laryngeal mask airway.

---

*See the S.T.A.B.L.E. – Cardiac Module PowerPoint presentation for two videos that explain Homeostatic Control of Respiration and Congestive Heart Failure.

Vital Signs – Heart Rate and Rhythm[119-121]

Normal

The neonatal heart rate is usually between 120 and 160 beats per minute, but may range between 80 or 90 beats per minute during sleep to 170 to 180 beats per minute when the infant is crying or in pain. When deeply asleep, some healthy term infants may have heart rates decline to as low as 70 beats per minute.

Abnormal

Bradycardia

A heart rate < 70 beats per minute in a neonate usually represents pathologic bradycardia.

Sinus bradycardia should be differentiated from complete heart block. In sinus bradycardia, a p wave precedes each QRS complex (see electrocardiogram (ECG) of sinus bradycardia in Figure 1.9). Underlying causes of sinus bradycardia include apnea, hypoxia, acidosis, hyperkalemia, hypercalcemia, hypothermia, hypertension, hypothyroidism, and increased intracranial pressure.

Hypoxemia and acidosis depress the conduction system and may lead to bradycardia. Therefore, any unwell neonate with a heart rate < 100 beats per minute should be assessed for signs of hemodynamic compromise. If shock is detected, bradycardia indicates the neonate is in severe crisis.

Heart Rate (HR)

Normal
- HR usually 120 – 160 beats/minute
- HR may range 80 – 180 beats/minute
  - Lower at rest
  - Higher with activity, crying, pain, fever
- Normal sinus rhythm

Abnormal
- Bradycardia → HR < 70 beats/minute
  - Usually pathologic
- Evaluate for shock
  - Hypoxemia and acidosis depress conduction system → can decrease heart rate
- Differentiate between
  - Sinus bradycardia
  - Complete heart block

Heart Rate (HR)

Sinus Bradycardia · Underlying Causes
- Apnea, hypoxia, acidosis
- Hyperkalemia, hypercalcemia
- Hypothermia, hypertension
- Hypothyroidism
- ↑ intracranial pressure

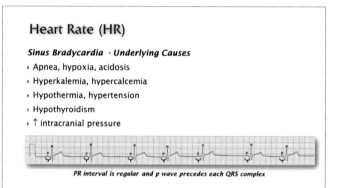

PR interval is regular and p wave precedes each QRS complex

*Complete Heart Block**

In complete heart block (also called third-degree atrioventricular block), the P waves are completely unrelated to the QRS complexes, indicating the atrial impulses are not conducted into the ventricle (see Figures 1.10 and 1.11). The ventricular (QRS) rate usually ranges from 45 to 80 beats per minute. The lower the rate, the more likely the infant will be critically ill.

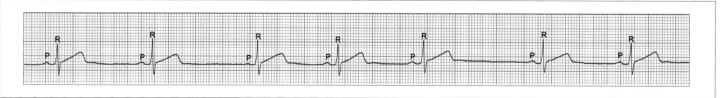

Figure 1.9. ECG of sinus bradycardia. The heart rate is 42 beats per minute. Note the QRS complex follows each p wave.

*See the S.T.A.B.L.E. – Cardiac Module PowerPoint presentation for a video that explains Complete Heart Block.

**Three primary causes of complete heart block
include the following:**

1) Structural heart disease (congenital).

2) Effects of maternal connective tissue
   (autoimmune) disorders such as systemic lupus
   erythematosus, Sjögren syndrome, rheumatoid
   arthritis, and other autoimmune disorders.

3) Complication of heart surgery (acquired).

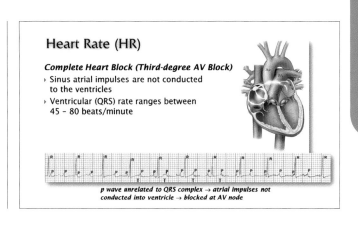

Heart Rate (HR)

Complete Heart Block (Third-degree AV Block)
- Sinus atrial impulses are not conducted
  to the ventricles
- Ventricular (QRS) rate ranges between
  45 – 80 beats/minute

*p wave unrelated to QRS complex → atrial impulses not
conducted into ventricle → blocked at AV node*

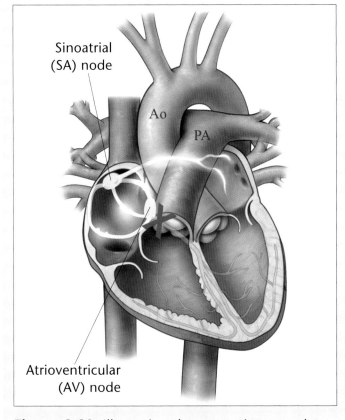

Figure 1.10. Illustration demonstrating complete
heart block and failure of the atrial impulse to be
conducted through the atrioventricular (AV) node
to the ventricles.

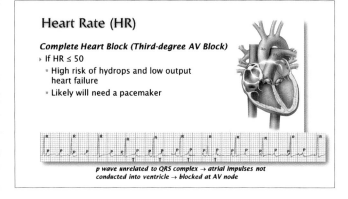

Heart Rate (HR)

Complete Heart Block (Third-degree AV Block)
- If HR ≤ 50
  - High risk of hydrops and low output
    heart failure
  - Likely will need a pacemaker

*p wave unrelated to QRS complex → atrial impulses not
conducted into ventricle → blocked at AV node*

Heart Rate (HR)

Complete Heart Block (Third-degree AV Block)
- Congenital or acquired
  - Structural heart disease [congenital]
  - Maternal connective tissue (autoimmune) disorders
    - Systemic lupus erythematosus, Sjögren syndrome,
      rheumatoid arthritis, and other autoimmune diseases
    - Affects fetal heart tissue → inflammation, calcification, fibrosis,
      and necrosis of conduction system / AV node
  - Complication of heart surgery [acquired]

*Infant with complete
heart block, HR 51*

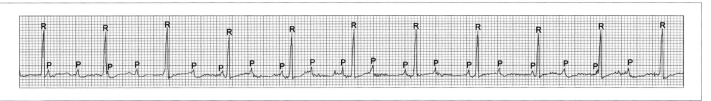

Figure 1.11. ECG of complete heart block. Note the P waves are regular (regular PP interval; atrial rate of
133 beats per minute), and the QRS complexes are regular (regular RR interval, ventricular rate of 68 beats
per minute). The P wave is unrelated to the QRS complex.

The etiology of injury to the conduction system in maternal autoimmune disease is that maternal antibodies are deposited in fetal heart tissue, which leads to inflammation, calcification, fibrosis, and necrosis of the conduction system. This injury is most often irreversible, and treatment involves placement of a pacemaker.[122]

Neonates who present at birth with hydrops fetalis (HF) secondary to complete heart block are critically ill. Hydrops is the descriptive term for the extravascular accumulation of fluid in two or more spaces, including the skin, abdomen, and pleural and/or pericardial cavities.[123] HF is a complex disorder with numerous etiologies; however, in the case of complete heart block, heart failure occurs inutero secondary to low output heart failure.

Cardiac output is heart rate times stroke volume (HR X SV). In complete heart block, stroke volume is usually normal. However, there are insufficient beats to provide adequate cardiac output, and the blood backs up in the lungs and venous side of the circulation. This imbalance between interstitial fluid production and lymphatic return leads to fluid accumulation in the interstitial spaces.[123]

Tachycardia

Sinus Tachycardia versus Supraventricular Tachycardia[124-126]

Crying or agitated neonates occasionally have heart rates that reach 200 to 220 beats per minute. However, a sustained heart rate > 180 beats per minute, in the absence of associated agitation, crying, pain, or fever, is abnormal.

Heart Rate (HR)

Normal
› HR usually 120 – 160 beats/minute
› HR may range 80 – 180 beats/minute
  ▪ Lower at rest
  ▪ Higher with activity, crying, pain, fever
› Normal sinus rhythm

Abnormal
› Tachycardia → sustained HR > 180 beats/minute at rest
› May indicate poor cardiac output, shock and/or congestive heart failure
› Investigate other causes:
  ▪ Anemia
  ▪ Fever
  ▪ Pain
  ▪ Medications → catecholamines, methylxanthines
  ▪ Arrhythmias

Heart Rate (HR)

Sinus Tachycardia → sustained HR 180 – 220 (or higher)
› Neonatal myocardium → has *limited* capacity to increase squeeze

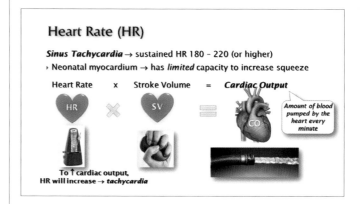

To ↑ cardiac output, HR will increase → *tachycardia*

Sinus Tachycardia[125]

Neonates in shock or CHF may have a sustained sinus tachycardia, with heart rates ranging between 180 and 220 beats per minute, or higher. Similar to why the infant breathes faster and deeper when trying to compensate for increased carbon dioxide (CO_2) levels, the heart rate will increase when the infant is trying to compensate for a low cardiac output. However, unlike the infant's ability to take a deeper breath when trying to compensate for increased CO_2 levels, the neonatal myocardium has poor capacity to increase the amount of blood that is ejected with each heartbeat (stroke volume [SV]), unless augmented with a medication and/or a volume infusion. Therefore, in order to increase cardiac output, the neonatal heart rate increases, resulting in tachycardia.

The formula for cardiac output (CO) is: heart rate (HR) X stroke volume (SV) = CO

Supraventricular Tachycardia (SVT)

Neonates with SVT usually have sustained heart rates > 220 beats per minute, although SVT may be present with sustained heart rates < 220 beats per minute. Due to the rapid heart rate, infants with SVT have insufficient diastolic filling time. Therefore, stroke volume is low and can lead to shock secondary to inadequate tissue perfusion and oxygenation. When an infant is in SVT, assess for signs of shock by evaluating perfusion, pulses, blood pressure, O_2 saturation, near infrared spectroscopy (NIRS; if available), respiratory status/effort, level of consciousness, development of metabolic acidosis and increased levels of lactate. Infants who poorly tolerate being in SVT include those with a history of hydrops or concurrent structural heart disease.

Heart Rate (HR)

Supraventricular Tachycardia (SVT)

🔊 Baseline HR 140 ↑ to 220 with onset of SVT

- Sustained HR > 220 (incidence 1: 250 neonates)
- ⚠ SVT may be present with HR > 180

Heart Rate (HR)

Supraventricular Tachycardia (SVT)

- Sustained HR > 220 (incidence 1:250 neonates)
- ⚠ SVT may be present with HR > 180
- SVT usually well tolerated initially *unless* associated hydrops or structural CHD

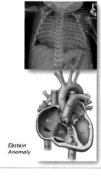

Ebstein Anomaly

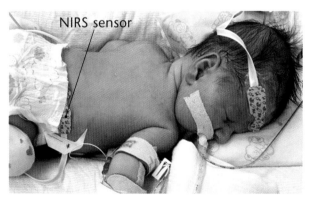

NIRS sensor

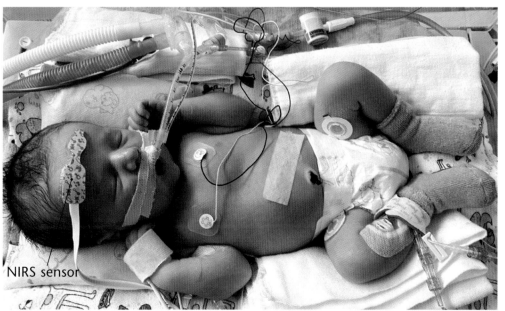

NIRS sensor

Term infant with critical COA, hypoplastic aortic arch (unrepaired), and congenital diaphragmatic hernia (post-operative day 10). Tissue oxygenation is being continuously monitored by cerebral and renal NIRS.

Treatment of SVT[119,126]

Vagal maneuvers to stop SVT. Mechanism of action: slows conduction through the AV node and interrupts a reentrant supraventricular tachycardia.

Option 1: Stimulate a gag.

Option 2: Suction the oropharynx.

Option 3: Apply crushed ice to the nose and forehead area.

Procedure for Performing the "Icing" Vagal Maneuver

- Place 1 cup of crushed ice in a plastic bag and add a little water to make the mixture slushy. Cover the plastic bag with a thin cloth before placing it on the face.

- If time allows, attach full-lead ECG equipment so that the episode may be captured, including while in SVT and if the infant converts to normal sinus rhythm (NSR). If time does not allow, use bedside defibrillator equipment and start a rhythm strip.

- Apply the ice bag to the upper half of the face (nose and forehead area) for approximately 15 seconds — or less if SVT stops. It is not necessary to obstruct the nose and mouth with the ice bag, although some cardiologists do recommend completely covering the face;[124] follow your institution's procedure for ice application.

- Be careful not to obstruct the airway with the ice bag.

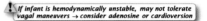

Termination of SVT

Vagal Maneuvers to Terminate SVT

› Stimulate gag

› Suction oropharynx

› Crushed ice applied to nose / forehead area → stimulates *diving reflex* → slows conduction through the vagal nerve and interrupts a reentrant SVT

⚠ *If infant is hemodynamically unstable, may not tolerate vagal maneuvers → consider adenosine or cardioversion*

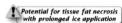

Termination of SVT

"Icing" Vagal Maneuver

❶ 1 cup crushed ice plus some water in plastic bag (slushy) and cover with thin cloth before applying to face

❷ Start rhythm strip → continue through conversion to normal sinus rhythm or for 1 minute if SVT continues

❸ Apply ice bag to nose / forehead area
  ▪ Remove bag if converts or after 15 seconds if SVT persists
  ▪ Not necessary to obstruct airway with ice bag → discuss desired procedure with cardiologist

❹ Monitor for conversion back to SVT

❺ If no response to ice → adenosine

⚠ *Potential for tissue fat necrosis with prolonged ice application*

- Continue the rhythm strip through the "break" to NSR or, if SVT continues, for 1 minute.

- When SVT stops, monitor the heart rate for conversion back to SVT.

- If SVT continues, notify the pediatric cardiologist or neonatologist for further instructions. At times, infants may need an additional medication (e.g., a beta blocker or propranolol) to prevent future episodes of SVT.[124]

Cautions

- The icing vagal maneuver procedure is not recommended for neonates experiencing severe cardiac compromise or shock. However, icing may be attempted while preparing to provide a more definitive treatment option such as adenosine administration or electrical cardioversion.

- If the neonate has a history of no response to ice, do not continue to attempt this maneuver. Proceed to adenosine administration.

- The application of ice may cause fatty tissue necrosis if the bag is applied over fatty tissue (cheeks) for a prolonged period of time (more than 15 to 20 seconds).[127,128]

- Discard the ice bag after one application. Refreezing the bag causes frost to form on the surface that will increase the probability of thermal injury of the infant's face if reapplied.

- Do not apply ocular pressure to stop SVT, as it can cause retinal injury.

- Do not apply carotid massage to stop the SVT, as it can damage the carotid body.

If the neonate is unstable or in shock, vagal maneuvers may be poorly tolerated and cardioversion may be the treatment of choice. The usual starting dose is 0.5 joule to 1 joule per kg. Attempt adenosine first and then, if the infant remains in SVT, proceed with cardioversion. If the infant is conscious, then pain medication is indicated (if at all possible) prior to cardioversion.

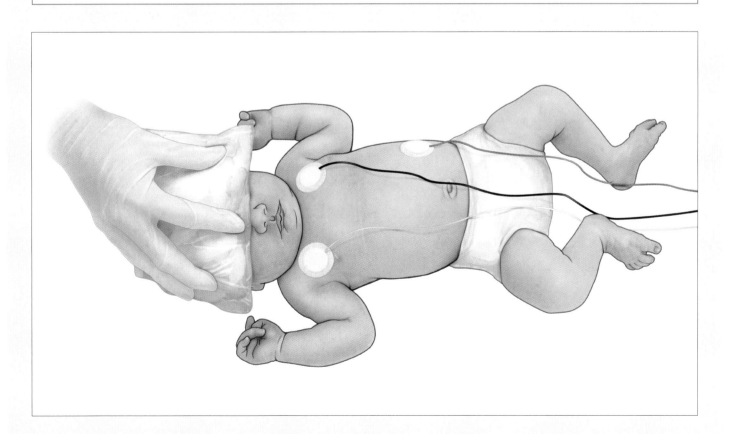

Adenosine[119,124,129]

Adenosine is an antiarrhythmic agent used to treat SVT. The goal of therapy is to restore NSR. Adenosine slows conduction through the atrioventricular (AV) node and interrupts the reentry pathway underlying this form of SVT (see Figure 1.12 on page 37). Within 10 seconds of entering the bloodstream, adenosine is rapidly metabolized by the red blood cells.

Patient Monitoring

- Notify medical providers involved with the infant's care of the onset of SVT.

- Begin a rhythm strip before administering adenosine, then continue the rhythm strip or ECG through the "break" to NSR (see Figure 1.12). If SVT continues, the recording can be stopped at the discretion of the medical team.

- If SVT terminates, monitor the heart rate for conversion back to SVT.

- When administration of adenosine 'breaks' the SVT, even for a few seconds before resumption of SVT, an additional antiarrhythmic agent may be indicated to keep the infant out of SVT. Repeated administration of adenosine in these cases will likely only transiently terminate the SVT.

Dose

Administer adenosine into a peripheral IV or central venous line closest to the heart. Do not use a central line if it is infusing an inotropic medication since boluses of those medications are contraindicated.

The initial adenosine dose is 0.1 milligrams per kilogram (mg/kg) rapid IV push over 1 to 2 seconds. Please note that some medication handbooks recommend a lower starting dose of 0.05 mg/kg.

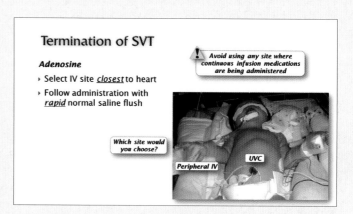

Termination of SVT

Adenosine
- Initial dose = 0.1 milligram/kilogram (0.1 mg/kg)
- Mechanism of action:
  - Slow conduction time through AV node
  - Interrupt reentry pathway through AV node
  - Restore normal sinus rhythm
- Onset of action: *rapidly metabolized* upon entering blood stream

! *Adenosine is not effective for treating atrial flutter or fibrillation, but when given, may reveal its presence*

Termination of SVT

Adenosine
- Select IV site *closest* to heart
- Follow administration with *rapid* normal saline flush

! *Avoid using any site where continuous infusion medications are being administered*

Which site would you choose?

Peripheral IV   *UVC*

- Follow the adenosine push immediately with a rapid bolus of 2 to 3 mL of sterile normal saline through the same IV catheter.

- If there is no response within 1 to 2 minutes, increase the dose by 0.1 mg/kg every 2 minutes until a maximum single dose of 0.3 mg/kg is given.

- If SVT continues, reevaluate how the adenosine is being administered and recognize that normal saline must be flushed as rapidly as possible (over seconds) following administration of adenosine.

- If the SVT breaks with adenosine administration and then resumes a few minutes later, do not increase the adenosine dose because the effect will still only last a brief time. Repeat the most recent adenosine dose and consult the neonatologist or pediatric cardiologist about starting additional antiarrhythmic treatment.

Adverse Reactions (including, but not limited to):

Cardiovascular

- AV heart block, chest pain or pressure, hypotension, transient or new arrhythmias including life-threatening arrhythmias, diaphoresis, flushing

Central Nervous System

- Irritability, headache

Gastrointestinal

- Nausea

Respiratory

- Dyspnea, hyperventilation

Termination of SVT

Adenosine

› Continue rhythm strip through "break" to normal sinus rhythm or 1 minute if SVT continues

› Monitor for conversion back to SVT
› If no response, reevaluate administration method
  - ↑ Dose by 0.1 mg/kg every 2 minutes
  - Maximum single dose 0.3 mg/kg
› Monitor patient stability while in SVT

⚠ *If hemodynamically unstable → synchronized cardioversion (0.5 to 1 joule/kg) – allows sinus node to resume normal pacemaker activity*

Warnings / Precautions

- Prior to giving adenosine, the defibrillator machine and defibrillator pads should be readily available in the event that an unstable rhythm develops after adenosine administration.

- Many warnings, contraindications, and adverse reactions accompany the use of adenosine. Therefore, it is the responsibility of the clinician to be familiar with these warnings before using adenosine.

- Adenosine is contraindicated in patients with second- or third-degree AV block, sick-sinus syndrome, asthma, and symptomatic bradycardia.

- Adenosine is not effective in atrial flutter, atrial fibrillation, or ventricular tachycardia (arrhythmias not due to reentry pathway through the AV or sinus node). In these cases, adenosine may slow the heart rhythm long enough to allow detection of the underlying rhythm. In this setting, adenosine aids in diagnosis of the abnormal rhythm, but it is not therapeutic for these abnormal rhythms.

Drug Interactions

- The effect of Adenosine may be decreased if the patient is on Caffeine or Theophylline derivatives.

- The effect of Adenosine may be increased if the patient is on Digoxin or Carbamazepine.

Adenosine effect

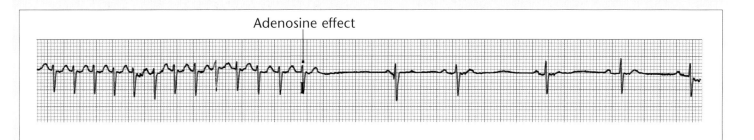

Figure 1.12. ECG of SVT treated with adenosine.

Vital Signs – Blood Pressure (BP)[107,130-141]

Normal

BP varies with gestational age, postmenstrual age, and weight. Arterial BPs in the first 12 hours after birth, in healthy preterm and term infants are shown in Figure 1.13.[140,141]

The 5-day trend of systolic, diastolic and mean BPs in hospitalized sick neonates of varying gestational ages increases steadily each day, regardless of changes in daily weight (see Figure 1.14 on page 39).[139]

Abnormal

Evaluation of BP is an important component of patient evaluation; however, the decision to treat shock should be based on history, physical exam, laboratory data, urine output, and patient condition – not just BP readings. In addition, in the early phase of shock, the BP may be in a normal range, but on exam the infant may have evidence of altered mental state and poor cardiac output such as a prolonged capillary refill time (CRT), weak pulses, and/or cool extremities.

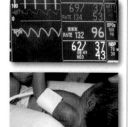

Blood Pressure (BP)

‣ Blood pressure varies with:
  ▪ Gestational age
  ▪ Postmenstrual age (gestational age plus age in days after birth)
  ▪ Weight
‣ Correlate BP readings with clinical exam and lab data

> ⚠ *Decision to treat shock should be based on history, exam, lab data, urine output, level of consciousness, not an isolated BP reading*

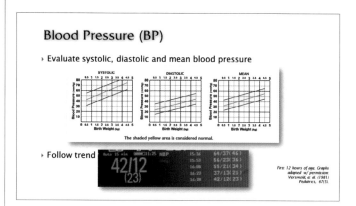

Blood Pressure (BP)

‣ Evaluate systolic, diastolic and mean blood pressure

The shaded yellow area is considered normal.

‣ Follow trend

First 12 hours of age. Graphs adapted w/ permission: Versmold, et al. (1981). Pediatrics, 67(5).

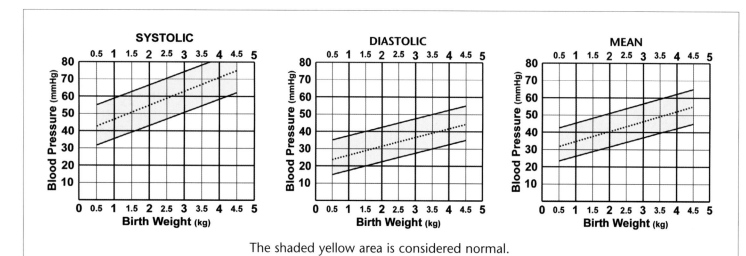

The shaded yellow area is considered normal.

Graphs adapted with permission from Versmold, HT, et al. (1981). Aortic blood pressure during the first 12 hours of life in infants with birth weight 610 to 4,220 grams. *Pediatrics*, 67(5), 607-613.

Figure 1.13. Average systolic, diastolic, and mean BPs during the first 12 hours of life in healthy preterm and term infants according to birth weight.

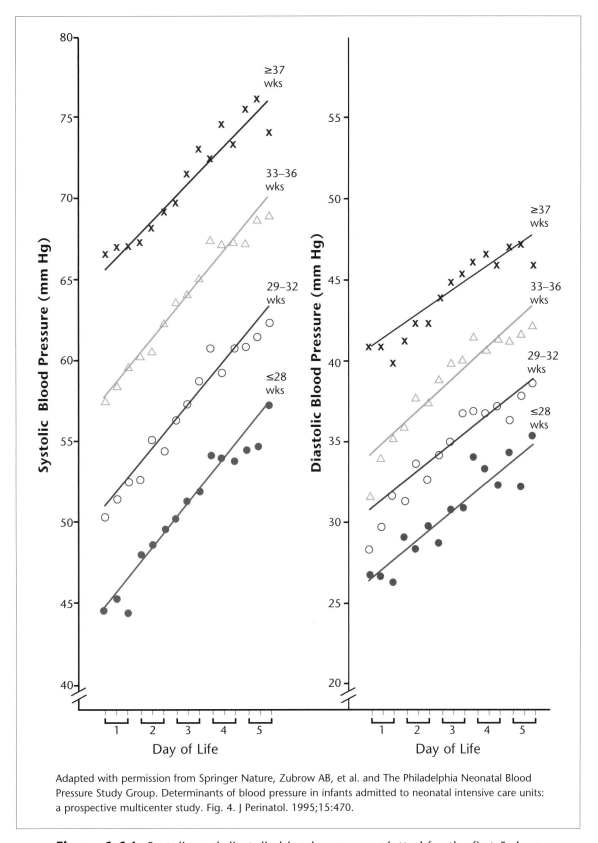

Adapted with permission from Springer Nature, Zubrow AB, et al. and The Philadelphia Neonatal Blood Pressure Study Group. Determinants of blood pressure in infants admitted to neonatal intensive care units: a prospective multicenter study. Fig. 4. J Perinatol. 1995;15:470.

Figure 1.14. Systolic and diastolic blood pressures plotted for the first 5 days of life, with each day subdivided into 8-hour periods. Infants are categorized by gestational age into 4 groups: ≤ 28 weeks (n = 33), 29 to 32 weeks (n = 73), 33 to 36 weeks (n = 100), and ≥ 37 weeks (n = 110).

Pulse Pressure[107,125,136,142-145]

Collectively, all three BP parameters (systolic, diastolic, and mean), provide important information, including information needed to calculate pulse pressure.[140,141] To determine the pulse pressure subtract the diastolic from the systolic measurement. Normal pulse pressures for preterm and term infants are shown in Table 1.4 and possible causes of a narrow or wide pulse pressure are shown in Figure 1.15 on page 41.

Gestation	Normal Pulse Pressure (mmHg)
Term	25 to 30
Preterm	15 to 25

Table 1.4. Normal pulse pressure in preterm and term infants.

Blood Pressure (BP)

Evaluate Pulse Pressure
‣ To calculate → systolic minus diastolic

Normal
‣ Term: 25 to 30 mmHg
‣ Preterm: 15 to 25 mmHg

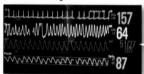

Example: 51 – 27 = 24
Pulse pressure = 24 mmHg

Blood Pressure (BP)

Narrow (Low) Pulse Pressure
‣ Causes may include:
  - Heart failure (low cardiac output, poor heart contractility)
  - Peripheral vasoconstriction
  - Compression on the heart
    - Pneumopericardium, pericardial effusion, tension pneumothorax, lung hyperinflation
  - Severe aortic valve stenosis
  - Significant tachycardia

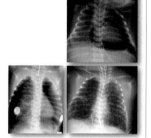

Blood Pressure (BP)

Wide (High) Pulse Pressure
‣ Causes may include aortic runoff lesions secondary to
  - Patent ductus arteriosus
  - Truncus arteriosus
  - Arteriovenous malformation
  - Aortopulmonary window
  - Aortic regurgitation
‣ Other → sepsis with vasodilated (warm) shock

Blood Pressure (BP)

Wide (High) Pulse Pressure
‣ Causes may include aortic runoff lesions secondary to

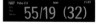

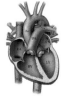 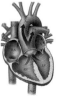 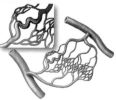

Patent Ductus Arteriosus (PDA)   Truncus Arteriosus   Arteriovenous Malformation (AVM)

Possible Causes of a Narrow or Wide Pulse Pressure

Narrow	
<ul><li>Heart failure – low cardiac output, poor myocardial contractility</li><li>Peripheral vasoconstriction</li><li>Compression on the heart – low cardiac output secondary to pneumopericardium, pericardial effusion, tension pneumothorax, lung hyperinflation</li></ul>	<ul><li>Severe aortic valve stenosis</li><li>Significant tachycardia</li></ul>

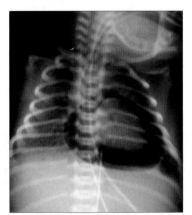 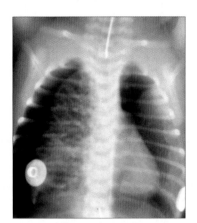 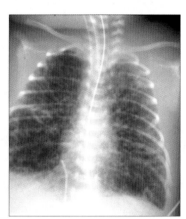

Pneumopericardium	Bilateral tension pneumothorax	Lung hyperinflation

Wide

Aortic runoff lesion that may be secondary to:

- Patent ductus arteriosus (PDA)
- Truncus arteriosus
- Arteriovenous malformation (AVM)

- Aortopulmonary window
- Aortic regurgitation

Other: sepsis with vasodilated (warm) shock

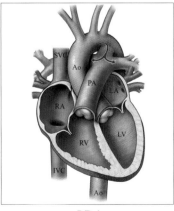 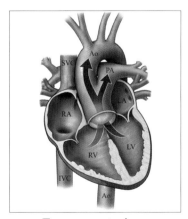 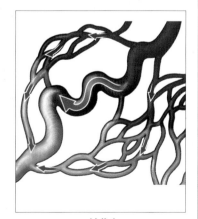

PDA	Truncus arteriosus	AVM

Figure 1.15. Possible causes of a narrow or wide pulse pressure.

Arm/Leg BP Measurement[107,136,146-150]

Four-extremity BP measurement is commonly performed when an infant is admitted to the neonatal intensive care unit (NICU). Thereafter, if concerned about a COA or an evolving coarctation, the right arm and either leg (calf) BP should be measured sequentially, with limited time between the two measurements, and with the infant as calm as possible. The brachial and femoral pulses, and temperature of the legs and feet should also be assessed at the same time as the BP. It is not necessary to evaluate 4 extremity BPs at this point.

If the right arm BP is more than 15 to 20 mmHg higher than the leg BP, especially if there are weak or absent femoral pulses, or if both upper extremity BPs are obtained and the right arm BP is significantly higher than the left arm BP, consider coarctation of the aorta (COA) or interrupted aortic arch (IAA) with a closing DA (see Figure 1.16 on page 45). It should be noted that not all arm/calf BP discrepancies of 15 mmHg or higher mean that an infant has a COA, as a small number of normal infants may also have this finding.[151] In addition, not all infants with a critical COA will have a right arm/leg BP discrepancy. Page 167 provides additional information regarding how to increase accuracy of oscillometric BP measurement.

Blood Pressure (BP)

› If concerned about CHD obtain 4 extremity BP → compare arm and leg

Normal
› Arm and leg systolic BP should be similar although leg BP may be slightly higher

If concerned about an evolving COA, continue to monitor right arm and calf BP

Abnormal
› Right arm BP 15 to 20 mmHg higher than leg BP → *may indicate closing ductus arteriosus in a ductal dependent lesion*
› Upper body pulses stronger than femoral/posterior tibialis/pedal pulses
› Weak or absent femoral pulses
› Cool or cold legs or feet
› Prolonged capillary refill time

Blood Pressure (BP)

As DA closes, right arm BP may be higher than the leg BP and right brachial pulse stronger than femoral pulse

Coarctation of the Aorta (COA)   Interrupted Aortic Arch (IAA, Type B)

EXAM TIP
The same cuff can be used when measuring BP on the arm and calf.

Shock[130-134,152]

Shock is a life-threatening condition that requires prompt recognition and treatment. The primary issue that leads to shock is inadequate delivery of oxygen to the tissues. In the early stages of shock, the infant will activate a complex response in order to maintain a normal blood pressure and to preserve blood flow to the heart, brain, and adrenal glands. However, the consequence is that blood is diverted away from what the body considers nonvital organs (liver, kidneys, gastrointestinal tract, muscles, and skin).*

As shock worsens, anaerobic metabolism leads to increased lactic acid production. The heart muscle weakens from lack of oxygen and the negative effects of acidosis. Failure to promptly recognize and treat shock may lead to cellular dysfunction, multiple organ failure, and even death. The treatment of shock centers around identifying and treating the underlying problem, as well as understanding how to improve and support heart function.

Shock · What is it?

› For cells to survive and function, they need oxygen
› Inadequate tissue perfusion and oxygen delivery to vital organs → *shock*

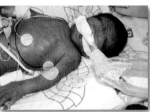

Shock

Early Stages of Shock

› Blood flow diverted from the liver, kidneys, gastrointestinal tract, muscles, skin to preserve blood flow to the heart, brain, and adrenal glands

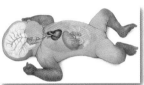

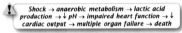
Shock → anaerobic metabolism → lactic acid production → ↓ pH → impaired heart function → ↓ cardiac output → multiple organ failure → death

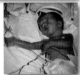

Shock · Review

Factors that Can Impair Cardiac Output

› Electrolyte, mineral or energy imbalances
› ↓ Venous return to heart *(preload)* → heart has less blood to "pump" with each contraction (↓ stroke volume)
› ↑ Systemic or pulmonary vascular resistance *(afterload)* → heart works harder to pump blood
› ↓ Myocardial contractility → heart squeezes poorly → less blood ejected with every beat

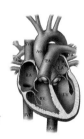

Because hypotension is a late sign of cardiac decompensation, BP may be normal when, in fact, the neonate is experiencing early stages of shock. If the exam indicates the infant is underperfused, base the decision to treat on the physical exam, heart rate, and history – not on an isolated BP measurement!

---

*See the S.T.A.B.L.E. – Cardiac Module PowerPoint presentation for a video that explains neonatal shock.

Patient Assessment

Bruit[153,154]

A bruit is a murmur-like sound that is heard in areas other than over the precordium. If a bruit is auscultated over the liver or anterior fontanelle, the infant should be evaluated for an arteriovenous malformation (AVM). Other signs of AVM include CHF, a hyperdynamic precordium, and liver enlargement.

Although some bruits over the carotid artery may be normal, a bruit heard in this area may indicate aortic stenosis (AS), especially if accompanied by a loud systolic ejection murmur at the right upper sternal border (RUSB).

Patient Assessment

Pulses[108,125,136,153,155,156]

Normal

- Brachial and femoral pulses are easy to feel (2+) and are equal in strength.

- Posterior tibial and/or pedal pulses are palpable, although they may be more difficult to locate than brachial and femoral pulses.

Pulses are usually classified using a numeric system:

0   Absent

1+ Weak or thready

2+ Normal, easily palpated

3+ Full or bounding

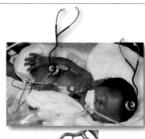

Bruit
- Murmur-like sound heard in other areas than over the precordium
- Auscultate over liver and anterior fontanelle
- If bruit heard → may indicate an *arteriovenous malformation (AVM)*

Other Signs of AVM
- Congestive heart failure
- Hyperdynamic precordium
- Liver enlargement

Pulses

Normal	Abnormal

▸ Brachial and femoral pulses
  ▪ Easy to feel
  ▪ Equal in strength
▸ Posterior tibialis and/or pedal pulses palpable
	▸ Difficult to palpate (weak or absent)
	  ▪ Evaluate for signs of shock
	▸ Brachial stronger than femoral
	  ▪ Consider COA and IAA
	▸ Right brachial stronger than left brachial
	  ▪ Consider COA and IAA

Classification of Pulses
0   Absent
1+ Weak or thready
2+ Normal, easy to feel
3+ Full or bounding

EXAM TIP
Palpate right and left brachial artery, then the femoral artery. To improve skill level, palpate pulses with every neonatal exam.

Pulses

Abnormal

Pulses difficult to feel

- May indicate poor cardiac output secondary to heart failure or shock.

- When brachial pulses are palpable, but femoral pulses are weak or absent, or when the right brachial pulse is stronger than the left brachial pulse, COA or IAA with a closing DA should be considered (see Figure 1.16).

Bounding pulses

- Bounding pulses with a wide pulse pressure may be found in PDA, AVM, truncus arteriosus, and severe aortic valve regurgitation.

- Septic/distributive shock is a noncardiac cause of bounding pulses.

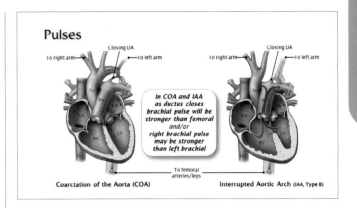

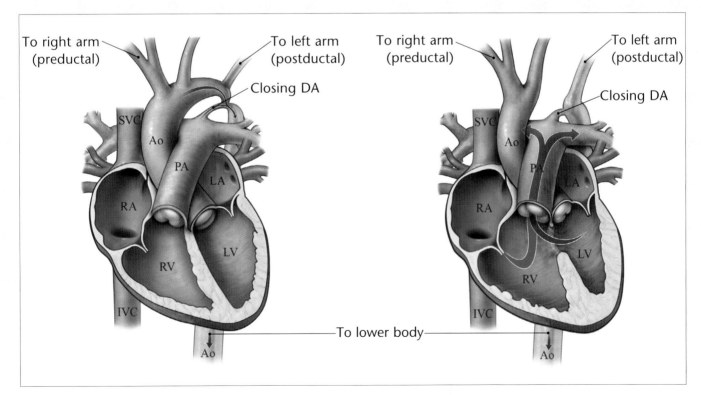

Figure 1.16. Illustrations of critical COA and IAA. With closure of the DA, the right arm BP may be higher than the leg BP and the right brachial pulse may be stronger than the femoral pulse.

Patient Assessment

Skin Perfusion and Appearance[36,108,125,157-160]

Normal

- CRT ≤ 3 seconds in neonates.
- CRT ≤ 2 seconds in older infants and children.
- Hands and feet are warm, pink, and well perfused.

Abnormal

- CRT ≥ 4 seconds may indicate peripheral vasoconstriction in response to shock.
- Pale, cool or cold extremities, or mottled skin may indicate vasoconstriction in response to shock.
- CRT > 2 seconds slower in the lower body compared to the upper body may indicate decreased distal perfusion secondary to a closing DA.
- Cold sweat on the forehead/scalp (diaphoresis) may be caused by increased sympathetic activity in response to decreased cardiac output.
- CRT < 2 seconds may be present with hypotensive, vasodilated ("warm") shock.

Note: Studies report variation in CRT because of gestational or postnatal age, skin temperature, ambient temperature, hydration status, polycythemia, duration of pressure applied to blanch the skin, and location where CRT was assessed.[158,161-165]

EXAM TIP
Since hypothermia may cause peripheral vasoconstriction, ensure the infant is normothermic when examined.

Skin Perfusion and Appearance

Reflects cardiac output
Normal

> Ensure infant is normothermic at time of exam since hypothermia causes peripheral vasoconstriction

- Capillary refill time (CRT) ≤ 3 seconds
- Hands and feet are warm, pink, well perfused

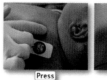

Press | Release | Count seconds until skin refills

Skin Perfusion and Appearance

- Compare upper to lower body

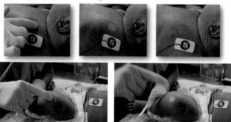

Skin Perfusion and Appearance

Abnormal

- Pale, cool or cold extremities, mottled skin
- CRT ≥ 4 seconds
- CRT more prolonged in lower body than upper body → may indicate closing DA in ductal dependent CHD
- Cold sweat on forehead/scalp (diaphoresis)
  - Caused by ↑ sympathetic activity in response to ↓ cardiac output

If CRT is brisk (≤ 2 seconds) evaluate for hypotensive, vasodilated "warm" shock

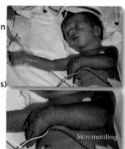

Skin mottling

EXAM TIP: Capillary Refill Time (CRT)

Assessment of CRT is subjective; therefore, use the same technique each time CRT is assessed.

- *Press firmly on a central (upper) and peripheral (lower) location.*

- *Use the same method to count how many seconds it takes for the skin to refill (e.g. "one-one thousand, two-one thousand, three-one thousand ...").*

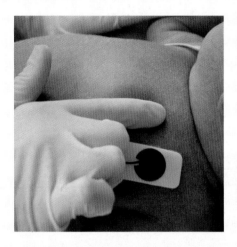

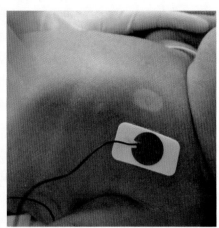

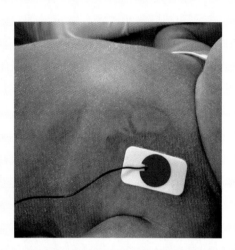

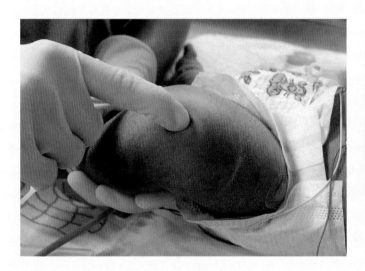

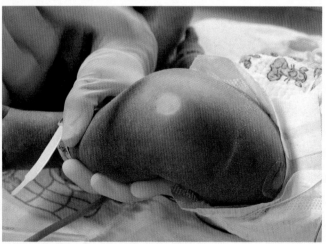

Patient Assessment

Precordial Activity[107,136,166]

Normal

- The heart lies underneath the area in the anterior chest called the precordium.

- In neonates, the point of maximal impulse (PMI) is located along the left lower sternal border (LLSB) in the 5th intercostal space.

- The PMI is generated by right ventricular dominance in the neonate.

- In newborns, the precordium may have a visible impulse, but within a few hours of age, the precordial impulse should be minimal.

- In preterm infants, the precordial impulse may be noticeable because of decreased subcutaneous fat.

Abnormal

Hyperactive precordium

- May be observed with various forms of CHD, including left-to-right shunt lesions with increased ventricular volume such as a PDA or large VSD.

If the PMI is located in the right chest, causes may include:

- Dextrocardia (heart located in the right chest)
- Left-sided tension pneumothorax
- Left-sided diaphragmatic hernia

If the PMI is located further lateral in the left chest than normal, consider:

- Right-sided tension pneumothorax

Precordial Activity

Normal
- Point of maximal impulse (PMI)
  - Left lower sternal border (LLSB)
  - 5th intercostal space

Abnormal
- Hyperactive precordium
  - May indicate L-to-R shunt lesions such as PDA or large VSD

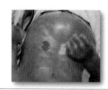

Newborn → Precordial impulse more noticeable secondary to right ventricular dominance
Preterm → Precordial impulse often noticeable because of decreased subcutaneous fat

Precordial Activity

Abnormal
- PMI shifted to the right

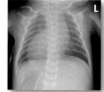 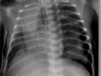 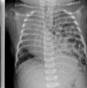

Dextrocardia   Tension left pneumothorax   Diaphragmatic hernia

Precordial Activity

Abnormal
- PMI shifted to the left
  - Tension right pneumothorax

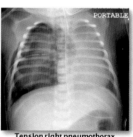

Tension right pneumothorax

Auscultation of the Heart[107]

Use a systematic approach to assess:

- Heart rate and regularity

- Heart sounds

- For any abnormal sounds, such as a click (may signify aortic or pulmonary valve stenosis)

- For presence or absence of a heart murmur

> *Muffled or distant heart sounds may indicate a pericardial effusion or tamponade, heart failure, or myocarditis.*

Patient Assessment

Heart Sounds[107,136,166,167]

Normal

First heart sound – S1

- Associated with closure of the mitral and tricuspid valves. After atrial systole, pressure in the ventricles exceeds pressure in the atria, and the mitral and tricuspid valves close.

- S1 is heard best at the apex of the heart or approximately the fifth intercostal space at the left midclavicular line (MCL) or the LLSB.

- Splitting of S1 may be normal but is infrequently heard.

Second heart sound – S2

- Associated with closure of the aortic and pulmonic valves. After ventricular systole, pressure in the great arteries exceeds the pressure in the ventricles, and the aortic and pulmonic valves close.

- S2 is heard best at the base of the heart or the mid- to left upper sternal border (LUSB).

Splitting of S2

- Two components of the second heart sound are audible with inspiration; closure of the aortic

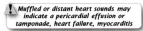

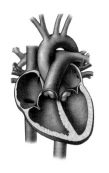

Auscultation

Use Systematic Approach to Assess:
- Heart rate and regularity
- Heart sounds
- For abnormal sounds such as a click
- Presence or absence of a heart murmur

> ⚠ *Muffled or distant heart sounds may indicate a pericardial effusion or tamponade, heart failure, myocarditis*

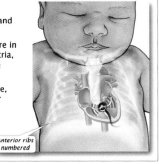

First Heart Sound – S1
- Associated with closure of mitral and tricuspid valves
  - After atrial systole, when pressure in ventricles exceeds pressure in atria, *mitral and tricuspid valves close*
- Heard best at apex of heart or approximately 5th intercostal space, left midclavicular line or left lower sternal border (LLSB)

Anterior ribs numbered

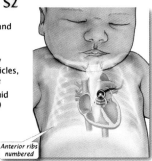

Second Heart Sound – S2
- Associated with closure of aortic and pulmonic valves
  - After ventricular systole, when pressure in aorta and pulmonary artery exceeds pressure in ventricles, *aortic and pulmonic valves close*
- Heard best at base of the heart, mid to left upper sternal border (LUSB)
- Aortic valve closes slightly before pulmonic valve → A2 / P2 ◀

Anterior ribs numbered

(A2), then pulmonic (P2) valves. S2 = A2, P2. S2 becomes a single sound with expiration.

- A single S2 is normal in the first several days of age because of increased PVR. It is also difficult to hear splitting of the second heart sound because of the infant's increased heart rate.

EXAM TIP:

Normally a physical exam is conducted from 'head to toe.' When listening to heart sounds, work in the opposite order. Start low with the stethoscope placed at approximately the fifth intercostal space, or the LLSB, left MCL. Next, move the stethoscope up slowly to the mid, then LUSB. The first heart sound will be louder in the low position and the second heart sound will be louder in the higher position. Note, the anterior ribs are numbered in the right chest.

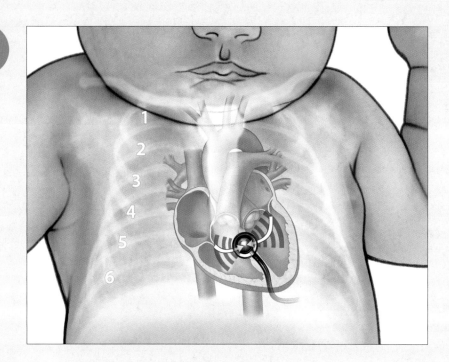

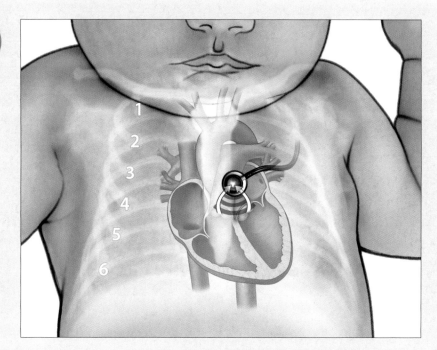

Abnormal

Single S2

- May represent absence of either the aortic (A2) or pulmonic (P2) valve component in the following forms of CHD:

  - Severe aortic stenosis or atresia

  - Severe pulmonary stenosis or atresia

  - Truncus arteriosus (single common truncal valve)

- May represent an inability to hear the pulmonary component in the following forms of CHD:

  - Transposition of the Great Arteries (TGA)

  - Tetralogy of Fallot (TOF)

- May be audible in neonates with elevated PVR because the pulmonary valve closes almost simultaneously with the aortic valve.

Narrowly split S2

May be a normal finding, but a narrowly split S2 may be associated with aortic stenosis or pulmonary hypertension.

Widely split S2

Can occur secondary to increased blood volume presented to the right ventricle (RV) secondary to an ASD with left-to-right shunting, or secondary to anomalous pulmonary venous return.

What happens to cause wide splitting of the S2? The increased blood volume flowing to the RV takes longer to empty into the pulmonary artery, thus causing the pulmonary valve to stay open longer. Causes of a widely split S2 in the neonate include pulmonary stenosis (pressure overload secondary to obstruction to right ventricular outflow) and an electrical delay (RV depolarization) secondary to right bundle

> ### Single S2
>
> › Single S2 → Normal in first few days of age with ↑ pulmonary vascular resistance
> › Splitting of S2 difficult to hear with higher heart rates
> ***Absence of Aortic (A2) or Pulmonic (P2) Valve Component***
> › Severe aortic stenosis or atresia
> › Severe pulmonary stenosis or atresia
> › Truncus arteriosus (single common truncal valve)
> ***Unable to Hear the Pulmonary Component***
> › Transposition of the Great Arteries, Tetralogy of Fallot
> › Pulmonary hypertension → pulmonary valve closes at same time as aortic valve

branch block. Later causes (months to years of age) include an ASD with L-to-R shunting or secondary to partial anomalous pulmonary venous return. In infants with an ASD, a soft systolic ejection murmur may be audible at the upper left sternal border secondary to the increased pulmonary blood flow.

EXAM TIP
The bell of the stethoscope picks up low-frequency events (e.g., a mid-diastolic rumble or a pulmonary regurgitation murmur), whereas the diaphragm picks up high-frequency events. Both the bell and diaphragm should be used to auscultate the chest.

Patient Assessment

Heart Murmur[2,107,136,168]

A heart murmur is sound caused by turbulent blood flow through the heart or adjacent blood vessels.

Blood forced through a stenotic valve

- Pulmonary stenosis
- Aortic valve stenosis

A softer murmur usually means the stenosis is less severe, whereas a louder murmur usually means the stenosis is more severe.

Regurgitation of blood through an incompetent valve

- Aortic, mitral, tricuspid, or pulmonary valve insufficiency

Blood forced through a narrowed area such as a ventricular septal defect (VSD)

- The more restrictive the VSD, the louder or higher pitched the murmur will sound
- Large, nonrestrictive VSDs may generate little to no murmur

Blood forced through stenotic systemic arteries

- Aortic coarctation

Murmur may be most prominent in the left paraspinal region.

Blood forced through stenotic pulmonary arteries

- Branch pulmonary stenosis
- Peripheral pulmonic stenosis

Murmur may be audible in one or both axillae and one or both posterior lung fields.

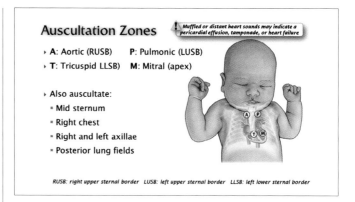

Auscultation Zones

Muffled or distant heart sounds may indicate a pericardial effusion, tamponade, or heart failure

- A: Aortic (RUSB)   P: Pulmonic (LUSB)
- T: Tricuspid LLSB   M: Mitral (apex)

- Also auscultate:
  - Mid sternum
  - Right chest
  - Right and left axillae
  - Posterior lung fields

RUSB: right upper sternal border   LUSB: left upper sternal border   LLSB: left lower sternal border

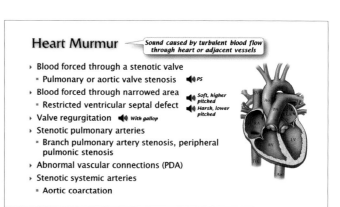

Heart Murmur — Sound caused by turbulent blood flow through heart or adjacent vessels

- Blood forced through a stenotic valve
  - Pulmonary or aortic valve stenosis PS
- Blood forced through narrowed area Soft, higher pitched
  - Restricted ventricular septal defect Harsh, lower pitched
- Valve regurgitation With gallop
- Stenotic pulmonary arteries
  - Branch pulmonary artery stenosis, peripheral pulmonic stenosis
- Abnormal vascular connections (PDA)
- Stenotic systemic arteries
  - Aortic coarctation

Increased blood flow across normal structures

- Increased RV blood volume secondary to left-to-right shunting of blood through an ASD. The increased RV blood volume generates sound as it passes through a normal pulmonary valve.

A murmur may be audible in anemic patients.

EXAM TIP: Systematic Approach to Auscultating for a Heart Murmur

When listening for a heart murmur, consider closing your eyes to tune out other sensory input. A systematic approach will help determine the following characteristics of a murmur: location, radiation, timing, intensity, quality, and pitch.

- **Location***
  - ◆ **A** = *Right upper sternal border (RUSB; aortic valve area)*
  - ◆ **P** = *Left upper sternal border (LUSB; pulmonary valve area)*
  - ◆ **T** = *Left lower sternal border (LLSB; tricuspid valve area)*
  - ◆ **M** = *Apex (mitral valve area)*
  - ◆ **Midsternum**

- **Radiation** (*auscultate the right chest, both axillae, and posterior lung fields*)
- **Timing** (*when the murmur is heard in the cardiac cycle*)
- **Intensity**
- **Quality** (*harsh, blowing, vibratory, machinery, to-and-fro*)
- **Pitch** (*high, medium, low*)

*In the setting of a normal heart position in the chest. Murmurs may be audible in more than one location, and timing, intensity, quality, and pitch may be different from one location to another.

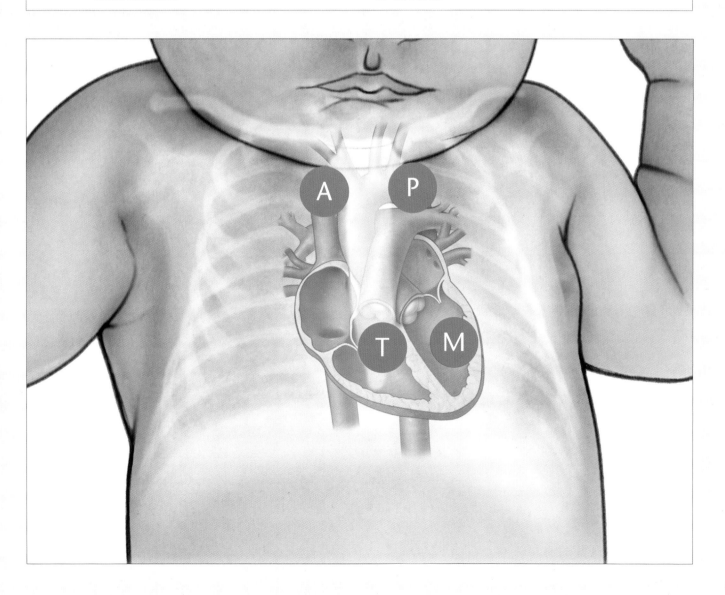

Heart Murmur

Timing

Systolic

- Heard after closure of the mitral and tricuspid valves during ventricular contraction (systole)

  ♦ Between the first and second heart sound — S1 and S2

  ♦ Majority of murmurs are systolic

Diastolic

- Heard after closure of the pulmonic and aortic valves during diastole

  ♦ Between the second and first heart sound — S2 and S1

Continuous

Heard throughout systole and extending into diastole

Loudness/intensity

Grade 1   Barely audible

Grade 2   Soft but audible

Grade 3   Moderately loud, no thrill

Grade 4   Loud and associated with a thrill

Grade 5   Audible with the stethoscope barely on the chest

Grade 6   Audible with the stethoscope not touching the chest

Thrill

A palpable vibratory sensation associated with a loud harsh murmur is known as a thrill. Presence of a thrill increases the grade of the murmur to 4. To detect a thrill, palpate the chest lightly with the palm of your hand or the more sensitive parts of your fingers.

Heart Murmur

Timing
› *Systolic* – after closure of mitral and tricuspid valves during ventricular contraction
  ▪ Heard between S1 and S2 of same beat
    ◦ S1 (*murmur*) S2   S1 (*murmur*) S2   S1 (*murmur*) S2
› *Diastolic* – after closure of pulmonic and aortic valves during diastole
  ▪ Heard between S2 and S1 of next beat
    ◦ S1, S2 (*murmur*)   S1, S2 (*murmur*)   S1, S2 (*murmur*)
› *Continuous*
  ▪ Heard throughout systole and extending into diastole

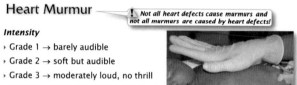

Heart Murmur — ! *Not all heart defects cause murmurs and not all murmurs are caused by heart defects!*

Intensity
› Grade 1 → barely audible
› Grade 2 → soft but audible
› Grade 3 → moderately loud, no thrill
› Grade 4 → loud, associated *with* thrill
› Grade 5 → audible with stethoscope barely on chest
› Grade 6 → audible without stethoscope on chest

When murmur is loud, palpate over the heart for a thrill – "vibratory sensation"

The base of the heart is the plane of the heart that lines up with the tricuspid, mitral, aortic and pulmonary valves. The apex of the heart is the tip of the left ventricle or the most pointed part of the ventricular mass. The apex lies to the left of the sternum, aiming forward and lying behind the fifth left intercostal space (see Figure 1.17 on page 56).

 An infant with NO heart murmur may still have significant cardiac disease, whereas an infant with a heart murmur may have NO structural heart disease.

Heart Murmur

Non Pathologic Murmurs

Peripheral Pulmonic Stenosis (PPS)

PPS is usually an innocent murmur secondary to flow through the branch pulmonary arteries that are mildly narrowed compared with the main pulmonary artery. In utero, the majority of right ventricular output is directed through the ductus arteriosus, leaving the branch pulmonary arteries to receive a reduced amount of pulmonary blood flow. After birth, the pulmonary blood vessels accommodate the entire RV output, sometimes resulting in turbulence and a murmur.

Characteristic qualities of a PPS murmur

- Heard loudest over both axillae and the back (posterior lung fields)
- Short systolic ejection murmur
- Grade 1-2/6
- May be intermittent
- Usually resolves by 6 months of age

Still's murmur[107,167,169]

- Innocent vibratory systolic ejection murmur
- Also described as musical or twanging string quality
- Grade 2-3/6
- Heard best along the LLSB and apex

Still's murmur was named after Dr. George Frederic Still, who first described it in the early 1900s. Especially common in school age children, the exact cause for a Still's murmur has not been determined.

Closure of the DA

- With closure of the DA, a grade 1-2/6 systolic ejection or continuous murmur may be audible.

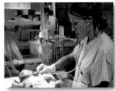

Heart Murmur

Non-Pathologic

› Peripheral pulmonic stenosis (PPS)
- Reflects mild narrowing of branch pulmonary arteries
- Heard loudest in axillae and back → listen to both right and left sides
- Short systolic ejection murmur
- Grade 1 - 2 / 6
- Usually resolves by 6 months of age

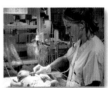

Heart Murmur

Non-Pathologic

› Still's murmur
- Innocent vibratory systolic ejection murmur
- Described as musical or twanging string quality
- Grade 2 - 3 / 6
- Heard best along lower left sternal border and apex

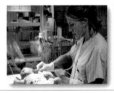

Heart Murmur

Non-Pathologic

› Systolic ejection or continuous murmur
- Often heard in first week after birth as pulmonary vascular resistance decreases and the ductus arteriosus closes
- Grade 1 - 2 / 6

Heart Murmur

Determining if a murmur is pathologic involves making an association to other signs of compromise that may include any of the following:

- Central cyanosis
- Respiratory distress
- Shock
- Weak or discrepant pulses (meaning the brachial pulses are palpable but the femoral pulses are weak or absent)
- Bounding pulses
- Abnormal heart size or pulmonary vascularity on chest x-ray

Heart Murmur

May be Pathologic if associated with:

- › Central cyanosis, respiratory distress, shock*
- › Weak or discrepant pulses
- › Bounding pulses
- › Abnormal heart size or pulmonary vascularity on chest x-ray
- › Loud grade 3 murmur within hours of birth
- › Gallop → evaluate for congestive heart failure
- › Diastolic murmur may be associated with abnormal aortic or pulmonary valve

Non-specific findings

Other abnormal findings that may indicate presence of a pathologic murmur

- A loud, grade 3 murmur within hours of birth
- Presence of a gallop that should prompt investigation for poor heart function and CHF
- A diastolic murmur is usually associated with abnormalities of the aortic or pulmonary valves

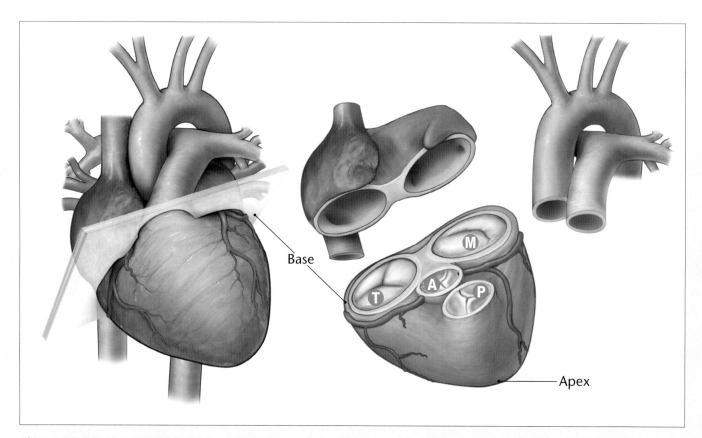

Figure 1.17. Anatomical display of the base of the heart, transected to show the location of the tricuspid (T), mitral (M), pulmonary (P), and aortic (A) valves.

Patient Assessment

Liver Size and Location

Normal

- Located in the right abdomen.
- Liver edge should be ≤ 2 cm below the right costal margin (RCM).
- Stomach bubble should be located in the left abdomen.

Abnormal

- Enlarged liver, > 2 cm below the RCM.
  - ◆ Evaluate for CHF, lung hyperinflation and liver disease.
- When the liver and the heart are on the same side, the infant should be evaluated for CHD or other abnormalities.

Misplaced liver

A midline location of the liver is seen with asplenia or polysplenia syndrome (see Table 1.5 on page 60).

Liver located in the left abdomen

When the liver is in the left abdomen and the heart is in the right chest, it may represent

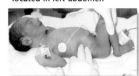

Liver Size and Location

Normal	*Abnormal*
▸ Located right abdomen	▸ Liver >2 cm below right costal margin
▸ ≤ 2 cm below right costal margin	• Evaluate for
▸ The stomach bubble should be located in left abdomen	Congestive heart failure
	Lung hyperinflation
	Liver disease
	▸ Location
	• Midline or left abdomen → implications for other abnormalities

Situs Inversus Totalis

Mirror Image Arrangement
- ▸ Heart and stomach on right side, liver on left side
- ▸ Approximately 3 – 5% incidence CHD

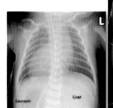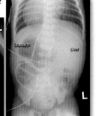

situs inversus totalis, and the heart may be structurally normal (see Figure 1.19 on page 59).

EXAM TIP

Palpate the liver when the infant is calm and the abdominal muscles are relaxed.

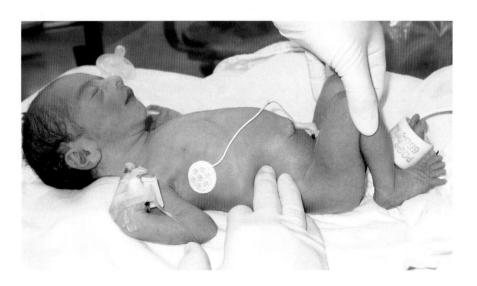

What does it mean? Situs solitus, situs inversus, and heterotaxy[2,66,170-175]

When the liver is in the left abdomen and the heart is in the left chest, complex CHD is most likely present.

In situs solitus, the abdominal viscera are in their normal, but asymmetric positions, and the cardiac structures are in their normal, but asymmetric configurations.

The right-sided organs are:

- Liver

- Gallbladder

- Trilobed right lung

- Right atrium that contains the sinoatrial node and receives deoxygenated systemic venous blood via the inferior and superior vena cava

- Tricuspid (3-leaflet) valve with chordae to ventricular septum that separates the right atrium from the right ventricle

- Right ventricle with trabeculated septum containing papillary muscles that attach via the chordae tendineae to the 3-leaflet tricuspid valve

- Infundibulum – a muscle bundle from which the pulmonary trunk arises

- Pulmonary (3-leaflet) valve that separates the right ventricle from the pulmonary artery

- Pulmonary artery that delivers blood to the right and left lungs

The left-sided organs are:

- Stomach

- Spleen

- Bilobed left lung

- Left atrium that receives oxygenated blood from four pulmonary veins

- Mitral (2-leaflet) valve that separates the left atrium from the left ventricle

- Left ventricle with a smooth-walled septum containing papillary muscles that attach via the chordae tendineae to the 2-leaflet mitral valve

- Aortic (3-leaflet) valve that separates the left ventricle from the aorta

- Aorta that delivers blood to the brain and body, left-sided aortic arch

Levocardia is the term used to describe a normal position of the heart in the left hemithorax with the apex pointing inferiorly and to the left.

Dextrocardia means the heart is located in the right hemithorax with the apex pointing inferiorly and to the right (Figure 1.18 on page 59).

Dextrocardia with situs inversus totalis means there is asymmetry of the abdominal organs and the lung lobes (as described in situs solitus), but they are swapped in a mirror image configuration (Figure 1.19 on page 59). Serious forms of CHD may be present, but the incidence is much lower.

Heterotaxy is the term used to describe failure of differentiation into right- and left-sided organs. This serious condition has implications for the organs and blood vessels that should normally be on the side that did not develop correctly. Two major variations are seen with heterotaxy. The first is **asplenia syndrome**, which is also called right isomerism or bilateral right-sidedness, and the other is **polysplenia syndrome,** which is also called left isomerism or bilateral left-sidedness. When asplenia is present, the cardiovascular effects are usually more severe. Table 1.5 on page 60 summarizes normal anatomy and the most common features of asplenia and polysplenia syndromes.

Dextrocardia with normal positions of the liver and stomach

Situs inversus totalis

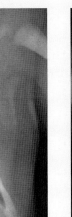
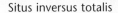
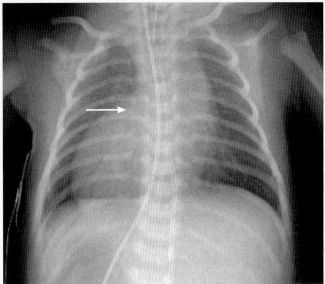
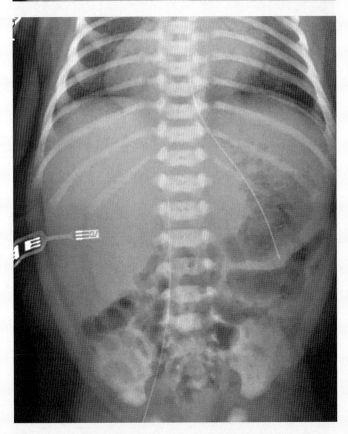
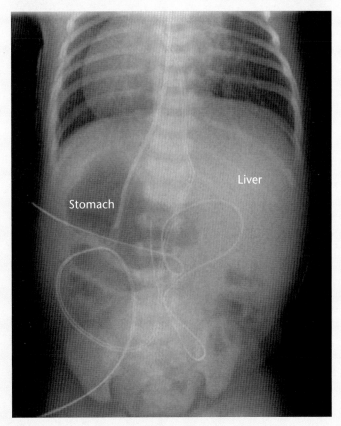

Liver

Stomach

Figure 1.18. Infant with dextrocardia and normal positions of the stomach and liver. The chest-xray demonstrates the UVC is too deep and needs to be repositioned. The gastric tube tip terminates in the stomach. The abdominal x-ray demonstrates a peripherally inserted central catheter (PICC) in the inferior vena cava. A near infrared spectroscopy (NIRS) monitor sensor is seen over the right flank.

Figure 1.19. Infant with situs inversus totalis. The heart is in the right chest and the liver is in the left abdomen. The umbilical venous catheter is malpositioned in the right atrium, or has passed through the foramen ovale to the left atrium (white arrow). The abdominal x-ray shows the gastric tube in the stomach (in the right abdomen) and the liver (in the left abdomen). The umbilical artery catheter tip is at lumbar vertebrae 2 (L2).

	Normal Anatomy	Asplenia Syndrome Right isomerism or bilateral right-sidedness	Polysplenia Syndrome Left isomerism or bilateral left-sidedness
Abdomen	Single spleen located in the left abdomen	Asplenia (no spleen) – has implications for severe immunocompromise	Polysplenia – multiple splenic tissues present (may have splenic dysfunction)
	Liver located in the right abdomen	Midline liver with 2 mirror image right lobes	Midline liver
	Gallbladder located in the right abdomen Patent biliary system	Gallbladder and biliary system not affected	May have hepatobiliary anomalies including biliary atresia
	Stomach located in the left abdomen Normal intestinal anatomy with appropriate mesenteric attachment	Stomach on the right or left side Intestinal malrotation may be present	Stomach on the right or left side Intestinal malrotation may be present
Lungs	Right lung trilobed Left lung bilobed	Bilateral trilobed (2 right lungs)	Bilateral bilobed (2 left lungs)
Heart & Vessels	Levocardia (normal position with a normal base-apex cardiac axis)	Dextrocardia (30 to 40% of cases), otherwise left chest (levocardia) or midline (mesocardia)	Dextrocardia (30 to 40% of cases)
	Atria Right atrium receives blood from the inferior and superior vena cava and is separated from the right ventricle by the tricuspid valve Left atrium receives blood from the 4 pulmonary veins and is separated from the left ventricle by a bileaflet mitral valve	Bilateral right atria, including two SA nodes Common AV valve (80 to 90% of cases)	Bilateral left atria and absent SA node Common AV valve (20 to 40% of cases)

	Normal Anatomy	Asplenia Syndrome Right isomerism or bilateral right-sidedness	Polysplenia Syndrome Left isomerism or bilateral left-sidedness
Ventricles Right ventricle has trabeculated septum and is separated from the pulmonary valve by a muscle bundle (infundibulum) Left ventricle has smooth-walled septum and is separated from the aorta by an aortic valve	Functionally single ventricle (40 to 50% of cases)	Two ventricles usually present	
Pulmonary veins 4 veins drain into the left atrium	TAPVC very common (obstructed in over half of cases)	Partial or total anomalous pulmonary venous connection (70% of cases)	
Great vessels Aorta originates from the left ventricle Left aortic arch Pulmonary artery originates from the right ventricle and branches to the right and left lungs	Transposition or malposition of the great arteries is common Pulmonary atresia or severe pulmonary stenosis (85% of cases)	Transposition (15% of cases) Coarctation of aorta (18% of cases) Pulmonary atresia or severe pulmonary stenosis (38% of cases)	
Systemic veins Inferior vena cava (IVC): drains into the right atrium Superior vena cava (SVC): drains into the right atrium	IVC usually present (may drain to right or left-sided atrium) Bilateral SVC (65% of cases)	Usually interrupted IVC at the suprahepatic segment with azygos or hemiazygos connection to SVC Bilateral SVC (33% of cases) Single right or left SVC (66% of cases)	

(Heart & Vessels (continued))

Table 1.5. Normal anatomy and the most common features of asplenia and polysplenia syndromes. Asplenia affects males more than females and occurs in 1% of newborns with symptomatic CHD. Polysplenia affects females more than males and occurs in <1% of all CHD.

Patient Assessment

Diagnostic tests

Chest X-Ray[168,176,177]

Diagnostic tests helpful in establishing a diagnosis of CHD include a chest x-ray, electrocardiogram, and echocardiogram. A chest x-ray is useful to evaluate heart size, shape, and location, pulmonary vascular markings, and any pulmonary pathology, such as pneumonia, that could account for an infant's presentation that includes respiratory distress.

Pulmonary Vascular Markings (PVM)

Determine whether PVM are decreased, normal, or increased. An infant with ductal dependent pulmonary blood flow may have decreased PVM, whereas an infant with excessive pulmonary blood flow may have increased PVM.

An increased heart size (cardiomegaly) with increased PVM or pulmonary edema may

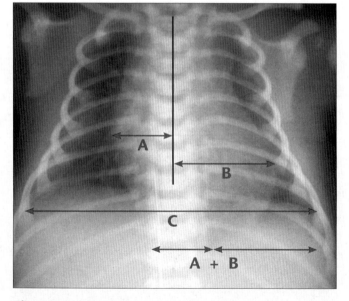

Evaluate Heart Size

Cardiothoracic Ratio

A = widest horizontal diameter of heart right of midline

B = widest horizontal diameter of heart left of midline

C = widest internal diameter of chest at or just below bottom of heart

⚠ *Ensure x-ray reflects good inspiration and infant is not rotated*

Normal in neonate = A + B < 60% of C

indicate heart defects with increased pulmonary blood flow or left-side obstruction and CHF. Cardiomegaly may also be seen following asphyxial injury to the myocardium or heart valves. In neonates, the cardiothoracic (CT) ratio should be < 60% of the thoracic diameter, and in infants, the CT ratio should be < 50% of the thoracic diameter. Figure 1.20 demonstrates the landmarks for measuring CT ratio.

1. Measure A + B
   A = widest horizontal diameter right of midline
   B = widest horizontal diameter left of midline

2. Measure C
   C = widest internal diameter of the chest at or just below the bottom of the heart

3. A + B divided by C equals the CT ratio

Normal
A + B < 60% of C
CT ratio < 60% in the neonate and < 50% in children and adults

Enlarged Heart
CT ratio > 60% in neonates and > 50% in children and adults

 Inadequate inspiration and rotation will make the heart appear enlarged. Ascertain that the x-ray being evaluated reflects a good inspiration and that the infant is not rotated.

Figure 1.20. The cardiothymic silhouette is measured and compared with the width of the chest at its largest dimension. To measure CT ratio, take the widest horizontal diameter right of midline (A), the widest horizontal diameter left of midline (B), and the widest internal diameter of the chest at or just below the base of the heart (C).

Electrocardiogram (ECG)[168]

An ECG is an essential test for evaluating and managing arrhythmias, and some ECG changes are suggestive of CHD. For example, an ECG often reveals left ventricular predominance in the setting of a hypoplastic right heart condition such as tricuspid atresia or pulmonary atresia with intact ventricular septum. Conclusive ECG findings may be difficult to ascertain with confidence; thus the ECG is best evaluated by a pediatric cardiologist.

Echocardiogram[168,179]

Echocardiographic imaging with color flow Doppler is a noninvasive test that allows for definitive diagnosis of congenital heart defects. Ultrasound beams identify cardiac structures, movement, and blood vessels entering and leaving the heart. Doppler including color mapping permits evaluation of blood flow, including assessment of valve regurgitation, valvular and vascular stenoses, and cardiac shunts. Ventricular function is also measured/estimated by an echocardiogram.

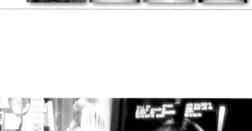

Diagnostic Tests

- Chest x-ray
  - ↑ or ↓ pulmonary vascular markings
  - Heart size, shape, location
- Electrocardiogram
- Echocardiogram
- Cardiac catheterization
- Lab tests → blood gas, lactate, genetics, other blood tests

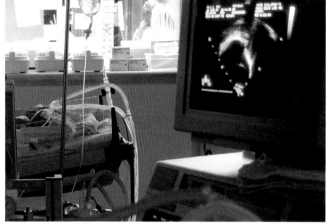

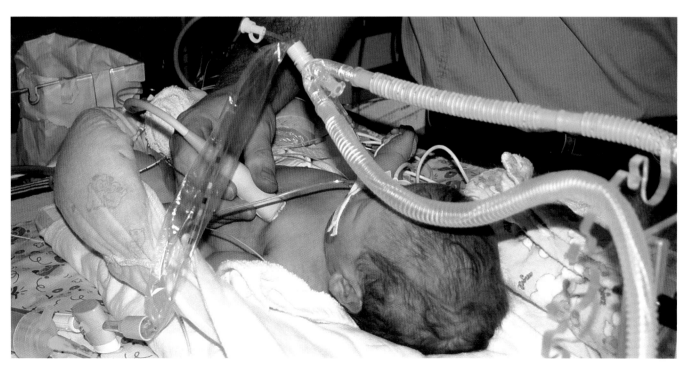

2-day old term infant with hypoplastic left heart syndrome.

Patient Assessment

Differential Diagnosis[169]

The clinical presentation of infants with CHD may be similar to other neonatal illnesses and respiratory conditions including sepsis, inborn error of metabolism, PPHN, congenital diaphragmatic hernia, transient tachypnea of the newborn, respiratory distress syndrome, meconium aspiration, pneumonia, or pneumothorax. PPHN occurs in approximately 10% of term and preterm infants with respiratory failure[110] and may present very similarly to cyanotic CHD. Infants with CHD usually present with one or more of the following:

- Tachypnea

- Cyanosis

- Signs of shock

- Heart murmur

- CHF

- Abnormal heart rhythm

- Abnormal heart size, shape, or location

It is important to recognize that infants with severe forms of CHD often have concurrent illnesses or conditions. Table 1.6 on page 65 contrasts key features of pulmonary versus cardiac disease to aid in differential diagnosis.

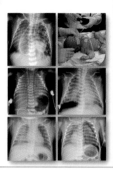

Differential Diagnosis for CHD

Pulmonary Causes of Respiratory Distress
- Persistent pulmonary hypertension (PPHN)
- Congenital diaphragmatic hernia (CDH)
- Transient tachypnea of newborn (TTN)
- Respiratory distress syndrome (RDS)
- Meconium aspiration
- Pneumonia
- Pneumothorax or other air leak

Other Causes of Respiratory Distress
- Sepsis, inborn error of metabolism

Differential Diagnosis for CHD

Neonates with CHD usually present with one or more of the following:
- Tachypnea
- Cyanosis
- Signs of shock
- Heart murmur
- Congestive heart failure
- Abnormal heart rhythm
- Abnormal heart size, shape, or location

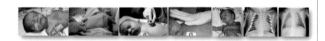

Differential Diagnosis for CHD

	Pulmonary	Cardiac
Cyanosis	Yes	Yes or No
Respiratory Rate	Tachypnea	Usually ↑ – may be "comfortable tachypnea"
Work of Breathing	↑ WOB: tachypnea, flaring, grunting, and/or retractions	Easy effort or ↑ WOB if in congestive heart failure
Acid / Base	↑ PCO_2 – respiratory acidosis or mixed acidosis if in shock	↓ PCO_2 – metabolic acidosis ↑ PCO_2 if CHF or lung pathology
Chest X-ray	Asymmetric pattern of infiltrates or other pulmonary pathology	↑ or ↓ pulmonary vascular markings, pulmonary edema*
Heart	Normal or cardiomegaly (especially if history of shock)	Normal or abnormal size, shape, location

May have infiltrates or other findings consistent with concurrent pulmonary disease

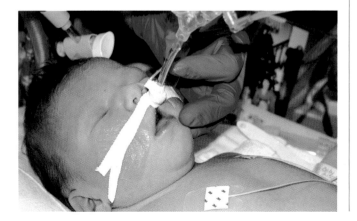

2-day old term infant with hypoplastic left heart syndrome.

	Pulmonary	Cardiac
Cyanosis	Yes	Yes or no
Respiratory rate	Usually increased	Usually increased and may be described as "comfortable tachypnea"
Work of breathing (WOB)	Increased WOB; may have nasal flaring, grunting, and/or retractions	Easy effort, but increased WOB if CHF has developed
Acid/base balance	Increased PCO_2 Respiratory acidosis or mixed acidosis if in shock	Decreased PCO_2 / metabolic acidosis Hypercarbia if CHF or concurrent pulmonary pathology*
Chest x-ray	May have asymmetric pattern of disease, infiltrates, or other pulmonary pathology	Increased or decreased pulmonary vascular markings; may have pulmonary edema*
Heart size, shape, location	Normal, or may have cardiomegaly if there is a history of shock	Normal, or may have an abnormal size, shape, or location

*May have infiltrates or other findings consistent with concurrent pulmonary disease.

Table 1.6. Key features of pulmonary versus cardiac disease to aid in differential diagnosis.

Infants with CHD may also have concurrent respiratory or other illnesses such as sepsis. Therefore, they may exhibit signs of both pulmonary and cardiac disease.

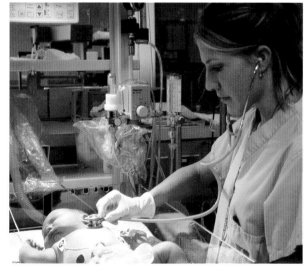
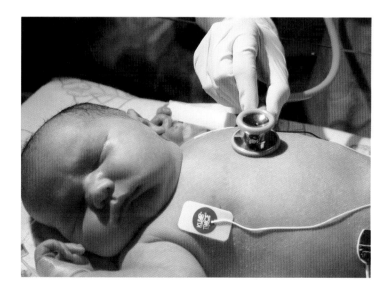

Late preterm, LGA, infant of a diabetic mother.

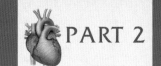

PART 2 Clinical Presentation and Stabilization of Neonates with Severe CHD

Part 2 of the S.T.A.B.L.E. – Cardiac Module is presented as follows:

1. Left-sided obstructive forms of CHD that are ductal dependent for systemic blood flow:

- Coarctation of the aorta
- Interrupted aortic arch
- Aortic valve stenosis
- Hypoplastic left heart syndrome

2. Cyanotic forms of CHD that are not ductal dependent for pulmonary blood flow:

- Tetralogy of Fallot*
- Tricuspid atresia*
- Truncus arteriosus
- Total anomalous pulmonary venous connection
- Ebstein anomaly*

3. Cyanotic forms of CHD that are ductal dependent for pulmonary blood flow:

- Pulmonary atresia with intact ventricular septum
- Pulmonary atresia with ventricular septal defect
- Transposition of the great arteries

_____

*Some forms may be ductal dependent

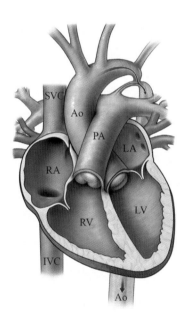
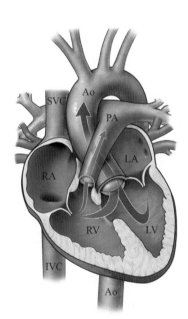
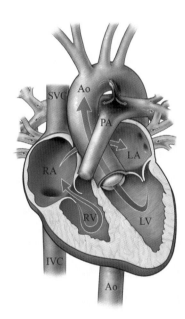

The Appendix on page 179 contains palliative and surgical options for the heart lesions presented in Part 2.

67

What does it mean?
Let's talk about CHD that is ductal dependent[82,83,169,180]

The ductus arteriosus (DA)

In utero, the placenta (not the lungs) is the site of gas exchange. In the fetus, most of the blood entering the right ventricle bypasses the lungs by flowing through a vessel that connects the pulmonary artery and aorta – the ductus arteriosus (DA). The DA is an artery that is lined with smooth muscle that normally closes shortly after birth. In most term infants, anatomic closure is by 4 days of age, but in some term infants, closure of the DA may be delayed or not happen spontaneously at all.

Factors contributing to vasoconstriction and closure of the DA include increased arterial oxygen content that occurs when the lungs take over gas exchange after birth, and removal of vasodilatory substances from the placenta upon cord separation.

Ductal dependent left-sided obstructive lesions

Infants with poor systemic perfusion secondary to critical left-sided obstructive lesions (coarctation of the aorta, critical aortic valve stenosis, interrupted aortic arch, hypoplastic left ventricle) will depend on a **right**-to-**left** shunt through the DA for systemic circulation. As the DA closes, poor cardiac output leads to shock.

Ductal dependent right-sided obstructive lesions

Infants with significantly decreased pulmonary blood flow secondary to right-sided obstructive lesions (pulmonary atresia with intact ventricular septum, severe pulmonary stenosis, tetralogy of Fallot with severe pulmonary stenosis or atresia, and tricuspid atresia with normally related great vessels, restrictive VSD and inadequate pulmonary blood flow), will depend on a **left**-to-**right** shunt from the aorta through the DA to the pulmonary arteries and lungs.

With transposition of the great arteries with an intact ventricular septum, maintaining ductal patency helps increase intercirculatory mixing by increasing the pressure in the left atrium to help drive oxygenated blood across the atrial septum to the right atrium, right ventricle, and out the aorta.

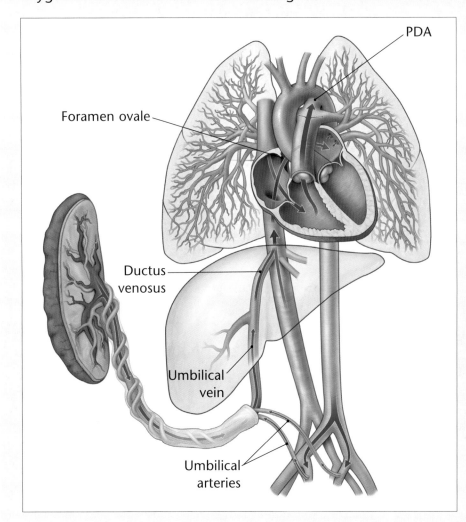

PDA

Foramen ovale

Ductus venosus

Umbilical vein

Umbilical arteries

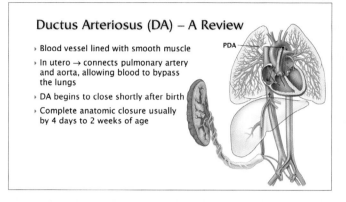

Ductus Arteriosus (DA) – A Review

- Blood vessel lined with smooth muscle
- In utero → connects pulmonary artery and aorta, allowing blood to bypass the lungs
- DA begins to close shortly after birth
- Complete anatomic closure usually by 4 days to 2 weeks of age

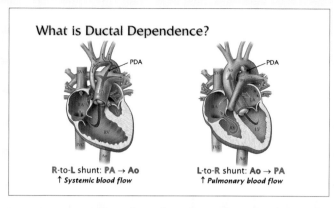

What is Ductal Dependence?

R-to-L shunt: PA → Ao
↑ *Systemic blood flow*

L-to-R shunt: Ao → PA
↑ *Pulmonary blood flow*

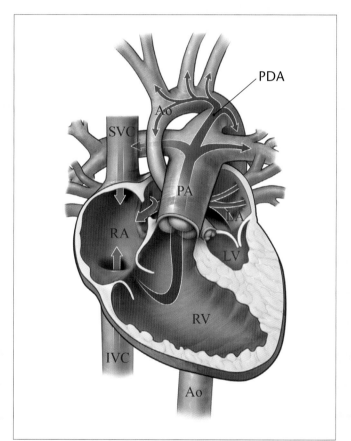

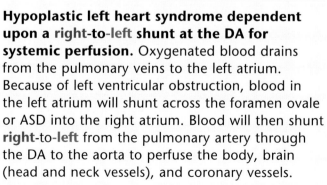

Hypoplastic left heart syndrome dependent upon a right-to-left shunt at the DA for systemic perfusion. Oxygenated blood drains from the pulmonary veins to the left atrium. Because of left ventricular obstruction, blood in the left atrium will shunt across the foramen ovale or ASD into the right atrium. Blood will then shunt **right**-to-**left** from the pulmonary artery through the DA to the aorta to perfuse the body, brain (head and neck vessels), and coronary vessels.

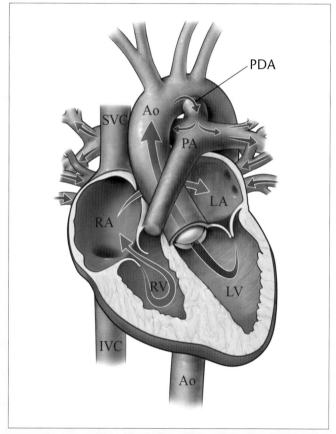

Pulmonary atresia dependent upon a left-to-right shunt at the DA for pulmonary perfusion. Because of outflow obstruction secondary to pulmonary valve atresia, blood that enters the right ventricle regurgitates back into the right atrium where it shunts across the foramen ovale or ASD to the left atrium, left ventricle, then into the aorta. To perfuse the lungs, blood shunts from the aorta, **left**-to-**right** through the DA, to the pulmonary arteries and lungs. In this setting, the orientation of the DA is reversed in comparison to the orientation of the normal DA with right-to-left flow in utero.

Pharmacology *Prostaglandin E1* (PGE, Alprostadil, Prostin)[129,181,182]

Indications

In the setting of ductal dependent left- or right-sided obstructive CHD, Prostaglandin E1 (PGE) is the life-saving medication used to dilate the DA and maintain ductal patency until either palliative or definitive intervention can be performed.

Action

- Causes vasodilation by direct effect on the smooth muscle in the DA and usually works within minutes to hours of starting the medication.
- PGE also dilates the pulmonary and systemic vascular beds so the infant should be monitored closely for hypotension.

Treatment Goals

- Improve BP and systemic perfusion in lesions dependent on the DA for systemic blood flow.
- Improve O_2 saturation and PO_2 in lesions dependent on the DA for pulmonary blood flow.

Dose

- The starting dose will vary depending on the age of the patient and clinical presentation. If ductal dependent CHD was diagnosed prenatally, the starting dose is usually lower because the PDA is widely open at the time of birth.
- If CHD is diagnosed after birth, the starting dose will depend on the infant's presenting signs and clinical stability.
- If the infant presents with CHD after 2 or 3 weeks of age, PGE infusion may not be as effective in opening the DA.

Prostaglandin E₁ (PGE)

Opens or Maintains Patency of the Ductus Arteriosus (DA)

> Action
  - Causes vasodilation by direct effect on smooth muscle in DA
  - Also dilates pulmonary and vascular bed → monitor for hypotension

> Treatment goals
  - Improve BP and systemic perfusion in lesions dependent on DA for systemic blood flow
  - Improve O_2 saturation and PO_2 in lesions dependent on DA for pulmonary blood flow

Prostaglandin E₁ (PGE)

Clinical Situation	Dose (mcg/kg/minute)
Prenatally diagnosed ductal dependent CHD, newborn (DA open)	0.01 – 0.03 mcg/kg/min
CHD *not* prenatally diagnosed (DA may not be open or is closing)	Usual starting dose is between 0.05 – 0.1 mcg/kg/min
Infant is critically ill (severe cyanosis or shock; DA is likely closed or very small)	Reasonable starting dose is 0.1 mcg/kg/min
NICU Management (echocardiogram demonstrates DA is widely open)	Titrate to 0.01 – 0.03 mcg/kg/min, based on side effects and institutional preference

⚠ *May cause apnea → be prepared to support breathing!*

Clinical Situation	PGE Dose (micrograms/kg/minute)
Prenatally diagnosed ductal dependent CHD and patient is a newborn (DA is open)	0.01 to 0.03 mcg/kg/minute
CHD was not prenatally diagnosed (DA may not be open or is closing)	Usual starting dose is between 0.05 to 0.1 mcg/kg/minute
Infant is critically ill (severe cyanosis or shock; DA is likely closed or very small)	Reasonable starting dose is 0.1 mcg/kg/minute
NICU Management (echocardiogram demonstrates DA is widely open)	Titrate to 0.01 to 0.03 mcg/kg/minute, based on side effects and institutional preference

Infusion Rules

- PGE has a short half-life and therefore must be administered as a continuous drip infusion.
- Infuse via a separate IV site, preferably a central line if one is available.
- PGE is compatible in D_5W, $D_{10}W$ or normal saline but is not compatible with many medications. Check with your pharmacist for medication compatibility.
- Prime the line effectively to ensure quick delivery and effect.

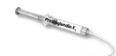

Prostaglandin E₁ (PGE)

Infusion Rules

- Continuous drip infusion
- Infuse via a separate IV site and via a central line if possible
- Compatible in D_5W, $D_{10}W$ or normal saline
- Check with pharmacist for medication compatibility → avoid using with any medications where rate may vary

Side Effects

Respiratory (usually dose dependent)

- Respiratory depression or apnea may occur.
- Apnea is usually seen within the first few hours of infusion, especially with higher doses and with administration of other sedating medications.
- Increased incidence of apnea is associated with preterm infants and infants who are < 2 kilograms.

Cardiovascular

- Hypotension, bradycardia, tachycardia.

Central Nervous System

- Fever, irritability, jitteriness, seizure-like activity.

Endocrine

- Hypocalcemia and hypoglycemia.

Gastrointestinal

- Stimulates intestinal smooth muscle and may cause diarrhea.

Hematologic

- Inhibits platelet aggregation, monitor for bleeding.

Bones

- Cortical hyperostosis and associated tenderness and bone pain with prolonged PGE exposure, especially when given for more than 30 days.[183,184]

 At all times, be prepared to offer positive pressure ventilation to support breathing

Underlying Concepts

With severe left-sided obstructive lesions, systemic perfusion is dependent upon a **right**-to-**left** shunt through the ductus arteriosus (DA). As the DA closes, blood flow to the tissues and organs is severely reduced which leads to CHF and shock. When the DA is re-opened with a PGE infusion, blood flows **right**-to-**left** from the pulmonary artery through the PDA to the aorta. In some cases, perfusion of the brain and coronary circulation depends on retrograde blood flow as follows: Pulmonary artery ➔ PDA ➔ retrograde into the aorta ➔ to the arterial branches perfusing the neck, brain, arms, and to the ascending aorta where the coronary arteries arise.

Left-Sided Obstructive Lesions

Ductal Dependent / Systemic Blood Flow

› Patent ductus arteriosus (PDA) *is* required for systemic perfusion

› R-to-L blood flow through ductal shunt
  ▪ PA → PDA → Ao

› If systemic blood flow is obstructed → infant will be in shock

The anatomic features and blood flow patterns of the left heart obstructive lesions will be presented first, followed by clinical presentation and stabilization

See the **Appendix** on page 183 for palliative and surgical options for the lesions discussed in this section.

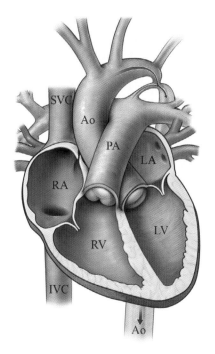

Coarctation of the aorta

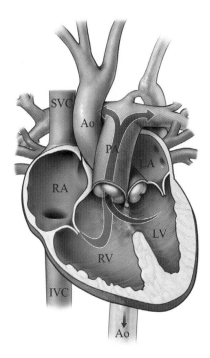

Interrupted aortic arch

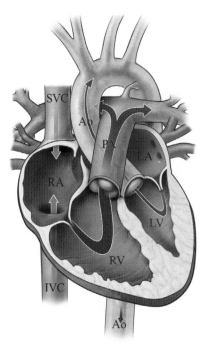

Aortic valve stenosis

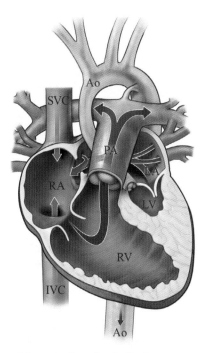

Hypoplastic left heart syndrome

Coarctation of the Aorta (COA)[73,185-188]

COA occurs in 0.3 to 0.4 per 1,000 live births or 5 to 8% of all cases of CHD.

COA is seen twice as often in males as in females. The incidence of COA in Turner's syndrome, which affects only females, is 30 percent.

COA is a discrete narrowing of the descending aorta often located just distal to the origin of the left subclavian artery and adjacent to the DA. The portion of the aorta beyond the left subclavian artery and right before the DA is called the aortic isthmus.

Ductal tissue often extends into the area of the coarctation and with ductal closure, the narrowing may become significant enough to impair systemic perfusion. In severe cases of COA, the left ventricle may be unable to pump blood past the narrowed area and the infant will develop CHF and shock.

The transverse aortic arch and isthmic area may also be hypoplastic. Associated cardiac defects include a bicuspid aortic valve (50% of cases) and ventricular septal defect.

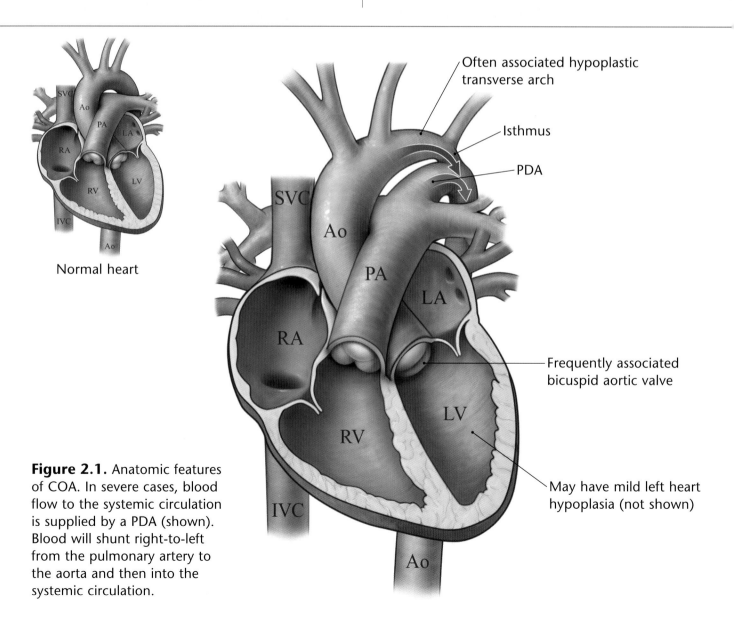

Normal heart

Often associated hypoplastic transverse arch

Isthmus

PDA

Frequently associated bicuspid aortic valve

May have mild left heart hypoplasia (not shown)

Figure 2.1. Anatomic features of COA. In severe cases, blood flow to the systemic circulation is supplied by a PDA (shown). Blood will shunt right-to-left from the pulmonary artery to the aorta and then into the systemic circulation.

Coarctation of Aorta

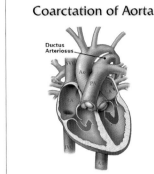

Coarctation "shelf" or "ledge" – seen on heart echo as the ductus arteriosus closes

Anatomic Features

▸ Juxtaductal narrowing of aorta
  ▪ Some ductal tissue in area of coarctation
▸ May have associated
  ▪ Hypoplastic transverse arch
  ▪ Bicuspid aortic valve *(shown)*

Coarctation of Aorta

Video Demonstrates

1) Initial PDA
2) PDA slowly closes → impairs systemic perfusion
3) PGE started to re-open the ductus arteriosus
4) Perfusion to systemic circulation improves

When an echocardiogram is performed, watch for mention of presence or absence of a posterior ridge or "shelf" in the juxtaductal region of the aortic arch. Presence of this finding should raise suspicion that there is a coarctation of the aorta. Additionally, aortic measurements more than 2-standard deviations below the mean for the patient's body size (z score less than -2) is consistent with clinically significant aortic hypoplasia that may require intervention.

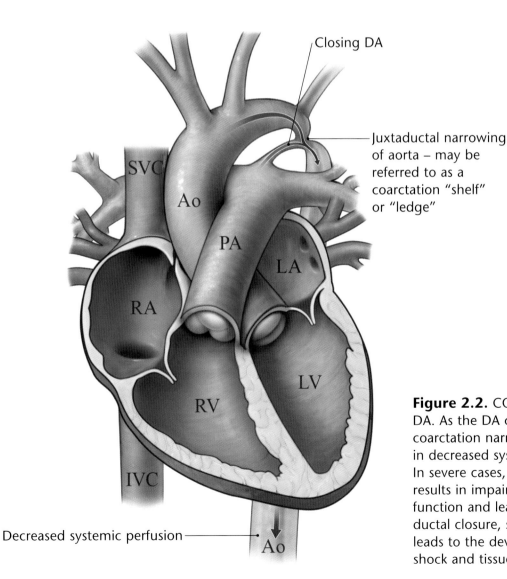

Figure 2.2. COA with a closing DA. As the DA closes, the area of coarctation narrows and results in decreased systemic blood flow. In severe cases, the narrowing results in impaired left ventricular function and leads to CHF. With ductal closure, severe coarctation leads to the development of shock and tissue hypoxia.

Interrupted Aortic Arch (IAA)[71,185,186,188,189]

IAA occurs in approximately 0.7 to 1.4% of all cases of CHD.

IAA is the most severe form of arch obstruction and is characterized by complete discontinuity of the proximal and distal portions of the aortic arch. A VSD is almost always present and allows oxygenated blood to shunt from the left to the right ventricle, to the pulmonary artery, to the PDA and into the aorta distal to the interruption. This right-to-left shunt through the PDA provides systemic perfusion beyond the interruption. Clinically, the infant may have differential cyanosis (higher O_2 saturation in the right hand and lower O_2 saturation in the foot).

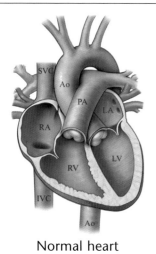

Interrupted Aortic Arch

Anatomic Features
▸ Type B (shown – most common)
▸ Ventricular septal defect (VSD)
▸ Varying degrees of
  ▪ Subaortic narrowing
  ▪ LV outflow tract hypoplasia

Evaluate for 22q11.2 DS

IAA can occur in one of three aortic locations (see page 77). Type B is most common.

22q11.2DS occurs in 50 to 80% of patients with IAA type B.

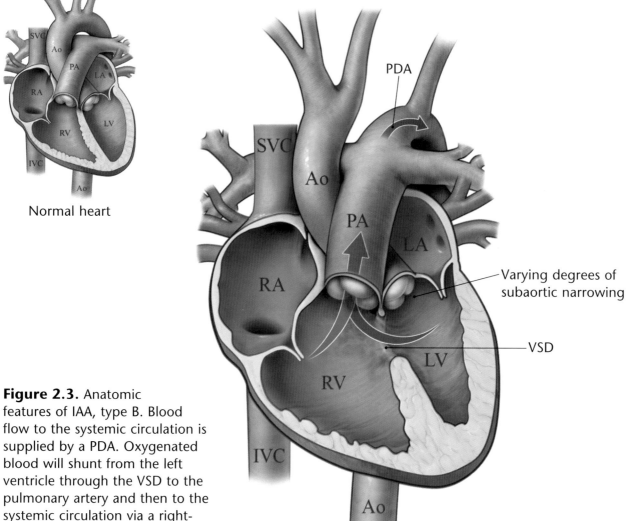

Normal heart

PDA

SVC

Ao

PA

LA

RA

Varying degrees of subaortic narrowing

VSD

LV

RV

IVC

Ao

Figure 2.3. Anatomic features of IAA, type B. Blood flow to the systemic circulation is supplied by a PDA. Oxygenated blood will shunt from the left ventricle through the VSD to the pulmonary artery and then to the systemic circulation via a right-to-left ductal shunt.

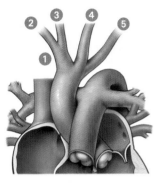

Type A: interruption of the aorta after the left subclavian artery and just proximal to the insertion of the DA. Occurs in approximately 30 to 44% of patients with IAA.

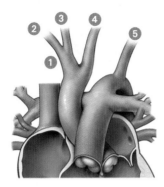

Type B: interruption of the aorta between the left carotid artery and left subclavian artery. Occurs in approximately 51 to 70% of patients with IAA.

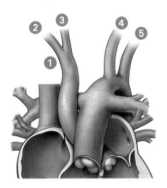

Type C: interruption of the aorta between the brachiocephalic artery and the left carotid artery. Occurs in approximately 1 to 5% of patients with IAA.

① Brachiocephalic (innominate) artery ② Right subclavian artery
③ Right carotid artery ④ Left carotid artery ⑤ Left subclavian artery

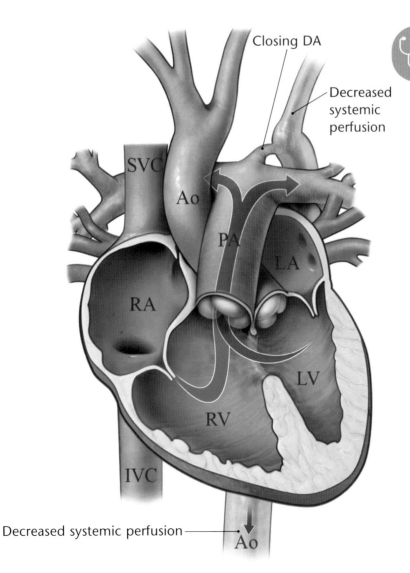

Figure 2.4. IAA with a closing DA. Depending on where the interruption occurs, blood flow to the area supplied by the right-to-left shunt through the DA will diminish, resulting in tissue hypoxia and shock.

EXAM TIP

Type A: With ductal closure, the right and left brachial pulses will be palpable and equal, while femoral pulses will feel decreased or absent.

Type B and C: With ductal closure, the right brachial pulse will be palpable. The left brachial pulse and femoral pulses will feel decreased or absent.

Memory tip! Type **C** occurs between the right and left **C**arotids.

Aortic Valve Stenosis (AS)[185,186,188,190,191]

AS accounts for approximately 3 to 6% of all cases of CHD, with males affected four times more often than females.

AS obstructs the flow of blood from the left ventricle to the aorta, compromising normal systemic perfusion. The aortic valve is abnormal and may be bicuspid (more common) or unicuspid. In severe cases, systemic perfusion depends upon a right-to-left shunt across the DA. In this case, the degree of AS is classified as "critical."

Associated heart defects may include:

- Left ventricular hypoplasia
- Mitral valve hypoplasia/stenosis
- VSD
- Coarctation of the aorta

Critical AS requires maintaining patency of the ductus arteriosus with a PGE infusion until the AS is treated. Less critical forms of AS can progress over time and therefore, close follow up is warranted. A systolic ejection murmur may be heard at the RUSB radiating toward the neck, and a systolic ejection click may be heard (often at the apex of the heart).

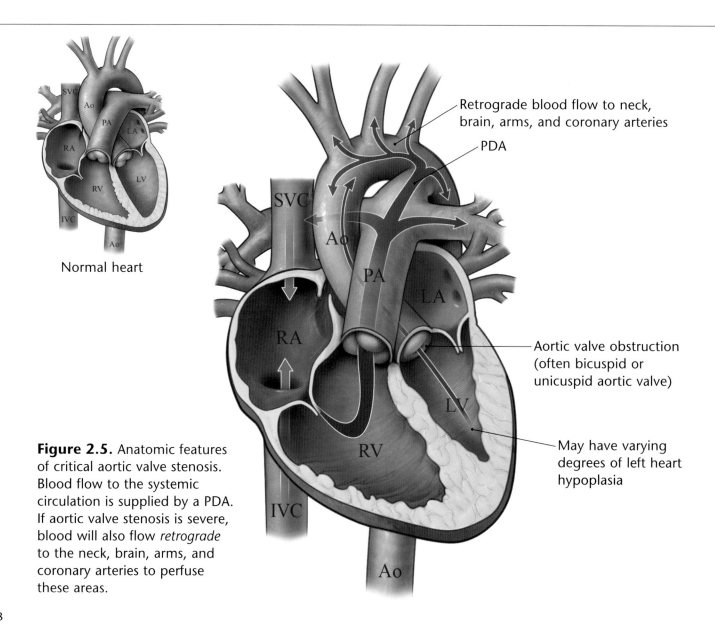

Normal heart

Retrograde blood flow to neck, brain, arms, and coronary arteries

PDA

Aortic valve obstruction (often bicuspid or unicuspid aortic valve)

May have varying degrees of left heart hypoplasia

Figure 2.5. Anatomic features of critical aortic valve stenosis. Blood flow to the systemic circulation is supplied by a PDA. If aortic valve stenosis is severe, blood will also flow *retrograde* to the neck, brain, arms, and coronary arteries to perfuse these areas.

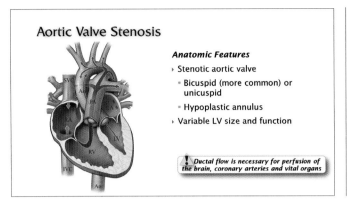

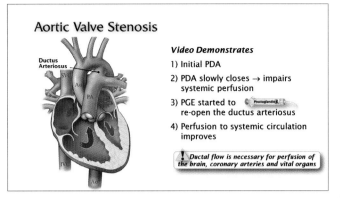

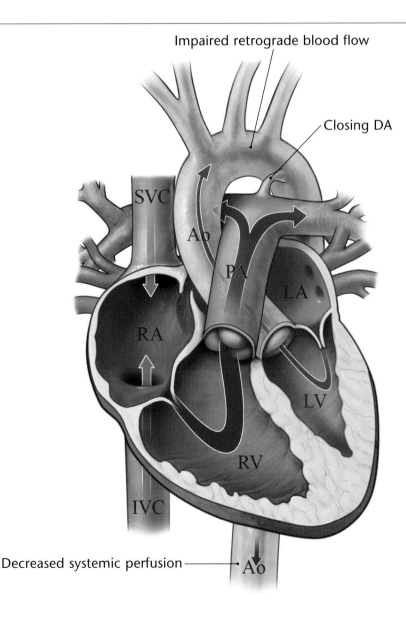

Figure 2.6. Critical aortic valve stenosis with a closing DA. Depending on the degree of aortic valve obstruction, a variable amount of blood will be ejected into the aorta. As the DA closes, systemic blood flow including retrograde aortic blood flow (to the neck, brain, arms, and coronary arteries), will significantly diminish.

Hypoplastic Left Heart Syndrome (HLHS)[170,186,187,190,192]

HLHS occurs in 1 in 5,000 live births and accounts for 1.4 to 3.9% of all cases of CHD. Males are affected more often than females.

HLHS is characterized by the following:

- A small left ventricle (hypoplasia)

- Either severe mitral valve stenosis or atresia, or severe aortic valve stenosis or atresia (any combination can exist)

- Hypoplastic ascending aorta and transverse aortic arch

- Coarctation of the aorta is a frequent finding and may be present in as many as 75% of patients

With HLHS, blood flow to all regions of the body is dependent on a right-to-left ductal shunt (pulmonary artery through the PDA to the aorta).

- To perfuse the brain and coronary arteries, blood must flow retrograde in the arch and ascending aorta.

- To perfuse the rest of the body, blood must flow antegrade down the descending aorta.

As the DA closes, perfusion is decreased to all organs, including the brain and heart.

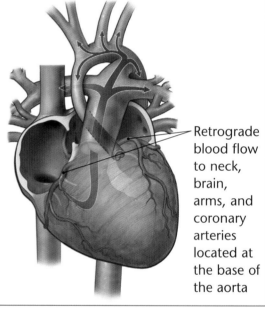

Retrograde blood flow to neck, brain, arms, and coronary arteries located at the base of the aorta

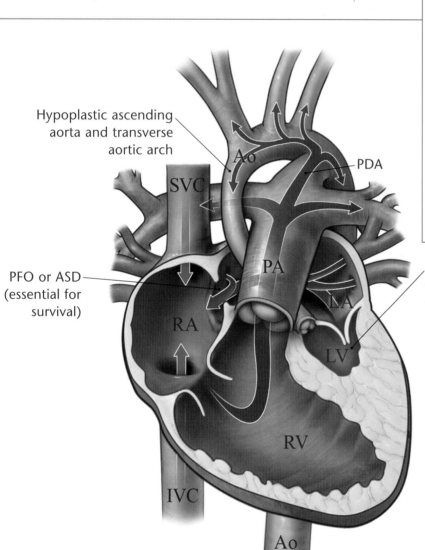

Hypoplastic ascending aorta and transverse aortic arch

Ao
SVC
PDA
PA
LA
PFO or ASD (essential for survival)
RA
LV
IVC
RV
Ao

Small left ventricle with associated aortic valve atresia/stenosis (shown) or mitral valve atresia/stenosis

Figure 2.7. Anatomic features of HLHS and the pattern of blood flow seen when PGE maintains ductal patency. Oxygenated blood will drain from the pulmonary veins to the left atrium where it will shunt left-to-right into the right atrium. Blood will then shunt right-to-left from the pulmonary artery through the DA to the aorta to perfuse the body, brain (head and neck vessels), arms, and coronary arteries (see illustration above). Coarctation of the aorta is a frequent finding (not shown).

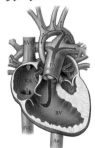

Hypoplastic Left Heart Syndrome (HLHS)

Anatomic Features

› Small left ventricle with associated aortic stenosis/atresia or mitral stenosis/atresia
› Hypoplastic aorta
  ▪ Coarctation is common (not shown)
› Atrial communication nearly always present
  ▪ If absent → severe cyanosis
› Systemic perfusion (including to the brain and coronary arteries) requires R-to-L shunting through DA

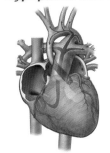

Hypoplastic Left Heart Syndrome (HLHS)

Anatomic Features

› PA → PDA → aorta → retrograde perfusion of arms, neck, brain, and coronary arteries

An atrial level shunt is *essential* to pulmonary blood flow by allowing oxygenated blood to shunt from the left atrium to the right atrium. A severely restricted atrial septal defect (ASD) or foramen ovale limits pulmonary blood flow, that leads to severe, life-threatening cyanosis, and respiratory distress, shortly after birth. However, most infants with HLHS have no restriction or mildly restricted flow at the foramen ovale or ASD, with signs of shock developing when the DA begins to close.

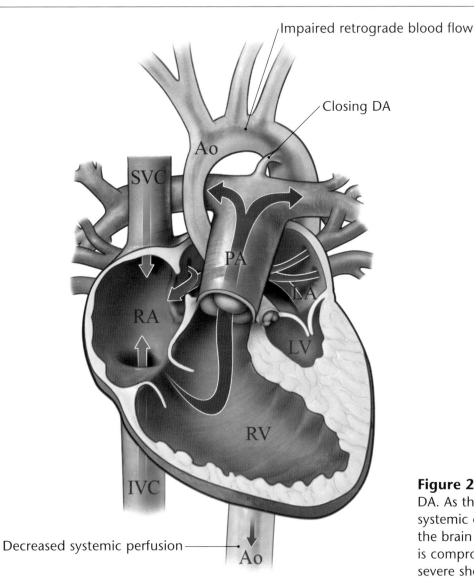

Impaired retrograde blood flow

Closing DA

Decreased systemic perfusion

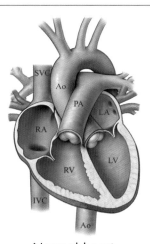

Normal heart

Figure 2.8. HLHS with a closing DA. As the DA closes, the entire systemic circulation (including to the brain and coronary arteries) is compromised, resulting in severe shock.

Left-Sided Obstructive Lesions[2,151,170,186,187,193]

Clinical Presentation

The clinical presentation for critical COA, IAA, critical AS, and HLHS is similar, and may mimic severe sepsis with low cardiac output. As the DA begins to close, the infant may present with tachypnea, cyanosis, poor feeding, a low urine output, and a change in level of consciousness.

Infants with COA and IAA often have a higher BP in the right arm compared to the legs. With all forms of left heart obstruction, further constriction of the DA reduces systemic blood flow and leads to signs of shock: weak pulses, a prolonged CRT, tachycardia, hypotension, metabolic acidosis and elevated lactate levels, dyspnea, and oliguria or anuria. Left untreated, most neonates with severe left heart obstruction will not survive long, and delayed recognition can result in organ damage and increased morbidity.

Cyanosis

May be an early presenting sign that triggers a diagnostic work-up. Differential cyanosis may be observed with right-to-left shunting through the DA (normal saturation in the right hand, lower saturation in the foot; postductal site).

Heart Sounds

An ejection click may be present with aortic valve stenosis, but there needs to be adequate flow across the aortic valve.

The second heart sound may be single.

With decreased ventricular function and heart failure, a gallop rhythm may be audible.

Murmur

In some cases, a systolic ejection murmur may be heard at the RUSB, while in other cases, no murmur is heard.

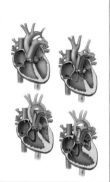

Left-Sided Obstructive Lesions

Clinical Presentation
- Symptoms coincide with closure of the ductus → usually first 10 days of life
- Early signs
  - Tachypnea
  - Poor feeding
  - Low urine output
  - Change in level of consciousness

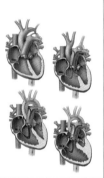

Left-Sided Obstructive Lesions

Clinical Presentation
- As ductus closes → signs of shock and congestive heart failure
  - Pulses diminish with ductal closure for all LVOT lesions
    - Coarctation, interrupted aortic arch leads to loss of femoral pulses
  - Tachycardia
  - Hypotension
  - Poor perfusion and tissue oxygenation → metabolic acidosis

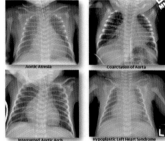

Left-Sided Obstructive Lesions

Chest X-ray
- May have normal or increased heart size
- Increased pulmonary vascular markings and pulmonary edema when CHF develops

Chest X-Ray

Heart Size

Cardiomegaly is common, but not uniformly observed.

Pulmonary Vasculature

Increased pulmonary vascular markings and pulmonary edema are observed when CHF develops.

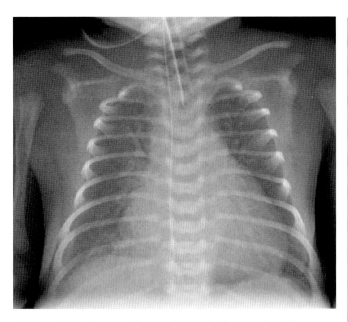

1-day old infant with aortic (valve) atresia. There are moderate diffuse bilateral granular opacities throughout the lungs; no pneumothorax or pleural effusion. The heart size is mildly enlarged. The ET tube tip is in good position. The gastric tube tip terminates in the lower thoracic esophagus.

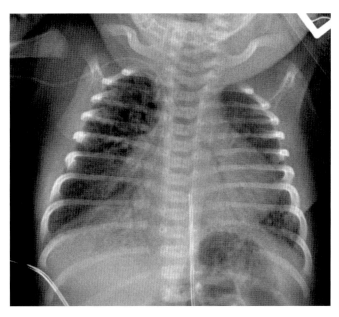

Neonate with COA. There is mild central atelectasis and a slightly cystic appearance of the right upper lung. No pneumothorax or pleural effusion. The cardiac silhouette is enlarged. The UAC tip projects at T7. The tip of the right upper extremity PICC overlies the mid SVC.

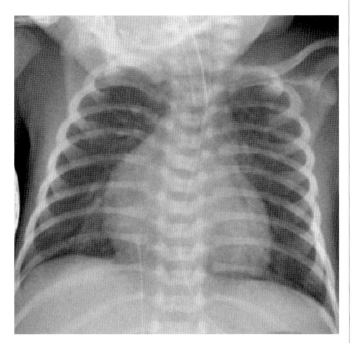

4-day old infant with IAA. The lungs are well expanded. There is no pneumothorax or pleural effusion. The cardiac silhouette is not enlarged. The endotracheal tube is in the mid-trachea. The tip of the lower extremity PICC terminates just above the IVC/right atrial junction. The gastric tube projects toward the stomach, but the tip is not visualized.

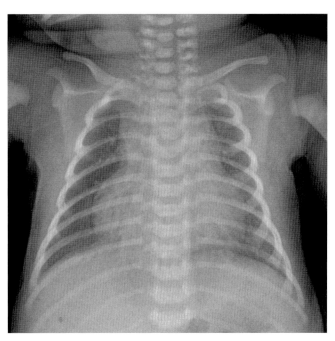

12-hour old term infant with HLHS. One hour prior to this x-ray, a loud murmur was heard by the infant's nurse, which prompted an exam by the neonatal nurse practitioner who ordered this chest x-ray and an ECG. There is mild cardiomegaly and mild diffuse opacities bilaterally. See the full case report on page 85.

Initial Stabilization

Treatment is aimed at improving systemic blood flow, reversing metabolic acidosis, providing respiratory support, balancing systemic with pulmonary blood flow, and assessing the degree of secondary organ damage suffered during any period of impaired organ perfusion.

Blood Pressure Support
- An infusion of PGE will help re-establish and maintain ductal patency and improve systemic perfusion. This usually relieves metabolic acidosis caused by tissue hypoxia.
- 5 to 10 mL/kg normal saline volume support may be useful to improve systemic perfusion.
- Inotropes (for example epinephrine, dopamine, milrinone) may improve myocardial function, but may also increase myocardial oxygen demand, which in the setting of decreased coronary perfusion can be detrimental.

Respiratory Support
- Endotracheal intubation and mechanical ventilation may be required to reduce the work of breathing and strain on the heart, or in cases of apnea secondary to PGE or sedating medications.
- Avoid hyperoxia and hypocarbia because both decrease PVR which promotes increased pulmonary blood flow at the expense of systemic circulation (right-to-left blood flow through the DA).
- Diuretics may be useful to treat systemic or pulmonary edema.

NICU Management
O₂ Saturation Goal

Once the infant is stable, consult cardiology or neonatology regarding the desired O_2 saturation range goal. An elevated arterial PO_2 should be avoided because of its constrictive effects on

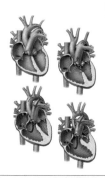

Left-Sided Obstructive Lesions

Stabilization
- Start PGE to establish and maintain ductal patency and improve systemic perfusion
- Provide respiratory support
  - Endotracheal intubation may be required
- ⚠ Avoid hyperoxia and hypocarbia → target O_2 saturation 75 – 85%
  - Elevated arterial PO_2
    - Constricts ductus arteriosus
    - Dilates pulmonary vasculature → increases pulmonary blood flow *at the expense of systemic perfusion*

Left-Sided Obstructive Lesions

Stabilization
- Cautious volume resuscitation as necessary
- Treat congestive heart failure → diuretics, inotropes
- Evaluate for and treat organ damage
  - Kidneys, liver, brain, intestine

ductal tissue and its vasodilatory effects on the pulmonary vasculature. Pulmonary vasodilation allows more blood to flow to the lungs at the expense of systemic blood flow.

Maintain the preductal O_2 saturation between 75 and 85% to help balance pulmonary blood flow (by increasing PVR) and promote systemic blood flow (via the right-to-left ductal shunt).

PGE Infusion
Once the DA is widely open, titrate the dose as able to 0.01 to 0.03 mcg/kg/minute. However, consultation with cardiology and neonatology should precede any titration of PGE.

 Because of the right-to-left shunt at the DA, use caution with central venous catheters (and peripheral IVs) to prevent emboli from reaching the systemic circulation.

An infant was born at term gestation to a 31-year-old, gravida 3, now para 3 woman whose pregnancy was complicated by gestational hypertension. The prenatal labs were all unremarkable except for a positive group B streptococcus (GBS) screening test at 36-weeks' gestation. There were no other known infectious risk factors, however the GBS was inadequately treated prior to delivery. An ultrasound at 20 weeks of gestation was normal. There was no family history of CHD. Labor was induced for maternal hypertension. Spontaneous rupture of membranes occurred 3 hours prior to delivery; the fluid was clear.

Apgar scores were 8 at one minute and 9 at five minutes. The infant transitioned well and maintained normal vital signs. He was breastfeeding without difficulty and the mother had no concerns.

At 11 hours of age, the nurse practitioner was asked to examine the infant because of a murmur that was heard by the nurse during a normal neonatal evaluation. On exam the infant was alert and in no distress. The exam was remarkable for a grade 3/6 holosystolic low pitched murmur loudest at the RUSB but radiating throughout the precordium and to the back, and a grade 2/6 high pitched short systolic murmur heard at the LLSB. The pulses were palpable and equal in the upper and lower extremities. The liver edge was palpable 1.5 cm below the right costal margin. Capillary refill was brisk and the lungs were clear to auscultation. There was easy respiratory effort without retractions or tachypnea. The pre and postductal saturations and upper and lower extremity blood pressures were obtained. A chest x-ray and electrocardiogram (ECG) were ordered. Echocardiography was not available at this facility. The chest x-ray is shown on page 83. The ECG reading was pending.

At 12 hours of age, the blood pressures were:
Right arm 63/39 MAP 48, preductal O_2 sat 99%
Left arm 60/43 MAP 49, preductal O_2 sat 99%
Right leg 67/43 MAP 52, postductal O_2 sat 100%
Left leg 65/42 MAP 50, postductal O_2 sat 100%

The infant remained with the mother who was advised to notify the nursing staff immediately if she had any concerns including tachypnea, increased work of breathing or any difficulty feeding.

At 19 hours of age, the mother was concerned for difficulty feeding and faster respirations. The respiratory rate was 74 breaths per minute, and the preductal O_2 sat was 100%. A postductal sat was not assessed at that time.

At 20 hours of age, the preductal O_2 sat was 99% (on room air) and the postductal O_2 sat was 88%. On exam, both murmurs persisted, but the liver edge had increased to 2 cm below the RCM. Brachial and femoral pulses were palpable and the capillary refill time was < 3 seconds. The lungs were clear to auscultation and there was no increased work of breathing. The blood pressures were assessed as follows:
Right arm 66/40 MAP 49
Left arm 55/45 MAP 48
Right leg 63/37 MAP 45
Left leg 59/34 MAP 42

A capillary blood gas was obtained: pH 7.36, PCO_2 39 (5.2 kPa), PO_2 35 (4.7 kPa), Base deficit -3. Blood cultures were drawn, and antibiotics were started. Two peripheral IV's were placed and PGE was ordered but not started per the transfer team's recommendations. On arrival to the Pediatric Cardiology unit following transfer, an echocardiogram revealed HLHS. PGE was then started.

Underlying Concepts

- Neonates with cyanotic congenital heart disease (CHD) have mixing of red (oxygenated, saturated) and blue (deoxygenated, desaturated) blood at the atrial and/or ventricular and/or ductal levels.

- Blood must flow through the pulmonary artery to the lungs to become oxygenated.

- When blood is diverted away from the pulmonary arteries and lungs by a right-to-left shunt at the atrial and/or ventricular level, a higher volume of blue blood will be ejected through the aorta — to the body — and the infant will appear cyanotic.

- In cases where the infant has reduced pulmonary blood flow, cyanosis will improve with improved pulmonary blood flow. As a larger volume of blue blood enters the lungs, a larger volume of oxygenated red

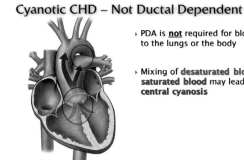

Cyanotic CHD – Not Ductal Dependent

› PDA is **not** required for blood flow to the lungs or the body

› Mixing of **desaturated blood** with **saturated blood** may lead to **central cyanosis**

blood will return via the pulmonary veins to the heart. Thus, the proportion of red to blue blood will increase and cyanosis will decrease or disappear.

See the **Appendix** on page 197 for palliative and surgical options for the lesions discussed in this section.

Stabilizing the Cyanotic Neonate with Suspected CHD

1. Administer blended oxygen and increase the FiO_2 to try and achieve a preductal O_2 saturation between 91 and 95%. Oxygen helps improve systemic oxygenation and decrease PVR. Infants with cyanotic CHD may not be able to achieve an O_2 saturation > 80% despite administration of 100% oxygen.

2. Optimize respiratory support.

3. Evaluate for physical and laboratory signs of shock and offer resuscitative treatment as indicated.

4. Evaluate for and treat any other causes of cyanosis such as pulmonary disease, sepsis, shock secondary to non-cardiac causes, metabolic derangements, and neurologic depression.

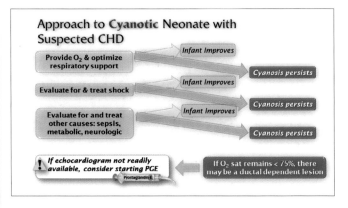

Approach to Cyanotic Neonate with Suspected CHD

Provide O_2 & optimize respiratory support → Infant Improves / Cyanosis persists

Evaluate for & treat shock → Infant Improves / Cyanosis persists

Evaluate for and treat other causes: sepsis, metabolic, neurologic → Infant Improves / Cyanosis persists

⚠ If echocardiogram not readily available, consider starting PGE (Prostaglandin E)

If O_2 sat remains < 75%, there may be a ductal dependent lesion

5. If CHD is suspected and the O_2 saturation remains < 75% after optimizing all support as outlined above, and if an echocardiogram is not readily available, then a PGE infusion should be considered to establish and then maintain ductal patency. See page 70 for more information about PGE dosing and side effects.

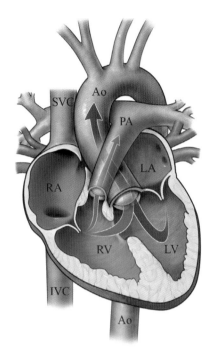

Tetralogy of Fallot*

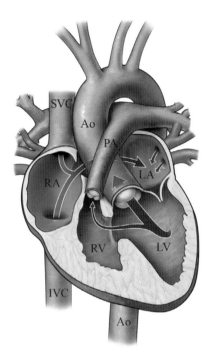

Tricuspid atresia*

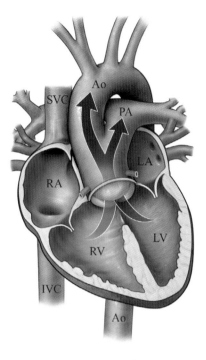

Truncus arteriosus

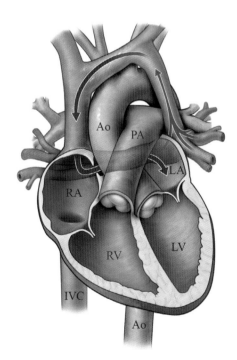

**Total anomalous
pulmonary venous
connection**

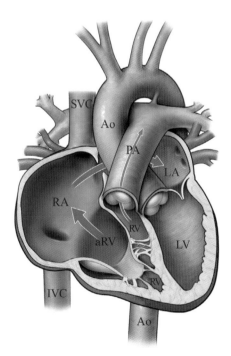

Ebstein anomaly*

*Some forms may be ductal
dependent

Tetralogy of Fallot (TOF)[71,73,171,186,188,194-196]

TOF affects approximately 10% of all infants with CHD and occurs in males slightly more than females. Four primary abnormalities characterize TOF:

- A large ventricular septal defect (VSD)
- RVOT obstruction secondary to infundibular (subvalvar) stenosis (most common) and/or pulmonary valve stenosis
- Aortic override of the ventricular septum
- Right ventricular hypertrophy secondary to systemic right ventricular pressure in the setting of a large VSD (i.e. the blood

pressures in the ventricles are equal, whereas without a VSD, the RV blood pressure should be much lower)

A right aortic arch is present in 25% of cases of TOF. The pulmonary valve annulus may be near normal in size to severely hypoplastic. The severity of cyanosis relates to the degree of RVOT obstruction. The most severe form of TOF, pulmonary atresia with a VSD, is described in more detail on page 132.

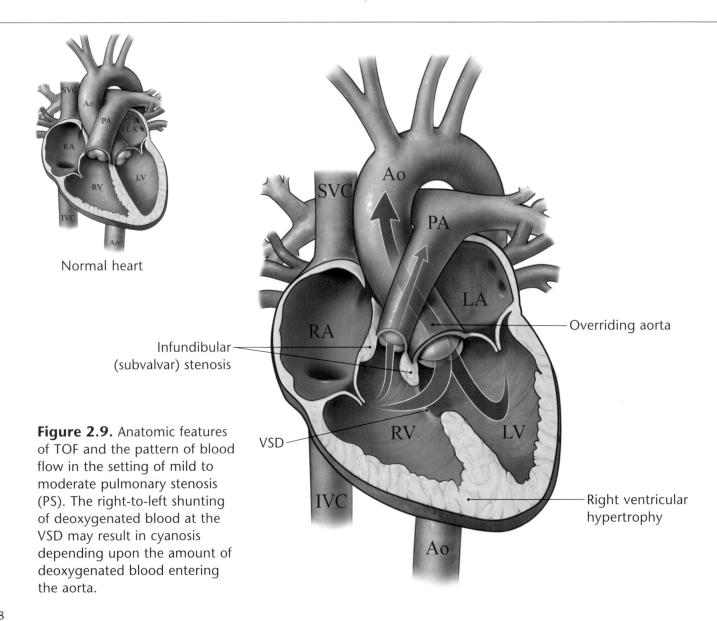

Normal heart

Figure 2.9. Anatomic features of TOF and the pattern of blood flow in the setting of mild to moderate pulmonary stenosis (PS). The right-to-left shunting of deoxygenated blood at the VSD may result in cyanosis depending upon the amount of deoxygenated blood entering the aorta.

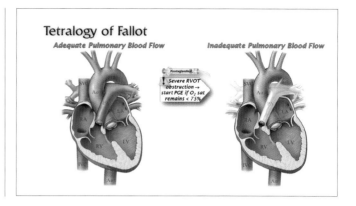

Tetralogy of Fallot

Anatomic Features

- Large ventricular septal defect (VSD)
- Right ventricular outflow tract (RVOT) obstruction
  - Infundibular (subvalvar) stenosis (*most common*) and/or pulmonary valve stenosis
- Overriding aorta
- Right ventricular hypertrophy
  - VSD results in equalized ventricular pressures

Tetralogy of Fallot

Adequate Pulmonary Blood Flow   *Inadequate Pulmonary Blood Flow*

Severe RVOT obstruction → start PGE if O₂ sat remains < 75%

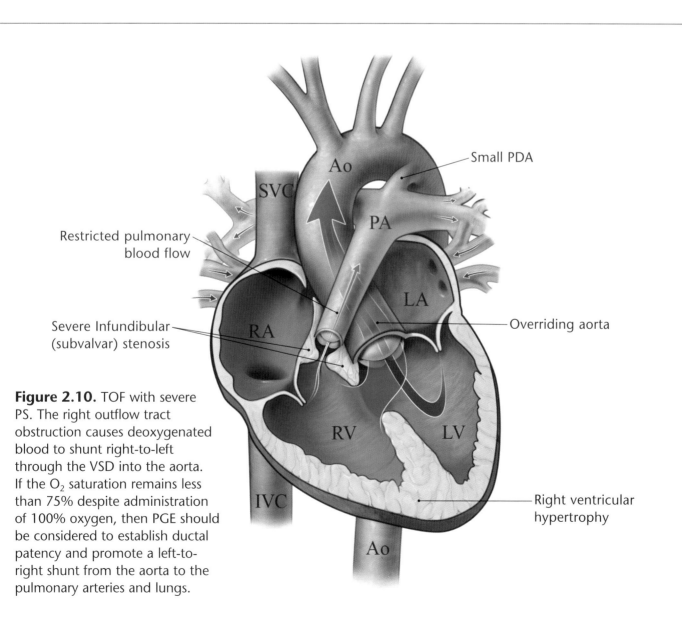

Figure 2.10. TOF with severe PS. The right outflow tract obstruction causes deoxygenated blood to shunt right-to-left through the VSD into the aorta. If the O₂ saturation remains less than 75% despite administration of 100% oxygen, then PGE should be considered to establish ductal patency and promote a left-to-right shunt from the aorta to the pulmonary arteries and lungs.

Tetralogy of Fallot (TOF)

Clinical Presentation

Cyanosis

- **Cyanotic tetralogy of Fallot ("Blue Tet").**
  As shown in Figures 2.9 and 2.10, with more pronounced pulmonary stenosis, cyanosis is moderate to severe because deoxygenated blood shunts right-to-left, from the right ventricle through the VSD and out the aorta.

- **Acyanotic tetralogy of Fallot ("Pink Tet").**
  As shown below, when RVOT obstruction is mild to moderate, pulmonary blood flow may be adequate, and cyanosis is mild or absent. When the right and left ventricles contract, blood shunts from the left ventricle through the VSD to the right ventricle, pulmonary arteries and lungs. This left-to-right shunting can cause pulmonary overcirculation. Signs/ symptoms of pulmonary overcirculation include tachypnea, diaphoresis, poor feeding, and poor weight gain. However, it is important to recognize that infants with pink tet may develop progressive obstruction to pulmonary blood flow and become cyanotic over time.

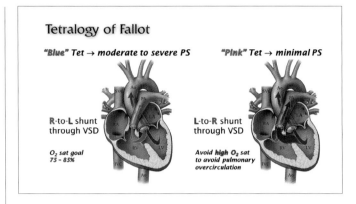

Tetralogy of Fallot

"*Blue*" Tet → moderate to severe PS   "*Pink*" Tet → minimal PS

R-to-L shunt through VSD

O₂ sat goal 75 – 85%

L-to-R shunt through VSD

Avoid **high** O₂ sat to avoid pulmonary overcirculation

Tetralogy of Fallot

Clinical Presentation
- Cyanosis relates to degree of RVOT obstruction
- Murmur
  - ↑ Intensity (loudness) = ↓ pulmonary stenosis
  - ↓ Intensity (loudness) = ↑ pulmonary stenosis

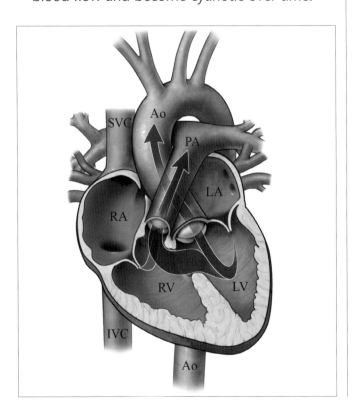

Heart Sounds

- The second heart sound is single because the pulmonary component (P2) is not audible (single S2).

Murmur

- The typical murmur is caused by the pulmonary stenosis (not the VSD) and is audible at birth.

- With a hypercyanotic episode ("tet spell"), the murmur is usually softer or even absent.

Chest X-Ray

Heart Size

- Heart size is usually normal.
- A right aortic arch is present in 25% of cases.

Heart Shape

- Concave main PA segment (secondary to a small PA) with an upturned apex secondary to right ventricular hypertrophy, creates the appearance of a "boot shaped" heart.

Pulmonary Vasculature

Variable pulmonary vascular markings:

- With decreased pulmonary blood flow (severe PS or atresia) the lung fields will appear dark (left x-ray)
- With adequate or increased pulmonary blood flow (mild PS), pulmonary vascularity may be increased (right x-ray)

Tetralogy of Fallot

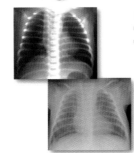

Chest X-ray
- ‣ Heart size usually normal
- ‣ Boot shaped heart
  - Concave main pulmonary artery segment
  - Upturned apex – secondary to RV hypertrophy
- ‣ Variable pulmonary vascular markings
  - Depends upon amount of pulmonary blood flow
  - ↓ With severe PS or pulmonary atresia

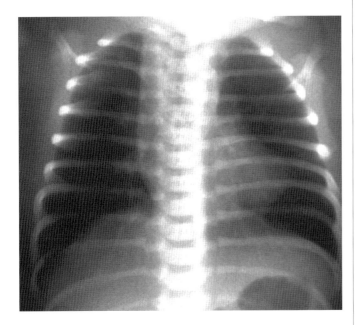

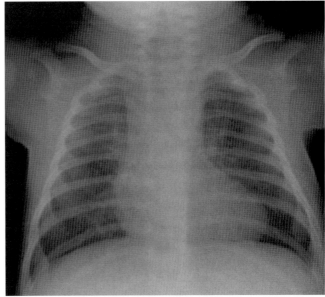

Initial Stabilization

1. Provide supplemental O_2 to treat hypoxemia and help relax the pulmonary vascular bed.

2. Cardiology consultation and echocardiography should be requested to allow further evaluation.

3. Most infants with TOF are not ductal dependent. If the O_2 saturation remains > 75%, the infant likely has adequate pulmonary blood flow.

4. If the O_2 saturation remains < 75% (on oxygen), the infant may have significant pulmonary stenosis or atresia. Until the diagnosis can be confirmed by echocardiogram, consider starting a PGE infusion to maintain ductal patency. See page 70 for PGE dosing and side effects.

5. Evaluate for 22q11.2DS; monitor for and treat hypocalcemia.

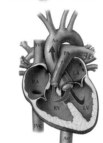

Tetralogy of Fallot

Initial Stabilization
- Provide O_2 to maintain O_2 sat > 75%
- Monitor O_2 sat as ductus arteriosus closes
- Evaluate for/treat hypocalcemia

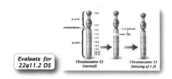

Evaluate for 22q11.2 DS

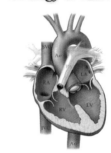

Tetralogy of Fallot

Initial Stabilization
- If O_2 sat remains < 75% after optimizing respiratory and cardiovascular support
  - May have severe RVOT obstruction/pulmonary valve stenosis
  - While awaiting echocardiogram, start PGE to maintain ductal patency

Prostaglandin E

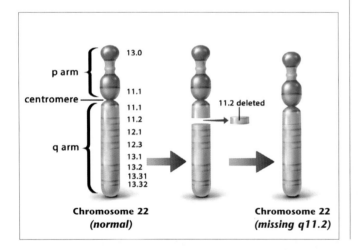

p arm	13.0	
centromere	11.1	
	11.1	
	11.2	11.2 deleted
	12.1	
q arm	12.3	
	13.1	
	13.2	
	13.31	
	13.32	

Chromosome 22 (normal) → **Chromosome 22 (missing q11.2)**

What does it mean?
Let's talk about hypercyanotic/tet spells[170,182,196-201]

What causes a hypercyanotic/tet spell?

Multiple theories have been proposed to explain the precise mechanism of hypercyanotic episodes ("tet spells"). A common explanation describes spasm of the already stenotic, muscular infundibular/subpulmonic area (Figure 2.11), but this theory is questionable given that tet spells can occur in infants without a significantly stenotic infundibular region. Most likely, the cause is multifactorial and includes catecholamine release and increased O_2 consumption that triggers an increase in pulmonary vascular resistance (PVR) in response to agitation, crying, or pain, (Figure 2.12 on page 94). Increased right-to-left shunting across the VSD may also result from a sudden decrease in systemic vascular resistance (SVR) secondary to hypovolemia, dehydration, or fever. Regardless of the actual cause of a tet spell, there is decreased pulmonary blood flow with increased shunting of blood from the right ventricle across the VSD and out the aorta.

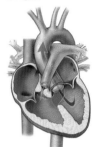

Tetralogy of Fallot – **Hypercyanotic / "Tet Spell"**

› Can occur prior to palliation or surgical intervention
› Acute decrease in pulmonary blood flow
  ▪ R-to-L shunt: **Right ventricle** → VSD → **Aorta**

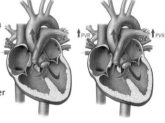

Tetralogy of Fallot – **Hypercyanotic / "Tet Spell"**

Multifactorial Causes

› Spasm of stenotic, muscular infundibular/subpulmonic area
› Catecholamine release and ↑ O_2 consumption in response to agitation, crying, pain → ↑ PVR and ↑ **R-to-L** shunting
› Sudden ↓ in SVR secondary to hypovolemia, dehydration, fever

SVR = systemic vascular resistance   PVR = pulmonary vascular resistance

(Continued on next page)

Cyanotic CHD
Not Ductal Dependent

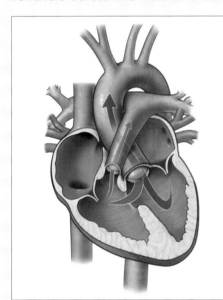
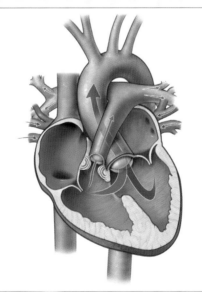
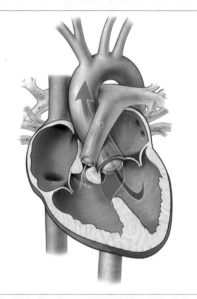

Figure 2.11. Pattern of blood flow seen during a hypercyanotic/tet spell. Severe right outflow tract obstruction causes most of the blood entering the right ventricle to shunt right-to-left through the VSD to the left ventricle, then out the aorta. Pulmonary blood flow is markedly reduced, resulting in severe hypoxemia and cyanosis.

What does it mean? Let's talk about hypercyanotic/tet spells (Continued)

Tet spells can be life threatening and the onset is usually sudden. Infants experiencing a spell become irritable, hypoxemic, pale, hyperpneic (increased rate and depth of respirations), flaccid, and in severe episodes, unconscious. A prolonged tet spell will lead to tissue hypoxia and ensuing metabolic acidosis that may severely impact the central nervous system and other organs.

Tet spells may occur at any time, beginning in the neonatal period and may worsen in frequency or severity because of clinical progression of the infundibular/subpulmonary stenosis and RV hypertrophy. Ideally, surgical correction of tetralogy of Fallot is performed before the onset of tet spells. In fact, given the potential morbidity of tet spells, the occurrence of documented spells is an indication for surgical intervention. Table 2.1 on page 97 summarizes the treatment steps when an infant is experiencing a tet spell.

Tetralogy of Fallot – Hypercyanotic / "Tet Spell"

Onset
- Can begin in the neonatal period and ↑ in frequency over next few months as subpulmonary stenosis and RV hypertrophy worsen

Signs of a Tet Spell
- Initially irritable
- Sudden and severe desaturation
- Hyperpnea (↑ rate and depth of respirations)
- Murmur becomes quieter or inaudible

EXAM TIP

If concerned about a tet spell, listen to the heart murmur to determine whether the murmur is less loud than usual. As blood flow through the pulmonary valve decreases, the systolic ejection murmur will be quieter or disappear altogether. As the spell resolves and pulmonary blood flow increases, the murmur will return to the baseline loudness.

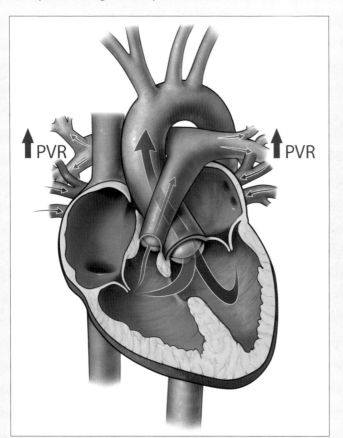

Figure 2.12. Tet spell secondary to increased PVR related to pain, agitation, or crying. As PVR increases, deoxygenated blood shunts right-to-left through the VSD, resulting in severe hypoxemia and cyanosis.

Hypercyanotic/Tet Spell – Treatment Principles

1. Calm the Infant
- To decrease oxygen demands and relieve anxiety, attempt to calm the crying irritable infant by non-pharmacologic methods initially.
- Avoid iatrogenic causes of agitation such as venipuncture (unless clinically indicated), or noxious stimuli (loud talking, painful procedures).
- Parental presence may be reassuring to the infant.

2. Improve Oxygenation
- Administer oxygen to help improve arterial saturation, which also helps decrease PVR. Recognize there may be little to no improvement until pulmonary blood flow increases given the obligate right-to-left shunt at the VSD, and that supplemental O_2 alone will not abort a spell.

3. Increase Systemic Vascular Resistance (SVR) to Decrease the Right-to-Left Shunt at the VSD *(this step is concurrent with number 2)*
- Place the infant in a knee-chest position. If the infant can tolerate being lifted, place the infant to your shoulder with the knees and hips drawn up toward the infant's chest. If lifting is not possible, press the knees up toward the chest (if lying supine), or lay the infant prone and tuck the knees up toward the chest. This position helps compress the femoral arteries and increase peripheral SVR, which will decrease the right-to-left shunt through the VSD and potentially improve/promote pulmonary blood flow.
- A 10 to 20 mL/kg IV normal saline fluid bolus can increase intravascular volume, improve preload, and prevent hypotension. However, this requires placement of an IV if none is already in place.

Tetralogy of Fallot – Hypercyanotic / "Tet Spell"
Treatment
- Attempt to calm infant
  - Non-pharmacologic methods initially
  - Avoid noxious stimuli – loud talking, painful procedures
- *Administer oxygen* to help improve oxygenation (done concurrently with next step)
  - Intubation and ventilatory support may be necessary

Tetralogy of Fallot – Hypercyanotic / "Tet Spell"
Treatment
- ↑ *SVR to ↓ R-to-L shunt at VSD* → help improve pulmonary blood flow
  - Place in knee-chest position
  - Normal saline fluid bolus to ↑ intravascular volume, improve preload, help prevent hypotension
  - Vasoconstrictor medications may be necessary (phenylephrine or norepinephrine)

- In severe cases where other maneuvers are not helping, administration of phenylephrine (Neo-Synephrine®) or norepinephrine increases SVR which helps reduce the right-to-left shunt at the VSD and therefore, promote pulmonary blood flow.
- Other medications that may be indicated for unremitting tet spells or to provide prophylaxis should surgical repair be delayed include beta blockers such as propranolol or esmolol. These medications lower the heart rate, improve diastolic ventricular filling and preload, and decrease O_2 consumption. Theoretically, beta blockers may also help lessen infundibular spasm or obstruction. It is important to ensure adequate intravascular volume/preload when initiating beta-blockade, as SVR will likely decrease, in addition to heart rate. (Continued on next page)

Cyanotic CHD Not Ductal Dependent

95

4. Attempt to Decrease Hyperpneic Respirations

- Hyperpnea, or an increased rate and depth of respirations, often accompanies the onset of a tet spell. During hyperpnea, the negative thoracic pump becomes more efficient and increases systemic venous return to the right heart. This in turn, increases the right-to-left shunt at the VSD.

- Strategies to eliminate hyperpneic respirations include administration of opioid or sedative medications including intramuscular (IM) ketamine or morphine. If an IV is already in place, morphine is commonly used. However, hypotension may occur with administration of morphine and complicate the situation by reducing SVR. If morphine is administered, it is important to ensure there is adequate intravascular volume and preload.

- Support ventilation with endotracheal intubation during prolonged and/or severe spells.

- Paralysis may also be necessary to reduce oxygen consumption. Severe hypoxemia from markedly decreased pulmonary blood flow will ultimately lead to tissue hypoxia and development of metabolic acidosis.

- Reverse acidosis (improve oxygenation and perfusion) as rapidly as possible to reduce the negative effects of acidosis on the respiratory center and pulmonary vasculature. In severe cases, sodium bicarbonate may be necessary to help correct acidosis, but ensure the patient is adequately ventilated before administration.

Tetralogy of Fallot – Hypercyanotic / "Tet Spell"

Treatment

🔴 *Medications that may be indicated*

- Beta blocker (esmolol, propranolol) → ↓ HR, ↑ diastolic ventricular filling and preload, ↓ O_2 consumption, and may ↓ infundibular spasm or obstruction
- To ↓ agitation and ↓ hyperpneic respirations
  - Intranasal versed
  - Morphine IM or IV — *Monitor closely for respiratory depression / hypotension ! Hypotension may worsen the situation!*
  - Ketamine IM or IV (also ↑ SVR)
  - Paralysis may be necessary to ↓ O_2 consumption
  - Sodium bicarbonate to treat severe acidosis — *Ensure adequate ventilation before administration!*

Tetralogy of Fallot – Hypercyanotic / "Tet Spell"

Treatment → Escalation of Care if Not Responding

🔴 *Options based on institutional preferences and resources*

- Extracorporeal membrane oxygenation (ECMO) support
- Emergency catheter intervention → stent the RV outflow tract
- Emergency surgical intervention → BT shunt or full cardiac repair

---

Other treatment options based on institutional preference include:

- Extracorporeal membrane oxygenation (ECMO) support.

- Stenting the RV outflow tract (catheterization procedure).

- Emergency placement of a Blalock-Taussig (BT) shunt to provide pulmonary blood flow (surgical procedure).

- Emergency surgical repair of the TOF.

Calm the infant	Parental presence, quiet environment, avoid painful stimuli
Administer oxygen	There may be little to no improvement until pulmonary blood flow increases. In severe cases, support breathing by intubating and providing ventilatory support.
Increase systemic vascular resistance (SVR) to decrease the R-L shunt at the VSD **Heart rate control to increase cardiac output** **Treat metabolic acidosis**	Knee-to-chest position. *If escalation in intervention is required:* Intravenous administration* - 10 to 20 mL/kg normal saline bolus: increase intravascular volume and prevent hypotension, maximize preload, improve cardiac output. - Beta blocker (esmolol, propranolol): lower the heart rate, improve diastolic ventricular filling and preload, decrease oxygen consumption, lessen infundibular spasm or obstruction. - Unremitting cases: systemic vasoconstrictor: phenylephrine or norepinephrine (increase SVR). - Sodium bicarbonate for worsening acidosis (and only if patient is adequately ventilated).
Decrease hyperpneic respiration **Treat pain and anxiety** **Decrease endogenous catecholamine release and decrease infundibular spasm**	IV is *not* present: - Midazolam (intranasal):[202] sedates infant and may help increase tolerance of IV insertion. - Morphine IM: reduces heart rate and respiratory rate, however hypotension may exacerbate the situation by increasing the R to L shunt at the VSD. - Ketamine IM: sedates infant and increases SVR. Onset of action is rapid. IV *is* present: - Morphine IV.
	*The pain from prolonged IV insertion attempts may further exacerbate the situation, so consider administering an intranasal or IM opioid or sedative medication before IV needle insertion.

Table 2.1. Treatment recommendations to break the vicious cycle of a hypercyanotic/tet spell.

What does it mean?
Let's talk about Double Outlet Right Ventricle (DORV)[71,170,186,203-207]

DORV occurs in approximately 0.06 per 1,000 live births and accounts for < 1% of all forms of CHD. There are multiple anatomic variants of DORV, leading to physiologic differences between the subtypes. Therefore, it is important to remember that the term DORV, without further anatomic description, does not define the physiology or the potential interventions that may be needed.

The primary anatomic features of DORV includes the following:

1. The pulmonary artery and the aorta arise mostly from the right ventricle.

2. There is usually a large VSD; oxygenated blood from the left ventricle shunts left-to-right through the VSD to the right ventricle where it mixes with deoxygenated blood. The blood is then ejected by the right ventricle into the aorta and pulmonary artery. The VSD is usually unrestricted.

3. The VSD location is described as subaortic (located close to the aorta), subpulmonary (located close to the pulmonary artery), doubly committed (aligned closely to both the aorta and pulmonary artery), or non-committed (located remotely from either great vessel).

4. Valvar or subvalvar pulmonary stenosis is common and may occur in about 50% of cases. However, in certain forms of DORV, there can be valvar or subvalvar aortic stenosis with associated arch hypoplasia/coarctation.

Double Outlet Right Ventricle

Anatomic features
› Pulmonary artery and aorta arise from right ventricle
› Large VSD (usually)
› May have valvar or subvalvar pulmonary or aortic valve stenosis

DORV with subaortic VSD and no PS

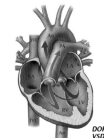

Double Outlet Right Ventricle

Anatomic Features
› VSD location affects clinical course
  ▪ Subaortic → close to Ao
  ▪ Subpulmonary → close to PA (*tetralogy-type; cyanosis*)
  ▪ Doubly committed → close to both Ao and PA (*transposition type; cyanosis*)
  ▪ Non-committed → remotely from either great vessel

DORV with subaortic VSD and no PS

Ao = aorta; PA = pulmonary artery

5. The position of the VSD in relation to the outlets (aortic and pulmonary valves), as well as the presence or absence of valvar or subvalvar obstruction determines the physiology.

6. Multiple other associated lesions may also be present depending upon the type of DORV including: ASD, PDA, right aortic arch, subvalvar, valvar or supravalvar aortic stenosis, mitral atresia, COA, IAA, coronary artery anomalies, and a left superior vena cava that drains to the coronary sinus or left atrium.

Types of DORV

DORV is categorized into different types based on the location of the VSD, the orientation of the great arteries to each other, and presence or absence of outflow tract obstruction.

- **_DORV with Subaortic VSD._** This is the most common type of DORV. It occurs in 45 to 55% of cases and can be further subclassified as being associated with or without subvalvar and/or valvar pulmonary stenosis.

- **_DORV with Subaortic VSD (without Pulmonary Stenosis)._** Clinically, this lesion presents like a large VSD and as PVR declines in the days and weeks after birth, these infants are at risk for developing CHF secondary to pulmonary overcirculation. This type of DORV is shown in Figure 2.13.

- **_DORV with Subaortic VSD and Pulmonary Stenosis (tetralogy-type of DORV)._** In as many as half of the cases in which there is a subaortic VSD, there is also valvar or subvalvar pulmonary stenosis, making this type of DORV similar to TOF. One commonly accepted diagnostic criterion to differentiate DORV from TOF, is that DORV is present when the aortic annulus overlies the RV by at least 50%. Like tetralogy of Fallot, these infants are at increased risk for experiencing hypercyanotic/tet spells. (Continued on next page)

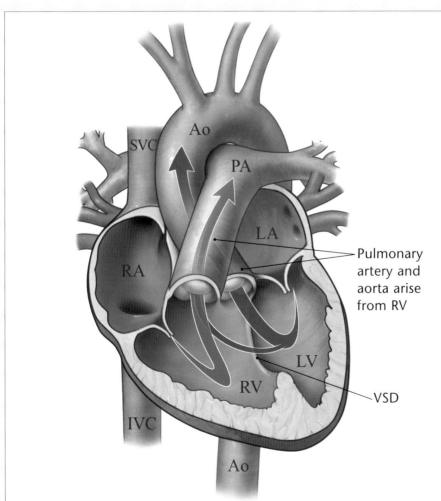

Figure 2.13. DORV with a subaortic VSD and no pulmonary stenosis. The pulmonary artery and aorta arise from the right ventricle and there is a large VSD. Oxygenated blood from the left ventricle shunts left-to-right to enter the aorta that arises from the right ventricle.

DORV with Subpulmonic VSD (also called transposition type or Taussig-Bing anomaly). This is the second most common form of DORV accounting for approximately 30 to 35% of cases. The VSD is subpulmonic and the aorta is pushed superiorly and anteriorly such that it lies rightward or even anteriorly of the pulmonary artery. This anatomy is 'transposition-like' because streaming of oxygenated blood allows shunting from the LV through the VSD to the RV to the pulmonary artery, and streaming of deoxygenated blood from the right atrium into the RV is ejected into the aorta. For these reasons, the degree of cyanosis is generally greater in these infants. Additionally, this lesion can be associated with valvar and/or subvalvar aortic stenosis and aortic arch hypoplasia/coarctation.

DORV with a Noncommitted VSD. This type of DORV occurs in approximately 10% of cases. With this variant, there may be conal tissue below both the aorta and pulmonary artery such that the VSD opens into the right ventricle but is not necessarily related to either of the great vessels. If there is no associated pulmonic stenosis, these infants may experience pulmonary overcirculation as PVR declines.

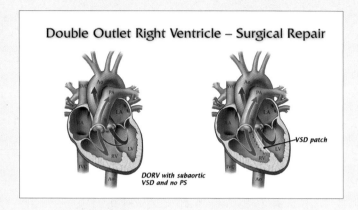

Double Outlet Right Ventricle – Surgical Repair

VSD patch

DORV with subaortic VSD and no PS

Surgical Repair of DORV

Surgical repair and timing of repair is based on the type of DORV and multiple other factors, including, but not limited to, the position and size of the VSD, the relationship of the great arteries, presence of pulmonary or aortic outflow tract obstruction, and coronary artery anatomy.

For the tetralogy type of DORV, a one-stage repair is usually done within the first 4 to 6 months of age. However, if a two-stage repair is required because of complex anatomy, initial palliation may involve placement of a systemic-to-pulmonary artery shunt or stenting of the DA to ensure adequate pulmonary blood flow, with complete repair after 6 months of age.

For the transposition type of DORV, repair is often in the neonatal period because of worsening cyanosis. This may involve a complex patch to close the VSD that also directs each ventricle to the appropriate great vessel or an arterial switch operation (as used in D-TGA).

For the noncommitted type of DORV, decision making is often complicated. Prior to complete repair, palliative options include either placement of a systemic-to-pulmonary artery shunt to increase pulmonary blood flow or placement of a pulmonary artery band to prevent pulmonary overcirculation. Some patients with DORV and a noncommitted VSD will be candidates for a biventricular repair that includes baffling of the VSD to the aorta. Others have anatomy that may not be amenable to a biventricular repair, and single ventricle palliation is required.

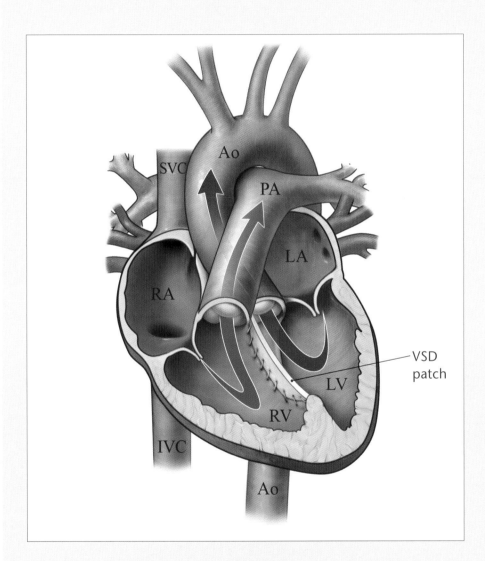

VSD patch

Figure 2.14. Repair of DORV with subaortic VSD and no pulmonary stenosis. This type of DORV is amenable to patching of the VSD to relocate the aorta into the left ventricle. This surgery usually occurs before 6 months of age to eliminate the left-to-right shunt that leads to pulmonary overcirculation.

Tricuspid Atresia[170,186,208,209]

Tricuspid atresia affects approximately 3% of all infants with CHD. Males and females are equally affected, unless there is an associated TGA, in which case males are more frequently affected. There are 3 classifications of tricuspid atresia:

- Tricuspid atresia with normally related great arteries (70 to 80% of cases; Figure 2.15)

- Tricuspid atresia with transposition of the great arteries (D-TGA) (approximately 10 to 25% of cases; Figure 2.16 on page 103).

- Tricuspid atresia with congenitally corrected transposition of the great arteries (L-TGA) (3 to 6% of cases; illustration not shown). See page 144 for more information about L-TGA.

Tricuspid Atresia with Normally Related Great Arteries (TA)

The tricuspid valve is absent, therefore, there is no direct communication between the right atrium and right ventricle and a VSD is almost always present (Figure 2.15). The size of the VSD influences the amount of pulmonary blood flow; the smaller the VSD, the smaller the amount of pulmonary blood flow. As many as 50% of patients with TA have a component of pulmonary stenosis, which ranges from mild to complete atresia. Neonates with a restrictive VSD and significant pulmonary stenosis may be ductal dependent for pulmonary blood flow (Figure 2.17 on page 105).

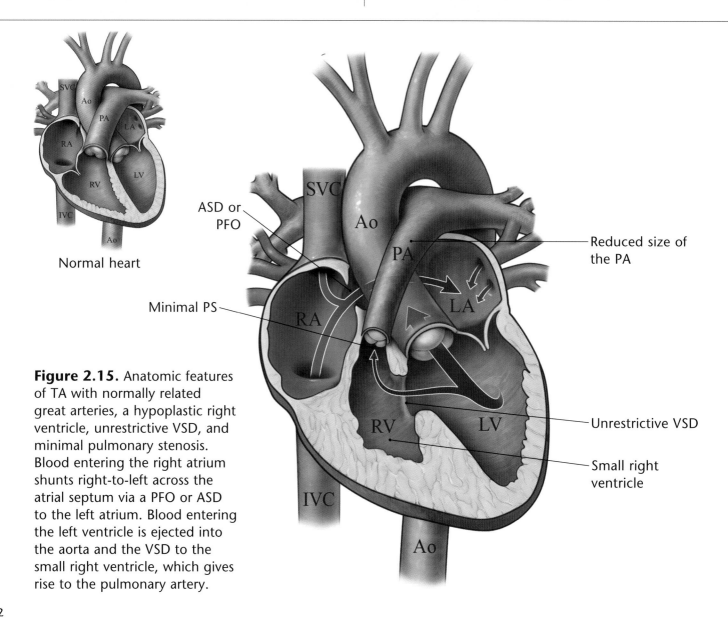

Normal heart

Figure 2.15. Anatomic features of TA with normally related great arteries, a hypoplastic right ventricle, unrestrictive VSD, and minimal pulmonary stenosis. Blood entering the right atrium shunts right-to-left across the atrial septum via a PFO or ASD to the left atrium. Blood entering the left ventricle is ejected into the aorta and the VSD to the small right ventricle, which gives rise to the pulmonary artery.

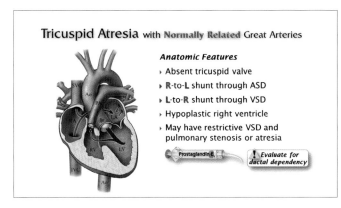

Tricuspid Atresia with **Normally Related** Great Arteries

Anatomic Features
▸ Absent tricuspid valve
▸ **R**-to-**L** shunt through ASD
▸ **L**-to-**R** shunt through VSD
▸ Hypoplastic right ventricle
▸ May have restrictive VSD and pulmonary stenosis or atresia

Prostaglandin E₁ **! Evaluate for ductal dependency**

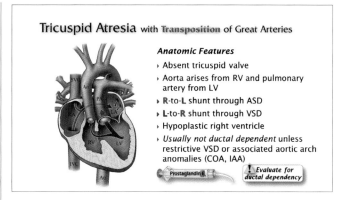

Tricuspid Atresia with **Transposition** of Great Arteries

Anatomic Features
▸ Absent tricuspid valve
▸ Aorta arises from RV and pulmonary artery from LV
▸ **R**-to-**L** shunt through ASD
▸ **L**-to-**R** shunt through VSD
▸ Hypoplastic right ventricle
▸ *Usually not ductal dependent* unless restrictive VSD or associated aortic arch anomalies (COA, IAA)

Prostaglandin E₁ **! Evaluate for ductal dependency**

Tricuspid Atresia with Transposition of the Great Arteries (TA-TGA)

In approximately 10 to 25% of cases, the great arteries are transposed (Figure 2.16). The size of the VSD dictates the adequacy of systemic blood flow; the smaller the VSD, the smaller the amount of blood ejected into the aorta. Infants with TA-TGA usually have increased pulmonary blood flow; therefore, cyanosis is less severe, and pulmonary overcirculation with CHF may develop. Other associated lesions may include COA or IAA. In the setting of aortic arch obstruction or a restrictive VSD that limits blood flow from the LV to the RV to the aorta, PGE is utilized to maintain ductal patency to support systemic perfusion.

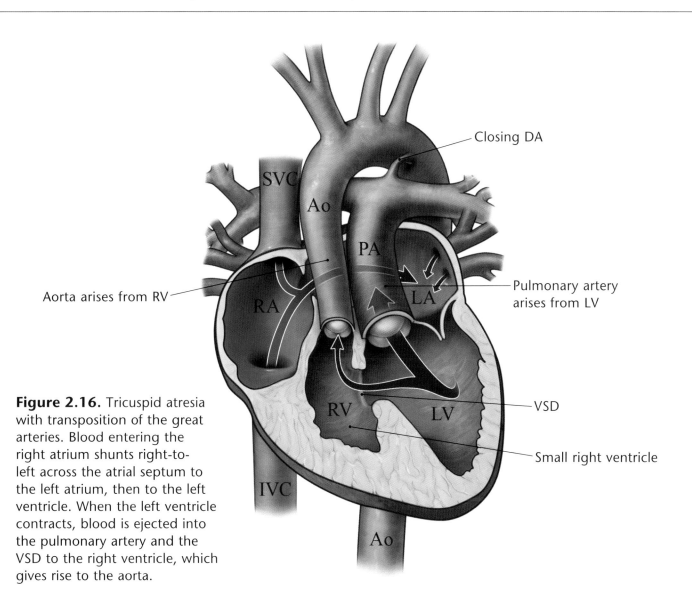

Figure 2.16. Tricuspid atresia with transposition of the great arteries. Blood entering the right atrium shunts right-to-left across the atrial septum to the left atrium, then to the left ventricle. When the left ventricle contracts, blood is ejected into the pulmonary artery and the VSD to the right ventricle, which gives rise to the aorta.

Tricuspid Atresia

Clinical Presentation

This discussion focuses primarily on the presentation and stabilization of neonates with tricuspid atresia with normally related great arteries. Presenting symptoms vary with the degree of restriction to pulmonary blood flow.

Cyanosis

- Initially, there may be little to no cyanosis in the setting of adequate pulmonary blood flow. However, the infant should be monitored closely for the first few weeks for progressive hypoxemia.

- There is moderate to severe cyanosis in cases of a restrictive VSD or severe pulmonary valve stenosis (Figure 2.17 on page 105).

Thrill

A thrill may be palpable if the VSD is restrictive or there is severe pulmonary or subpulmonary stenosis. Presence of a thrill increases the grade of the murmur to a 4.

Heart Sounds

The second heart sound is usually single.

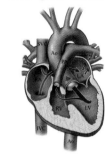

Tricuspid Atresia

Clinical Presentation
- Tachypnea
- Varying degrees of cyanosis
  - Unrestricted VSD and adequate pulmonary blood flow → minimal to no cyanosis
  - Restrictive VSD and/or pulmonary stenosis/atresia → cyanosis
- Single S2 is usually present
- Murmur is usually present

Murmur

- A grade 2-3/6 holosystolic VSD murmur may be heard at the LLSB.

- A systolic ejection murmur may be heard if pulmonary stenosis is present.

- A continuous PDA murmur may be present.

Pulses

Brachial and femoral pulses can be felt, unless COA or IAA is present, in which case femoral pulses may be difficult to feel as the DA closes. COA and IAA are usually associated with TA-TGA.

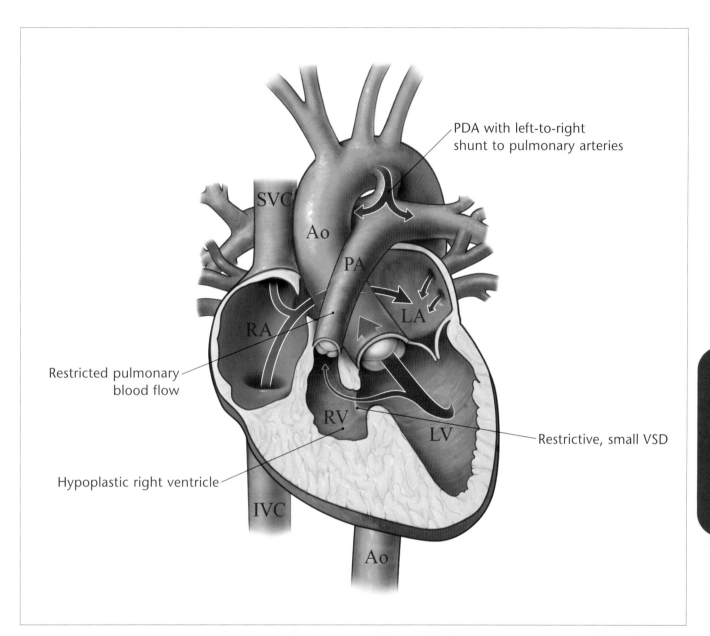

Figure 2.17. TA with a restrictive VSD, hypoplastic RV and decreased pulmonary blood flow. Initiation of a PGE infusion promotes ductal patency and allows blood to shunt left-to-right from the aorta to the pulmonary arteries, thus increasing pulmonary blood flow. The increased pulmonary blood flow results in increased oxygenated blood returning to the left atrium and left ventricle, leading to improved systemic O_2 saturation.

Tricuspid Atresia

Chest X-Ray

Heart Size

- The heart size is normal or slightly increased. With unrestricted pulmonary blood flow, the heart size is moderately enlarged.

- A right aortic arch is present in 3 to 8%.

- In TA-TGA, the mediastinum may be narrow secondary to the transposed arteries.

Pulmonary Vasculature

Pulmonary vascularity varies with the degree of restriction to flow across the VSD or RVOT.

Increased pulmonary vascular markings are seen with TA-TGA or in TA when there is a large VSD and minimal to no pulmonary stenosis.

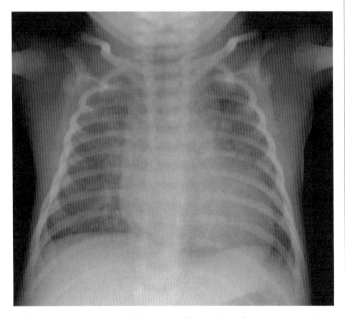

Tricuspid Atresia

Chest X-ray
› Heart size
  - May be normal or slightly increased
  - Unrestricted PBF → moderately enlarged
› Pulmonary vascularity varies with degree of restriction to flow across the VSD or right ventricular outflow tract
› TA-TGA and TA with large VSD
  - ↑ Pulmonary vascular markings

PBF = pulmonary blood flow

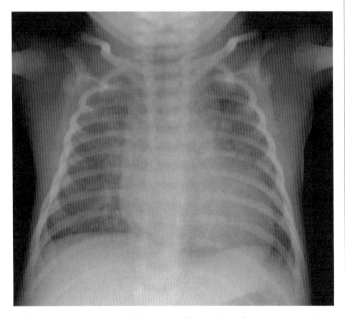

Tricuspid atresia with normally related great arteries

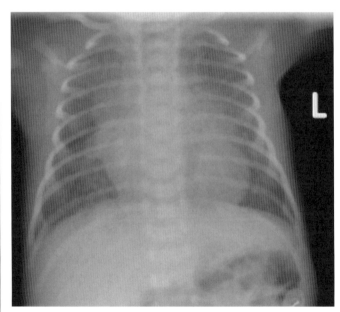

Tricuspid atresia with D-TGA (TA-TGA)

1. Provide supplemental O_2 to treat hypoxemia and help relax the pulmonary vascular bed. Maintain the O_2 saturation > 75%.

2. Cardiology consultation and echocardiography should be requested to allow further evaluation.

3. Most infants with TA are not ductal dependent. Monitor closely as the DA closes. If the O_2 saturation remains > 75%, the infant most likely has adequate pulmonary blood flow.

4. If the O_2 saturation is < 75% (on oxygen), the infant may have a restrictive VSD and/or pulmonary valve stenosis with decreased pulmonary blood flow. Until echocardiography confirmation, consider starting a PGE infusion to maintain ductal patency. See page 70 for PGE dosing and side effects.

5. For infants with unrestricted pulmonary blood flow, monitor for development of pulmonary edema and CHF.

6. For infants with TA-TGA, monitor the upper and lower extremity pulses and blood pressures closely for signs of poor systemic perfusion and/or aortic arch obstruction as the DA closes. If these signs are observed, then PGE may be necessary to establish ductal patency.

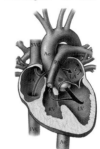

Tricuspid Atresia with **Normally Related** Great Arteries

Initial Stabilization
- Provide O_2 → target O_2 sat > 75%
- **If O_2 sat remains < 75%** → may have restrictive VSD and/or pulmonary stenosis

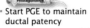
- Start PGE to maintain ductal patency

PDA

Restrictive VSD and ↓ PBF

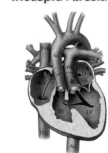

Tricuspid Atresia with **Transposition** of Great Arteries

Initial Stabilization
- Provide O_2 → target O_2 sat > 75%
- Monitor upper and lower extremity pulses and BP for signs of poor systemic perfusion and/or aortic arch obstruction

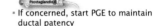
- If concerned, start PGE to maintain ductal patency

Cyanotic CHD Not Ductal Dependent

Truncus Arteriosus[170,210-212]

Truncus arteriosus affects approximately 1 to 3% of all neonates with CHD.

The primary anatomic features of truncus arteriosus include:

- A single great vessel arises from the heart and gives rise to the aorta, pulmonary, and coronary arteries

- A single truncal valve with a variable number of leaflets

  - Trileaflet is the most common, followed by quadricuspid, then bicuspid

  - The truncal valve may be stenotic or incompetent (causing regurgitation)

- A large VSD

  - Allows for mixing between the right and left ventricles

  - When the ventricles contract, blood is ejected from both ventricles into the common great vessel

- The DA is absent in 50% of patients with truncus arteriosus

- Coronary artery anomalies may be present and may have implications for surgical repair

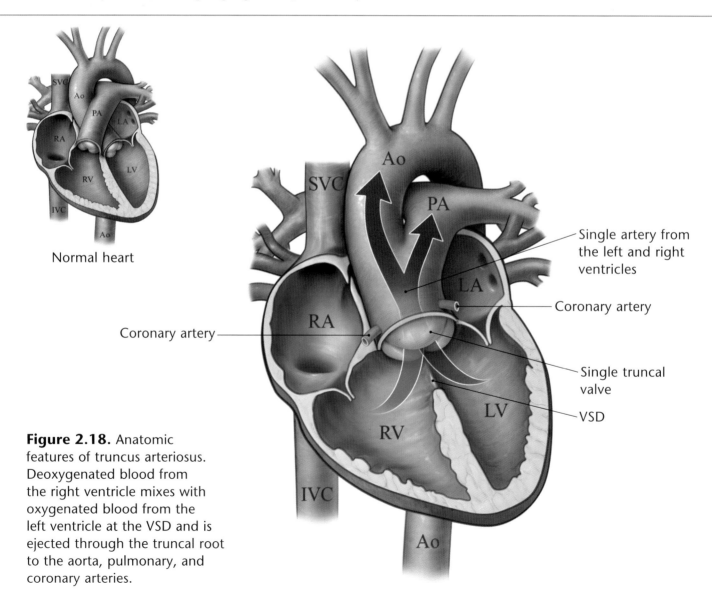

Normal heart

Figure 2.18. Anatomic features of truncus arteriosus. Deoxygenated blood from the right ventricle mixes with oxygenated blood from the left ventricle at the VSD and is ejected through the truncal root to the aorta, pulmonary, and coronary arteries.

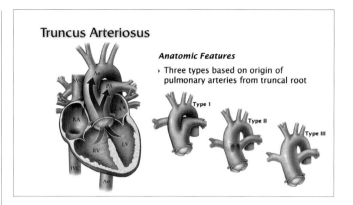

Truncus Arteriosus

Anatomic Features
- Single great vessel from left and right ventricles → provides circulation to aorta, pulmonary and coronary arteries
- Single truncal valve
  - May be stenotic or incompetent
- Ventricular septal defect (VSD)
- Ductus arteriosus often absent
- Coronary artery anomalies may be present

Truncus Arteriosus

Anatomic Features
- Three types based on origin of pulmonary arteries from truncal root

Three main subtypes of truncus arteriosus are described based on the origin of the pulmonary arteries from the truncal root. Type I and Type II account for 85% of cases of truncus arteriosus. The most common associated anomalies include a right aortic arch (approximately 33% of patients), IAA, and secundum ASD. If IAA is present, systemic blood flow beyond the interruption is dependent upon the DA, and a PGE infusion will be necessary to maintain ductal patency and systemic perfusion.

Type I	Type II	Type III

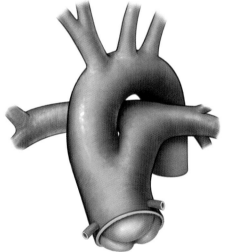 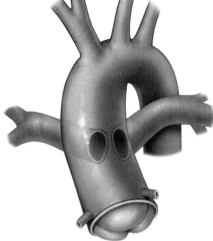 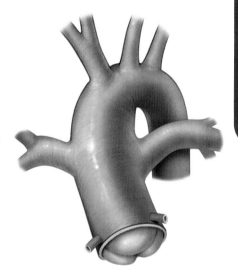

A short main pulmonary artery segment gives rise to both branch pulmonary arteries.

The branch pulmonary arteries arise from the common truncal root, adjacent to each other with a small rim of truncal tissue between them. There is no common pulmonary artery segment like in Type I.

The pulmonary arteries arise from either side of the truncal root and are distant from one another. There is no common pulmonary artery segment like in Type I.

Truncus Arteriosus

Clinical Presentation

Cyanosis

In the early neonatal period, PVR is increased and there is usually mild cyanosis. As PVR decreases, pulmonary blood flow increases and the O_2 saturation usually reaches 90% or more. Because of the negative effects of pulmonary overcirculation, the goal O_2 saturation, when possible, is 75 to 85%.

Congestive Heart Failure (CHF)

As PVR decreases, blood flow to the lungs increases and leads to pulmonary overcirculation and CHF. Signs of CHF include tachypnea, tachycardia, diaphoresis, increased work of breathing, and poor feeding. With increased diastolic runoff into the pulmonary circulation, or in the setting of truncal valve insufficiency, pulses may be bounding and the pulse pressure widens secondary to a reduced diastolic arterial pressure.

Heart Sounds

- Loud single S2
- An ejection click may be audible

Murmur

- A loud pansystolic murmur may be audible
- Diastolic flow into the pulmonary arteries may be audible

Chest X-Ray

Heart Size

- Moderate cardiomegaly is usually apparent
- A right-sided aortic arch is present in 30 percent of cases

Pulmonary Vasculature

- Increased pulmonary vascular markings are common

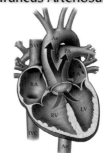

Truncus Arteriosus

Clinical Presentation
- Mild cyanosis initially
- Tachypnea
- As pulmonary vascular resistance ↓
  → pulmonary blood flow ↑
  → pulmonary overcirculation
  → congestive heart failure (CHF)
- Signs of CHF: tachypnea, tachycardia, diaphoresis, ↑ work of breathing, poor feeding

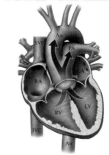

Truncus Arteriosus

Clinical Presentation
- Heart sounds
  - Loud single S2
  - May have ejection click
- May have systolic and/or diastolic murmur

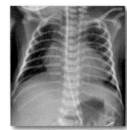
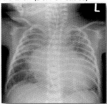

Truncus Arteriosus

Chest X-ray
- Moderate cardiomegaly is common
- Right-sided aortic arch (30% of cases)
- ↑ Pulmonary vascular markings

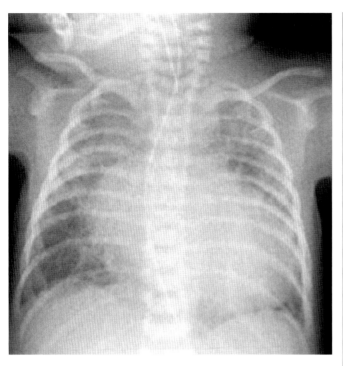

7-day old infant with truncus arteriosus. There is significant cardiomegaly and increased pulmonary vascular markings secondary to pulmonary overcirculation and CHF.

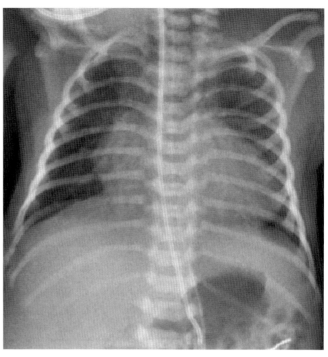

4-day old infant with truncus arteriosus. There is mild cardiomegaly.

Initial Stabilization

1. If possible, maintain O_2 saturation between 75 to 85%. Avoid giving supplemental O_2 if saturations are in the goal range since O_2 promotes pulmonary vasodilation and increased pulmonary blood flow.

2. PGE is not necessary unless the infant also has an interrupted aortic arch.

3. Evaluate for 22q11.2DS; monitor for and treat hypocalcemia.

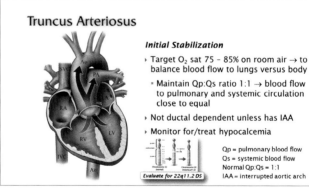

Truncus Arteriosus

Initial Stabilization

› Target O_2 sat 75 - 85% on room air → to balance blood flow to lungs versus body

  ▪ Maintain Qp:Qs ratio 1:1 → blood flow to pulmonary and systemic circulation close to equal

› Not ductal dependent unless has IAA

› Monitor for/treat hypocalcemia

Evaluate for 22q11.2 DS

Qp = pulmonary blood flow
Qs = systemic blood flow
Normal Qp:Qs = 1:1
IAA = interrupted aortic arch

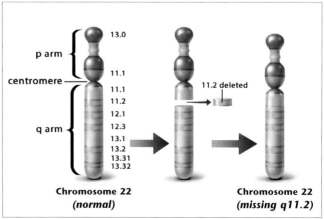

p arm
centromere
q arm

13.0
11.1
11.1
11.2
12.1
12.3
13.1
13.2
13.31
13.32

11.2 deleted

Chromosome 22
(normal)

Chromosome 22
(missing q11.2)

Total Anomalous Pulmonary Venous Connection (TAPVC)[71,170,187,213-216]

TAPVC (also called total anomalous venous return; TAPVR) affects 1 to 1.5% of all infants with CHD. Males and females are equally affected except in the case of infracardiac TAPVC that affects males four times more often than females.

Normally, four pulmonary veins (two from each lung) drain oxygenated blood to the left atrium. In TAPVC, the pulmonary veins have no direct connection with the left atrium. Instead, they drain oxygenated blood directly or indirectly to the right atrium. The blood must then shunt across the foramen ovale or ASD to reach the

left atrium and left ventricle. A right-to-left atrial level shunt is essential for survival. Only 2 to 10% of cases of TAPVC are prenatally diagnosed.

The three most common types of TAPVC are shown in Figure 2.19. A fourth type, mixed, is not shown. In mixed TAPVC, the pulmonary veins drain in two different locations that may be superior or inferior to the diaphragm. For example, two pulmonary veins might drain via a supracardiac pathway and two pulmonary veins might drain via an infracardiac pathway. Mixed TAPVC occurs in approximately 10% of cases

Supracardiac

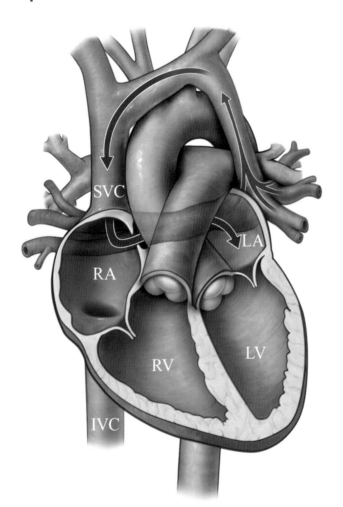

Cardiac

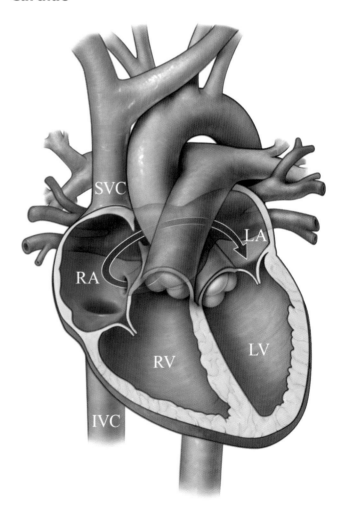

Figure 2.19. The three most common types of TAPVC – supracardiac, cardiac, and infracardiac.

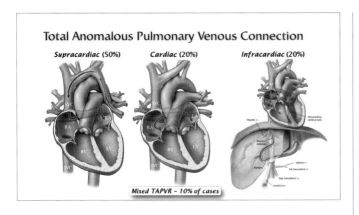

of TAPVC. Partial anomalous pulmonary venous return (PAPVR) is the term used to describe when some, but not all, of the pulmonary veins drain anomalously. PAPVR is generally well tolerated and clinically behaves more like an ASD.

Infracardiac

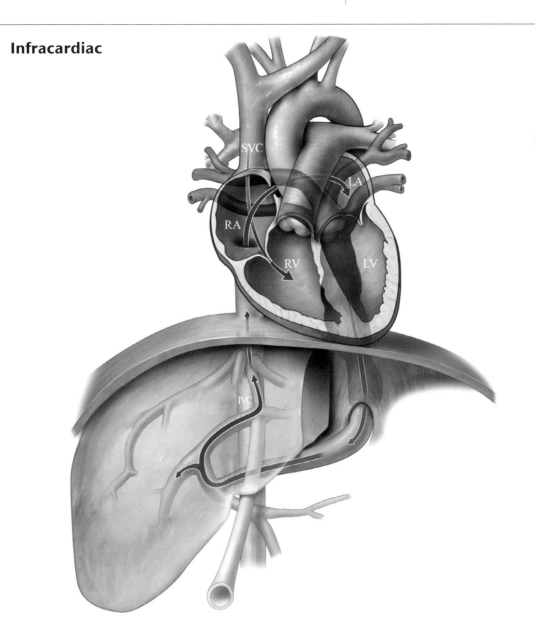

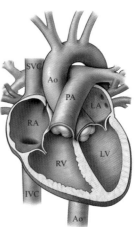

Normal heart

Supracardiac TAPVC

Approximately 50% of cases of TAPVC. The four pulmonary veins drain oxygenated blood to a confluence or collecting chamber behind the left atrium, to a left vertical vein, to the innominate vein, to the superior vena cava, and then to the right atrium. When the oxygenated pulmonary venous blood enters the right atrium, it mixes with deoxygenated blood returning from the body. The partially oxygenated blood must then shunt right-to-left across the foramen ovale or ASD to reach the left atrium, left ventricle, and aorta.

The usual pathway of the vertical vein is anterior to the left pulmonary artery and mainstem bronchus. At times, however, the ascending vertical vein courses between the left pulmonary artery and left mainstem bronchus resulting in obstructed blood flow (Figure 2.21 on page 115). With obstructed pulmonary veins, the infant will have severe cyanosis and signs of decreased systemic perfusion. Other sites of obstruction can be at the atrial septum, or in the case of anomalous connection directly to the SVC, obstruction can occur between the right pulmonary artery and trachea. Infants with unobstructed pulmonary veins usually present with tachypnea and mild cyanosis.

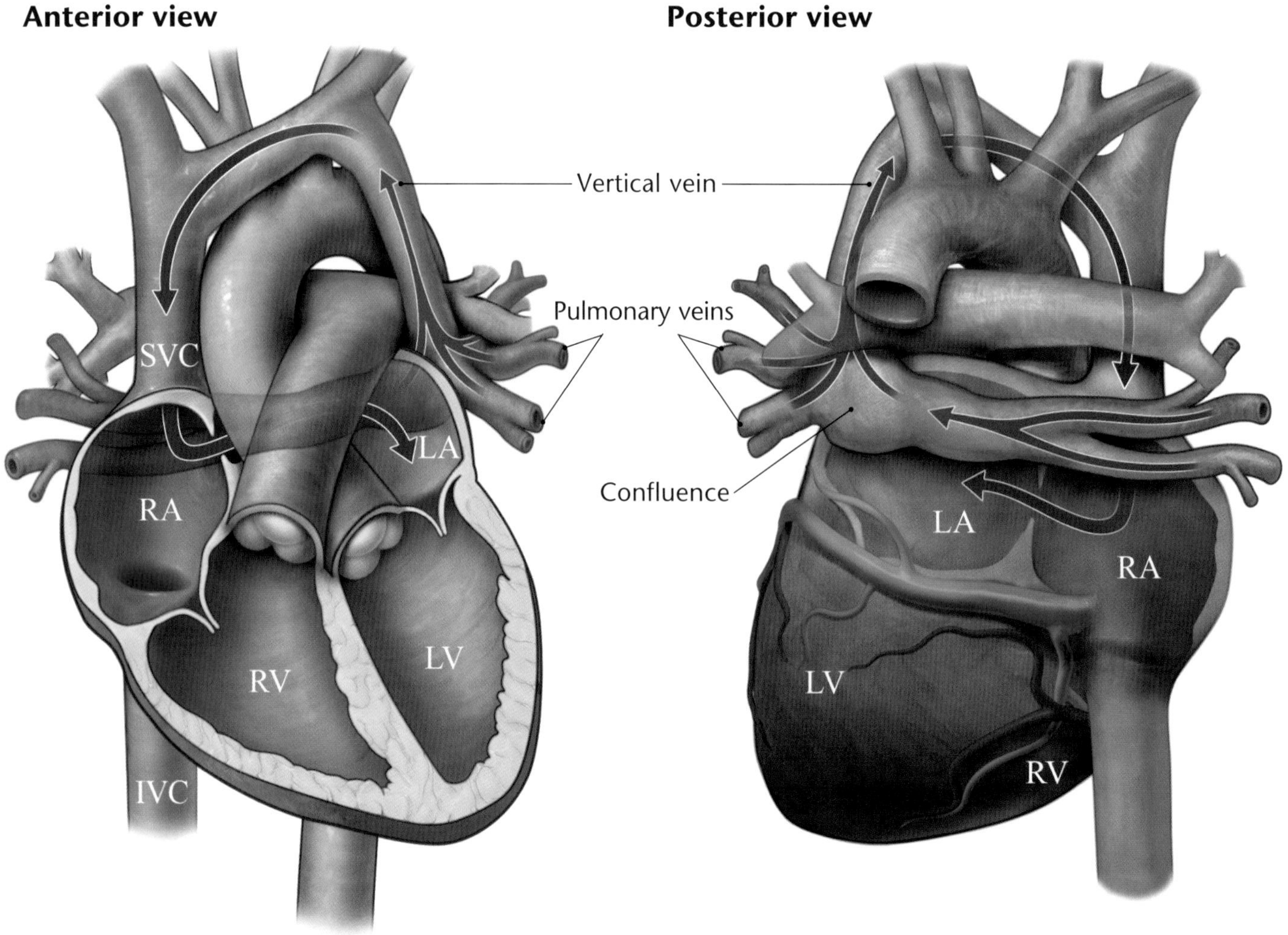

Anterior view

Posterior view

Figure 2.20. Blood flow pattern in supracardiac TAPVC. Oxygenated blood from the pulmonary veins drain to a confluence behind the left atrium, to a left vertical vein, to the innominate vein, to the superior vena cava, and then to the right atrium where it shunts right-to-left to the left atrium.

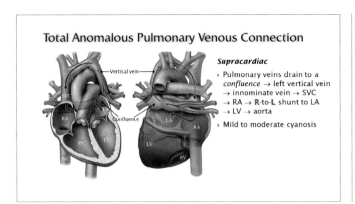

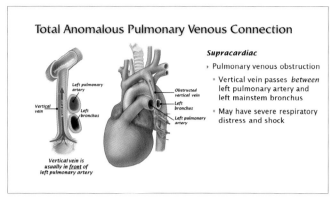

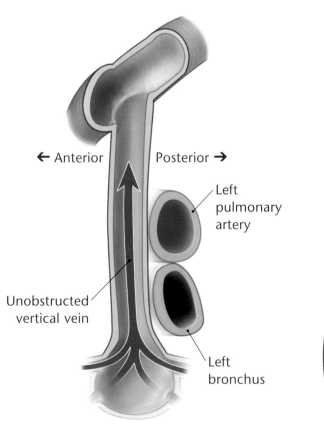

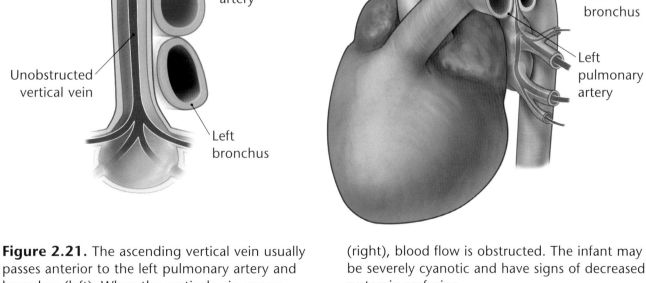

Figure 2.21. The ascending vertical vein usually passes anterior to the left pulmonary artery and bronchus (left). When the vertical vein passes *between* the left pulmonary artery and left bronchus (right), blood flow is obstructed. The infant may be severely cyanotic and have signs of decreased systemic perfusion.

Cardiac TAPVC

Approximately 20% of cases of TAPVC. The
four pulmonary veins drain to a confluence
that then connects to the coronary sinus. The
coronary sinus normally drains blood from the
coronary veins in the heart to the right atrium.
Obstruction to blood flow is rare, but it can
occur. These infants will usually present with
tachypnea and mild cyanosis.

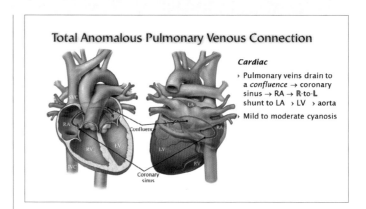

Total Anomalous Pulmonary Venous Connection

Cardiac
› Pulmonary veins drain to
a *confluence* → coronary
sinus → RA → R-to-L
shunt to LA › LV › aorta
› Mild to moderate cyanosis

Anterior view   **Posterior view**

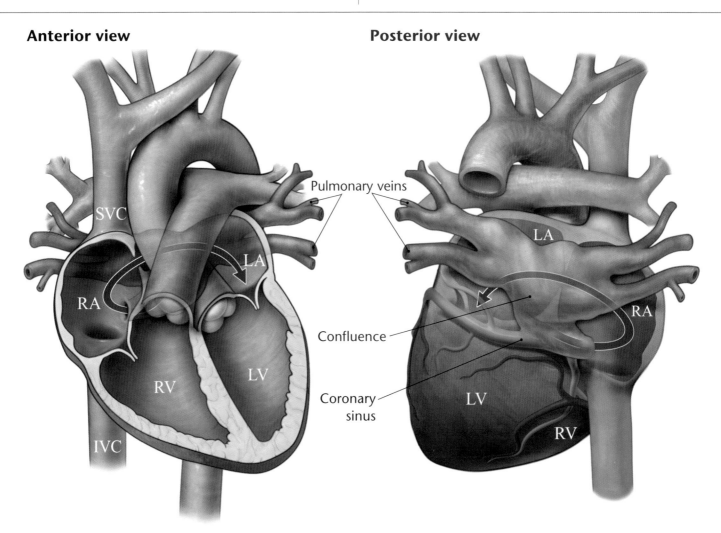

Figure 2.22. Blood flow pattern in cardiac TAPVR.
The pulmonary veins drain to a confluence behind the
left atrium that then connects to the coronary sinus.

The blood enters the right atrium and shunts right-
to-left to the left atrium.

Infracardiac TAPVC (also called infradiaphragmatic)

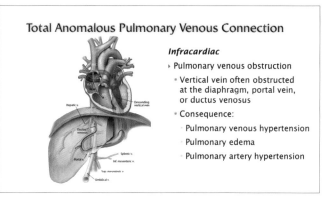

Total Anomalous Pulmonary Venous Connection

Infracardiac
- › Pulmonary veins drain via a descending vertical vein → through the diaphragm → then connects to:
  - ▪ Portal vein, ductus venosus, hepatic vein, or the IVC
  - ▪ Blood flows to IVC → RA → R-to-L shunt to LA → LV → aorta

Total Anomalous Pulmonary Venous Connection

Infracardiac
- › Pulmonary venous obstruction
  - ▪ Vertical vein often obstructed at the diaphragm, portal vein, or ductus venosus
  - ▪ Consequence:
    - · Pulmonary venous hypertension
    - · Pulmonary edema
    - · Pulmonary artery hypertension

Approximately 20% of cases of TAPVC. The four pulmonary veins drain to a confluence behind the left atrium, to a descending vertical vein that traverses anterior to the esophagus and through the diaphragm at the esophageal hiatus, where it connects near the liver to the portal vein or less frequently, to the ductus venosus, a hepatic vein, or the IVC. Infracardiac TAPVC is commonly obstructed, resulting in pulmonary venous congestion, elevated PVR (pulmonary hypertension), decreased pulmonary blood flow, and severe cyanosis.

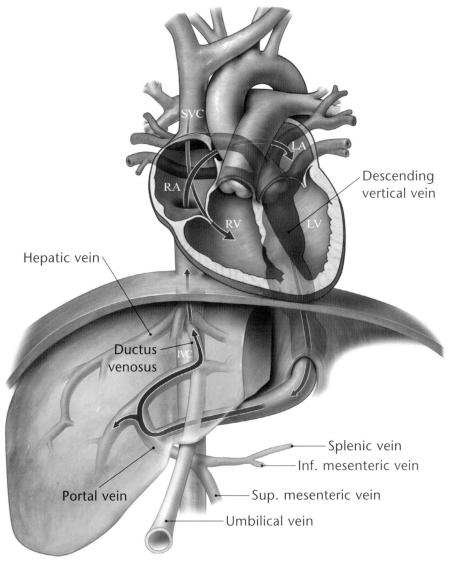

Sites of obstruction include:

- Compression of the descending vertical vein at the level of the diaphragm.

- Stenosis of the descending vertical vein at the junction with the portal vein.

- Obstruction in the liver if the ductus venosus is no longer patent.

Figure 2.23. Blood flow pattern in infracardiac TAPVC. Oxygenated blood from the pulmonary veins drain via a descending vertical vein, through the diaphragm, and to the portal venous system. Deoxygenated blood in the portal venous system mixes with the oxygenated pulmonary venous blood before entering the right atrium.

Total Anomalous Pulmonary Venous Connection (TAPVC)

Clinical Presentation

TAPVC without Obstruction

The infant may only exhibit minimal symptoms and mild cyanosis at birth because of adequate mixing of oxygenated and deoxygenated blood and right-to-left shunting at the atrial level. However, as PVR decreases in the days and weeks after birth, the infant may develop signs of pulmonary overcirculation and CHF. Volume and pressure overload of the right heart may lead to dilation of the right atrium and ventricle. A diuretic is usually required to treat CHF. Surgical correction is necessary for survival.

TAPVC with Obstruction

The infant will be profoundly ill shortly after birth. The presentation of obstructed TAPVC mimics PPHN which increases the risk of misdiagnosing the patient. Signs of poor cardiac output and severe respiratory distress (tachypnea, retractions, and intense cyanosis) are common. Usually, no murmur is present. Emergency corrective surgery is required as soon as possible after diagnosis.

> Use of PGE in patients with TAPVC is controversial.
>
> **Pros** for use include potential dilation of the ductus venosus in the setting of infracardiac TAPVC with obstruction secondary to closure of the ductus venosus.
>
> **Cons** include promotion of a right-to-left shunt through the DA that then reduces pulmonary blood flow.
>
> Use of PGE should be guided by cardiology and echocardiography.

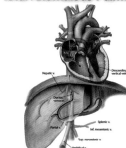

Total Anomalous Pulmonary Venous Connection

Infracardiac – Clinical Presentation
- Profoundly ill shortly after birth
- Mimics severe lung disease and persistent pulmonary hypertension
  - Severe respiratory distress, cyanosis, tachypnea, retractions
- May have severe shock
- Usually no murmur

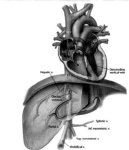

Total Anomalous Pulmonary Venous Connection

Infracardiac – Initial Stabilization
- Airway support
  - 100% O_2, endotracheal intubation
- Treat shock
  - Volume infusion
  - Inotropic medication
- Emergency corrective surgery
  - Anastomose pulmonary venous confluence to LA and ligate common collector

Chest X-Ray

TAPVC without Obstruction

May show cardiomegaly and increased PVM. Supracardiac TAPVR without obstruction may show the classic "snowman" heart configuration, but this finding is not usually observed in the neonatal period. The snowman shape is caused by the dilated left vertical vein and dilated superior vena cava (upper half of the snowman) and the enlarged heart (lower half of the snowman).

TAPVC with Obstruction

The heart size is small or normal on chest x-ray with a diffuse reticular pattern and hazy lung fields (secondary to pulmonary edema), that may be confused as respiratory distress syndrome, pneumonia, pulmonary lymphangiectasia, or meconium aspiration.

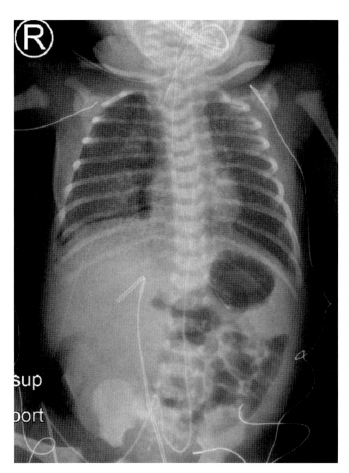

Neonate with infracardiac TAPVC and a right pneumothorax. The heart size appears small. The UAC tip is at T7. The UVC is malpositioned in the portal venous system.

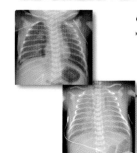

Total Anomalous Pulmonary Venous Connection

Chest X-ray

> Without pulmonary vein obstruction

- May have cardiomegaly and increased pulmonary vascular markings
- Supracardiac → "snowman" configuration is a later finding

> With pulmonary vein obstruction

- Small or normal heart size
- Diffuse reticular pattern of pulmonary edema (hazy lung fields) → may be confused with RDS or pneumonia

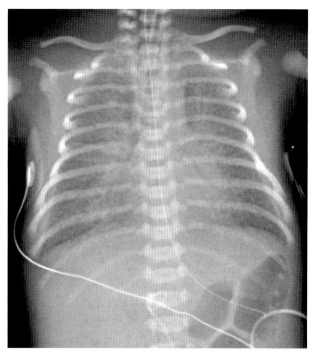

Neonate with infracardiac TAPVC. The heart size appears small. There is a diffuse reticular pulmonary venous pattern secondary to pulmonary edema.

Initial Stabilization

TAPVC *without* Obstruction

- The infant may be asymptomatic at birth, although mild cyanosis may be apparent.
- Offer normal neonatal care, including standard respiratory and nutritional care.
- Anticipate pulmonary overcirculation as PVR declines in the days and weeks after birth.
- Corrective surgery will be required in the neonatal period.

TAPVC *with* Obstruction

- Severe respiratory distress is treated with 100% oxygen, endotracheal intubation, and mechanical ventilation.
- An inotropic medication may be necessary to treat hypotension.
- In severe cases of cardiorespiratory compromise, ECMO support may be necessary until corrective surgery can be accomplished. Surgery will establish patency between the pulmonary veins and the left atrium.

Ebstein Anomaly[84,168,170,171,192,208,217]

Ebstein anomaly (also referred to as Ebstein's anomaly) occurs in < 1% of infants with CHD. Males and females are equally affected. Ebstein anomaly may be mild, moderate, or severe.

Anterior, septal, and posterior (sometimes called inferior) leaflets comprise the tricuspid valve. In Ebstein anomaly, the septal and posterior leaflets are displaced apically and attached abnormally to the RV which prevents the tricuspid valve from being able to close normally (also called a coaptation defect). This coaptation defect causes tricuspid valve regurgitation. Abnormal apical attachment of

the tricuspid valve also causes the portion of the RV above the valve to become incorporated into the right atrium (the 'atrialized' portion of the RV; Figure 2.24). The volume of the RV below the tricuspid valve is smaller than normal, which contributes to less blood being ejected into the lungs. An ASD or PFO with a right-to-left shunt is always present. In severe cases, there is extreme cardiomegaly primarily due to right atrial enlargement. In the fetus, severe cardiac enlargement may lead to lung hypoplasia, hydrops fetalis secondary to increased right atrial pressures, and fetal demise.

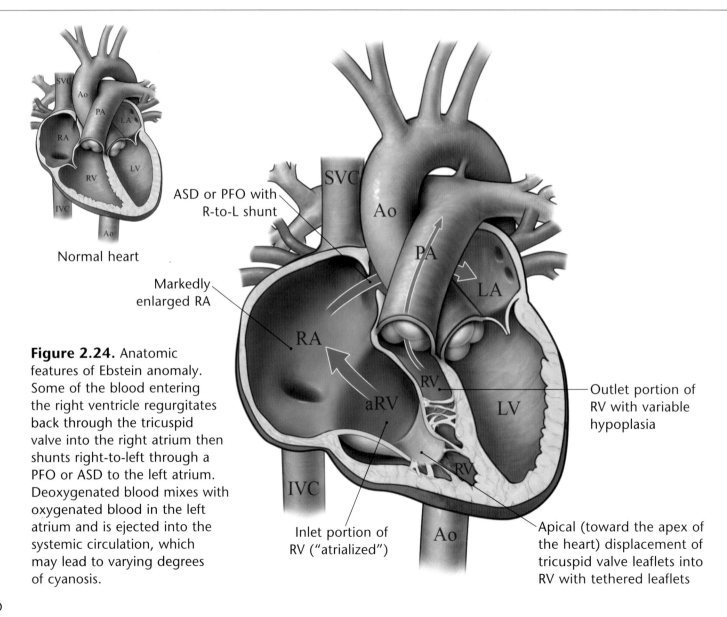

Normal heart

ASD or PFO with R-to-L shunt

Markedly enlarged RA

Outlet portion of RV with variable hypoplasia

Inlet portion of RV ("atrialized")

Apical (toward the apex of the heart) displacement of tricuspid valve leaflets into RV with tethered leaflets

Figure 2.24. Anatomic features of Ebstein anomaly. Some of the blood entering the right ventricle regurgitates back through the tricuspid valve into the right atrium then shunts right-to-left through a PFO or ASD to the left atrium. Deoxygenated blood mixes with oxygenated blood in the left atrium and is ejected into the systemic circulation, which may lead to varying degrees of cyanosis.

Associated defects may include:

- Pulmonary outflow tract obstruction that is either anatomic (pulmonary valve stenosis or atresia), or functional (the RV is unable to generate enough force to open the pulmonary valve in systole)

- VSD

- Abnormal conduction system leading to arrhythmias

- Pulmonary hypoplasia secondary to massive cardiomegaly

- Coarctation of the aorta (rare)

Maternal exposure to lithium early in the pregnancy has been associated with development of Ebstein anomaly. Supraventricular tachycardia (SVT) occurs in approximately 20% of infants with Ebstein anomaly.

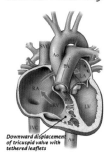

Ebstein Anomaly

Anatomic Features
- Malformation of tricuspid valve and right ventricle (RV)
- Tricuspid valve has 3 leaflets:
  - Anterior, septal and inferior (posterior)
    - Septal and posterior leaflets apically displaced and tethered to RV
  - Shortened chordae tendineae
  - Tricuspid valve not able to close → *"coaptation defect"* → tricuspid regurgitation

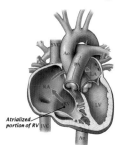

Ebstein Anomaly

Anatomic Features
- RV divided into 2 regions
  - Inlet portion → functionally associated with the right atrium
    - "Atrialized" portion of the RV (aRV)
  - Outlet portion → functional RV
- Variable RV hypoplasia
  - Less blood is ejected into lungs
  - May have "functional" pulmonary atresia or pulmonary valve stenosis or atresia

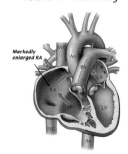

Ebstein Anomaly

Anatomic Features
- Markedly enlarged RA
- ASD or PFO
  - R-to-L atrial shunt
- Associated defects:
  - VSD with or without pulmonary atresia
  - Abnormal conduction system
  - Coarctation of the aorta (rare)
  - Lung hypoplasia secondary to massive cardiomegaly

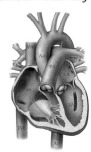

Ebstein Anomaly

Anatomic Features
- Markedly enlarged RA
- ASD or PFO
  - R-to-L atrial shunt
- Associated defects:
  - VSD with or without pulmonary atresia
  - Abnormal conduction system
  - Coarctation of the aorta (rare)
  - Lung hypoplasia secondary to massive cardiomegaly

Ebstein Anomaly

Clinical Presentation

The clinical presentation varies with the severity of the Ebstein anomaly. Symptoms depend on the degree of tricuspid valve regurgitation, the ability of the RV to pump blood to the pulmonary arteries, and the severity of the RA enlargement. Mild forms of Ebstein anomaly may be asymptomatic in the neonatal period.

Cyanosis

- Infants with little right-to-left shunting at the atrial level and good pulmonary blood flow may have only minimal decrease in O_2 saturation.

- In severe cases, significant tricuspid regurgitation and decreased pulmonary blood flow leads to severe cyanosis.

Congestive Heart Failure (CHF)

- Symptoms of CHF and hepatomegaly are present in severe cases.

Heart Murmur and Arrhythmias

- A systolic murmur can vary from soft to loud, depending upon the degree of tricuspid regurgitation and pulmonary artery pressure.

- SVT occurs in approximately 20% of patients secondary to the presence of extra conduction tissue (accessory pathway).

- Wolff-Parkinson-White syndrome is a common cause of SVT in these patients.

- Severe RA enlargement can contribute to development of atrial tachycardia or atrial fibrillation.

Chest X-Ray
Heart Size and Shape

- The heart size can be normal in mild cases to massively enlarged in severe cases.
- The heart can appear "wall-to-wall" or "balloon-shaped."

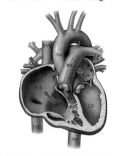

Ebstein Anomaly

Clinical Presentation
- Mild to severe cyanosis
- CHF in severe cases
- Murmur
  - Gallop is common
  - Soft to loud murmur depending on degree of tricuspid regurgitation and pulmonary artery pressure
- SVT → approximately 20% of cases

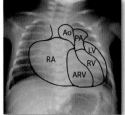

Ebstein Anomaly

Chest X-ray
- Mild cases → heart size may be normal
- Severe cases → massive cardiomegaly due to RA enlargement
- "Balloon-shaped" heart
- ↓ Pulmonary vascular markings with ↓ pulmonary blood flow

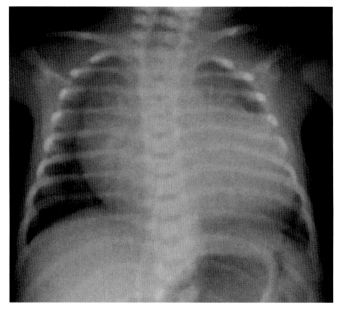

One-day old infant with Ebstein anomaly and massive cardiomegaly.

Pulmonary Vasculature

- Decreased pulmonary vascular markings are seen when pulmonary blood flow is decreased.

1. Provide oxygen to help lower the PVR and over time, improve pulmonary blood flow.

2. In some cases, inhaled nitric oxide can help reduce PVR.

3. Severe respiratory distress is treated with endotracheal intubation and mechanical ventilation.

4. Inotropes may be necessary to treat hypotension and CHF, but may exacerbate any associated arrhythmias.

5. Correct metabolic acidosis to reverse the negative effect of acidosis on the pulmonary vasculature.

6. Treat SVT if it occurs. SVT may be poorly tolerated, so be prepared to promptly administer adenosine or proceed with synchronized cardioversion if the infant is unstable.

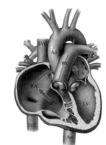

Ebstein Anomaly

Initial Stabilization

- Provide O₂ to help ↓ PVR and ↑ pulmonary blood flow
- Inhaled nitric oxide may help ↓ PVR
- Severe respiratory distress → endotracheal intubation
- Inotropes → hypotension and CHF
- Treat SVT with adenosine or cardioversion if indicated
- Extreme forms may be ductal dependent
  - If O₂ sat < 75%, consider PGE

7. Assess for ductal dependence.

- Neonates with severe Ebstein anomaly may be ductal dependent for pulmonary blood flow because of either functional pulmonary atresia, or pulmonary stenosis or atresia. If the O₂ saturation is persistently < 75% while being given 100% oxygen and appropriate respiratory support, a PGE infusion should be strongly considered to support pulmonary blood flow.

- Inhaled nitric oxide might also be useful in this situation to decrease PVR and promote antegrade flow from the right ventricle to the pulmonary arteries.

Cyanotic CHD
Not Ductal Dependent

Underlying Concepts

This next section will review cyanotic congenital heart lesions that are dependent on the DA for pulmonary blood flow or to improve intercirculatory mixing as in transposition of the great arteries.

- When blood flow to the lungs is reduced because of severe narrowing or atresia of the pulmonary outflow tract, blood must enter the lungs via an aorta-to-pulmonary artery shunt, that is, a **left-to-right** shunt via the PDA.

- With right-sided obstructive lesions, as the DA closes, blood flow to the body remains adequate, but blood flow to the lungs is reduced. Once the DA is re-opened with a PGE infusion, pulmonary blood flow improves.

- The color of the blood in the aorta correlates with the color of skin (e.g., deoxygentated dark blood correlates with cyanotic, blue-hued skin). If the lungs are functioning normally, as pulmonary blood flow improves, O_2 saturation and cyanosis should also improve.

- Transposition of the great arteries (TGA) is a special situation. In TGA, the aorta arises from the right ventricle and the pulmonary artery arises from the left ventricle. Although blood flow to the lungs is not decreased, cyanosis is observed because the deoxygenated blood

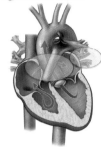

Cyanotic CHD

Ductal Dependent for Pulmonary Blood Flow

› PDA is required to improve pulmonary blood flow
or
To improve intercirculatory mixing as in Transposition of Great Arteries

› ↓ Pulmonary blood flow = ↓ pulmonary venous return

› Mixing of **desaturated** blood with **saturated** blood leads to **cyanosis**

returning from the body enters the RV only to be pumped back out to the body through the aorta without going to the lungs for oxygenation. Similarly, the oxygenated blood returning from the lungs is pumped right back to the lungs. An intracardiac defect (ASD) is essential to allow mixing of the oxygenated blood returning from the lungs with the deoxygenated blood returning from the body. A PDA alone does not allow sufficient mixing, but it does help drive mixing between the atria. If the atrial septum is restrictive, an emergency balloon atrial septostomy is indicated to enlarge the ASD.

See the **Appendix** on page 207 for palliative and surgical options for the lesions discussed in this section.

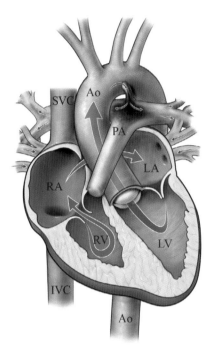 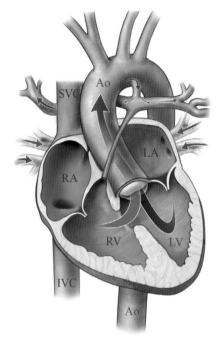 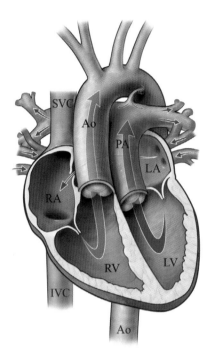

| **Pulmonary atresia with intact ventricular septum** | **Pulmonary atresia with ventricular septal defect** | **Transposition of the great arteries** |

Stabilizing the Cyanotic Neonate with Ductal Dependent Pulmonary Blood Flow

1. Administer blended oxygen and increase the FiO_2 to try and achieve a preductal O_2 saturation between 91 and 95%. Oxygen helps improve systemic oxygenation and decrease PVR. Infants with cyanotic CHD may not be able to achieve an O_2 saturation > 80% despite administration of 100% oxygen.

2. Optimize respiratory support.

3. Evaluate for physical and laboratory signs of shock and offer resuscitative treatment as indicated.

4. Evaluate for and treat any other causes of cyanosis such as pulmonary disease, sepsis, shock secondary to non-cardiac causes, metabolic derangements, and neurologic depression.

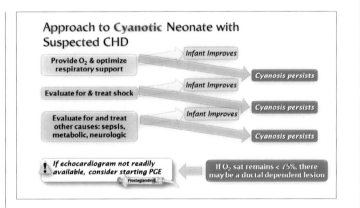

5. If CHD is suspected and the O_2 saturation remains < 75%, after optimizing all support as outlined above, and if an echocardiogram is not readily available, then a PGE infusion should be considered to establish and then maintain ductal patency. See page 70 for more information about PGE dosing and side effects.

Pulmonary Atresia with Intact Ventricular Septum (PA-IVS)[71,170,186,218-220]

PA-IVS affects just under 1% of infants with CHD and occurs in approximately 0.6 per 10,000 live births. Males and females are affected at similar rates.

Characterized by a either a membranous or muscular atretic pulmonary valve and a hypertrophied, variably hypoplastic right ventricle, pulmonary blood flow is dependent upon a left-to-right shunt from the aorta through the PDA to the pulmonary arteries. The tricuspid valve is usually anatomically abnormal, variably hypoplastic, and variably regurgitant. At times, the tricuspid valve may be severely stenotic, in which case all blood in the right atrium shunts directly across a PFO or ASD to the left atrium.

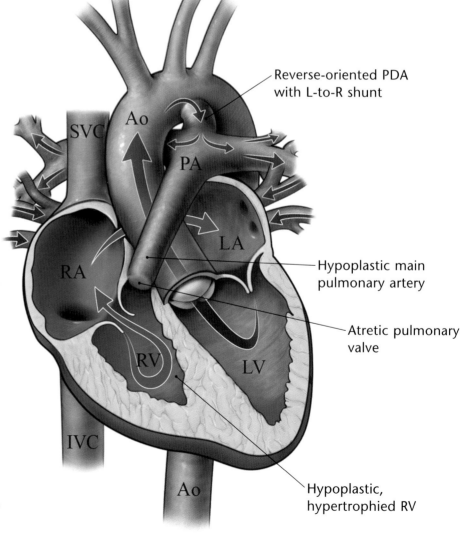

Figure 2.25. Anatomic features of PA-IVS with a PDA. There is no direct communication between the RV and pulmonary artery. The main pulmonary artery is hypoplastic and the right ventricle is hypertrophied and variably hypoplastic. There is a right-to-left atrial level shunt. Blood flow to the lungs is dependent upon a left-to-right shunt from the aorta through the PDA to the pulmonary arteries. When the DA is open, cyanosis is still apparent, but hypoxemia should be less because of improved pulmonary blood flow and the return of oxygenated blood to the left atrium.

Labels on figure: Reverse-oriented PDA with L-to-R shunt; Ao; SVC; PA; LA; RA; Hypoplastic main pulmonary artery; Atretic pulmonary valve; RV; LV; IVC; Ao; Hypoplastic, hypertrophied RV

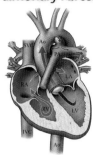

Pulmonary Atresia with Intact Ventricular Septum

Anatomic Features

- Pulmonary valve atresia → no direct communication between RV and PA
- Hypoplastic main PA
- RV hypertrophied and variably hypoplastic → RV size correlates with size of tricuspid valve
- R-to-L shunt through ASD or PFO

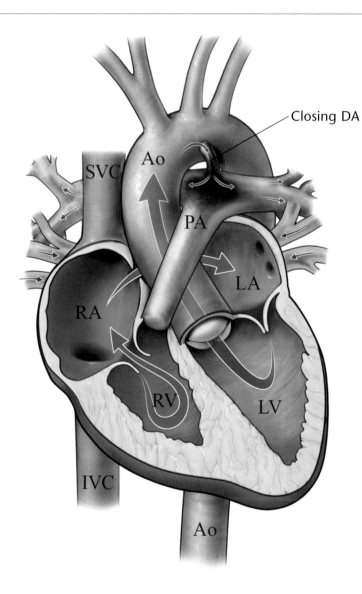

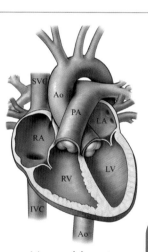

Normal heart

Figure 2.26. PA-IVS with a closing DA. As the DA closes, pulmonary blood flow is significantly decreased. Severe hypoxemia leads to hypoxia and metabolic acidosis. A PDA is essential for survival.

Pulmonary Atresia with Intact Ventricular Septum (PA-IVS)

Clinical Presentation

Infants with PA-IVS usually present at birth or shortly after birth with varying degrees of cyanosis and tachypnea.

Cyanosis

Cyanosis is usually apparent after birth and worsens dramatically as the DA closes. Initially, the infant may display "comfortable tachypnea," but respiratory distress increases as severe hypoxemia leads to hypoxia and anaerobic metabolism. Without the DA, there is no pulmonary blood flow, risking imminent death.

Heart Sounds

Single second heart sound because the pulmonary component is not present.

Murmur

May have no murmur or may have a pansystolic murmur secondary to tricuspid regurgitation (TR). In some cases, a thrill may be palpable.

Chest X-ray

Heart size

Mild to severe heart enlargement secondary to right atrial enlargement. Pulmonary vascular markings are usually reduced secondary to poor pulmonary blood flow.

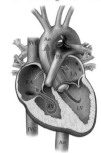

Pulmonary Atresia with **Intact Ventricular Septum**

Clinical Presentation
- May initially have "comfortable" tachypnea
- With ductal closure, ↓ in pulmonary blood flow → **severe cyanosis**
- Single S2
- May have no murmur or pansystolic murmur secondary to tricuspid regurgitation

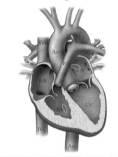

Pulmonary Atresia with **Intact Ventricular Septum**

Stabilization
Video Demonstrates
1) Closed ductus arteriosus (PDA)
2) PGE started to re-open the ductus arteriosus
3) PDA slowly opens
4) Provide O_2 to maintain O_2 sat > 75%

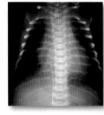
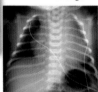

Pulmonary Atresia with **Intact Ventricular Septum**

Chest X-ray
- Cardiomegaly if RA is enlarged
- Decreased pulmonary vascular markings

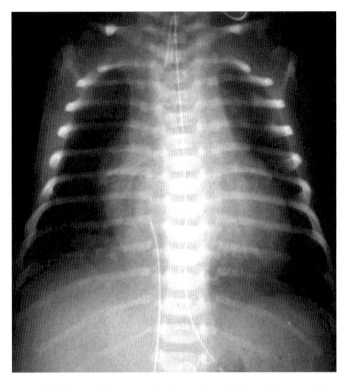

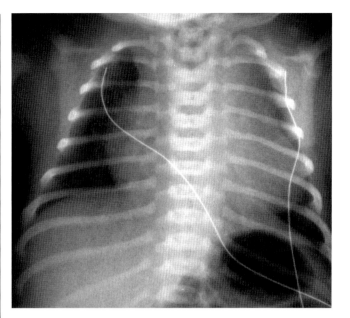

Term infant with PA-IVS. The lungs are not well inflated and there is cardiomegaly. Pulmonary vascular markings are decreased.

Term infant with PA-IVS. There is mild cardiomegaly. Pulmonary vascular markings are decreased. The endotracheal tube is at the thoracic inlet and the umbilical venous catheter tip is in the right atrium.

Initial Stabilization

Treatment is aimed at ensuring pulmonary blood flow and reversing the effects of severe hypoxemia and acidosis. The approach to cyanotic neonates with suspected CHD remains the same as discussed previously:

1. Begin an infusion of PGE to re-establish and maintain ductal patency.

2. Begin oxygen to improve systemic oxygenation and decrease PVR.

3. Maintain O_2 saturation > 75%.

What does it mean?
Let's talk about PA-IVS and Ventriculocoronary Connections

30 to 50% of patients with PA-IVS develop connections between the high-pressure right ventricle and the coronary arteries. These ventriculocoronary connections (also called coronary artery sinusoids or coronary sinusoids; Figure 2.27 on page 131) affect blood flow into the coronary arteries and therefore the overall health of the entire heart. Management of these patients can be especially challenging because procedures that reduce the pressure within the RV can affect blood flow to the coronary arteries. For example, opening of the atretic pulmonary valve in the cardiac catheterization lab or in the operating room can be expected to lower the pressure in the RV. Consequently, blood in the coronary arteries can then drain through the ventriculocoronary connections into the RV without supplying normal blood flow to the myocardium. The outcome of this can be cardiac ischemia, myocardial infarction, and life threatening arrhythmias. Thus, determining the status of the ventriculocoronary connections in the setting of PA-IVS (done by cardiac catheterization and angiography) is critically important prior to any palliative procedures such as radiofrequency perforation or surgical valvotomy.

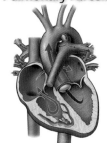

Pulmonary Atresia with **Intact Ventricular Septum**

Ventriculocoronary Connections

› 30 – 50% develop *ventriculocoronary connections* between high-pressure RV and the coronary arteries

! *Relieving pressure in RV by radiofrequency perforation or surgical valvotomy allows blood in coronary arteries to flow into RV instead of into myocardium → ischemia / infarct*

› Cardiac catheterization necessary to define coronary artery anatomy

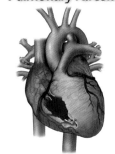

Pulmonary Atresia with **Intact Ventricular Septum**

Ventriculocoronary Connections

› 30 – 50% develop *ventriculocoronary connections* between high-pressure RV and the coronary arteries

! *Relieving pressure in RV by radiofrequency perforation or surgical valvotomy allows blood in coronary arteries to flow into RV instead of into myocardium → ischemia / infarct*

› Cardiac catheterization necessary to define coronary artery anatomy

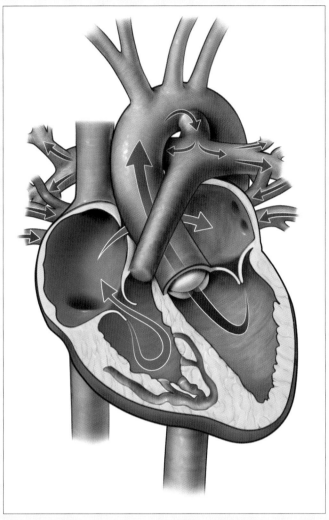 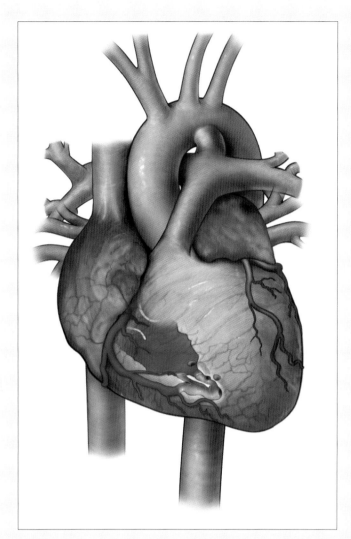

Figure 2.27. Anatomic features of PA-IVS and RV-dependent coronary circulation (ventriculocoronary connections). As the RV contracts, blood is forced through the myocardial sinusoids into the coronary circulation and myocardium. During diastole, blood typically flows from the aorta toward the same coronary circulation.

Pulmonary Atresia and Ventricular Septal Defect (PA-VSD)[221-225]

PA-VSD can be considered a severe form of TOF. Pulmonary atresia occurs in approximately 15 to 20% of cases of TOF. Pulmonary blood flow is supplied by the DA (Figure 2.28) and/ or major aortopulmonary collateral arteries (MAPCAs) that arise from the aorta or branches of the aorta (Figure 2.30 on page 134). MAPCAs are present in approximately 30% of cases of PA-VSD.

The anatomic features of PA-VSD include:

- Atretic pulmonary valve
- Main and branch pulmonary artery hypoplasia
- Overriding aorta
- Right ventricular hypertrophy
- Reverse-oriented ductus arteriosus

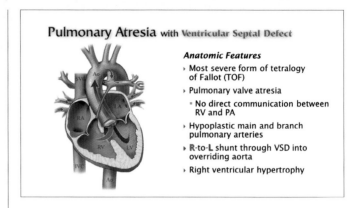

Pulmonary Atresia with Ventricular Septal Defect

Anatomic Features
- Most severe form of tetralogy of Fallot (TOF)
- Pulmonary valve atresia
  - No direct communication between RV and PA
- Hypoplastic main and branch pulmonary arteries
- R-to-L shunt through VSD into overriding aorta
- Right ventricular hypertrophy

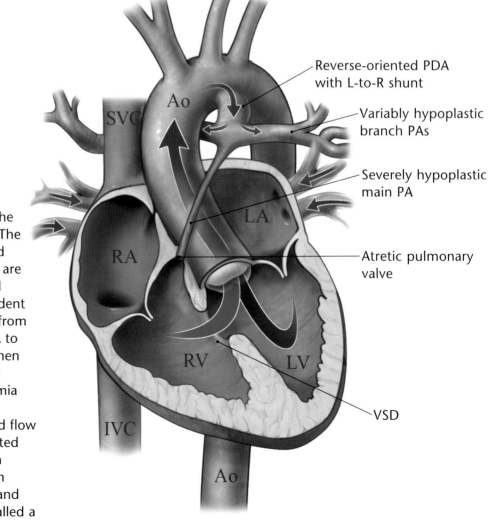

Figure 2.28. Anatomic features of PA-VSD with a PDA. There is no direct communication between the RV and pulmonary artery. The main pulmonary artery and branch pulmonary arteries are variably hypoplastic. Blood flow to the lungs is dependent upon a left-to-right shunt from the aorta through the PDA to the pulmonary arteries. When the DA is open, cyanosis is still apparent, but hypoxemia should be less because of improved pulmonary blood flow and the return of oxygenated blood to the left atrium. In PA-VSD, the DA arises from the transverse aortic arch and courses downward (also called a 'reverse-oriented' ductus).

Labels on figure: Reverse-oriented PDA with L-to-R shunt; Variably hypoplastic branch PAs; Severely hypoplastic main PA; Atretic pulmonary valve; VSD; Ao; SVC; LA; RA; RV; LV; IVC; Ao

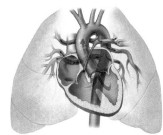

Pulmonary Atresia with **Ventricular Septal Defect**

Video Demonstrates
1) DA has closed and **cyanosis** severe
2) PGE started to re-open the DA

Prostaglandin E₁

3) Blood flow to lungs improves and O₂ saturation increases

Pulmonary Atresia with **Ventricular Septal Defect**

Anatomic Variation
- Major aortopulmonary collateral arteries (MAPCAs) present in approximately 30% of cases
- Collateral arteries arise from aorta or branches of aorta
  - Supply pulmonary blood flow
- May or may not have PDA

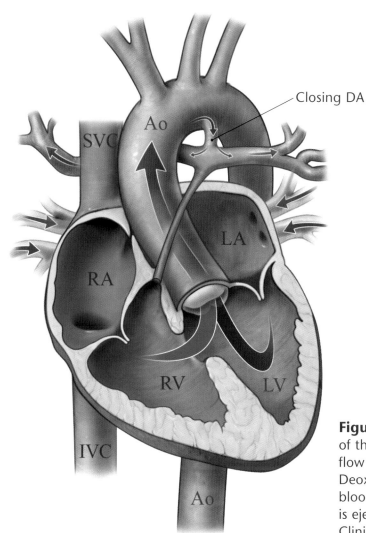

Closing DA

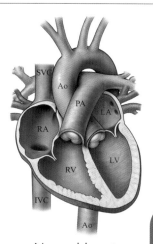

Normal heart

Figure 2.29. With closing of the DA, pulmonary blood flow decreases significantly. Deoxygenated and oxygenated blood that mixes at the VSD is ejected into the aorta. Clinically, the infant will be more desaturated and cyanotic.

Pulmonary Atresia and Ventricular Septal Defect (PA-VSD)

Clinical Presentation

Infants usually present at birth with varying degrees of cyanosis and respiratory distress. In the absence of MAPCAs, as the DA closes, pulmonary blood flow may become non-existent and the risk of dying is high.

Cyanosis

No MAPCAs

Cyanosis is usually apparent at birth. Cyanosis worsens significantly with constriction of the DA.

With MAPCAs

Cyanosis may be apparent at birth; however, these infants may have adequate pulmonary blood flow even with ductal closure.

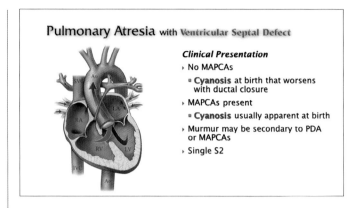

Pulmonary Atresia with **Ventricular Septal Defect**

Clinical Presentation
› No MAPCAs
  ▪ **Cyanosis** at birth that worsens with ductal closure
› MAPCAs present
  ▪ **Cyanosis** usually apparent at birth
› Murmur may be secondary to PDA or MAPCAs
› Single S2

Heart Sounds

Single second heart sound because the pulmonary component is not present.

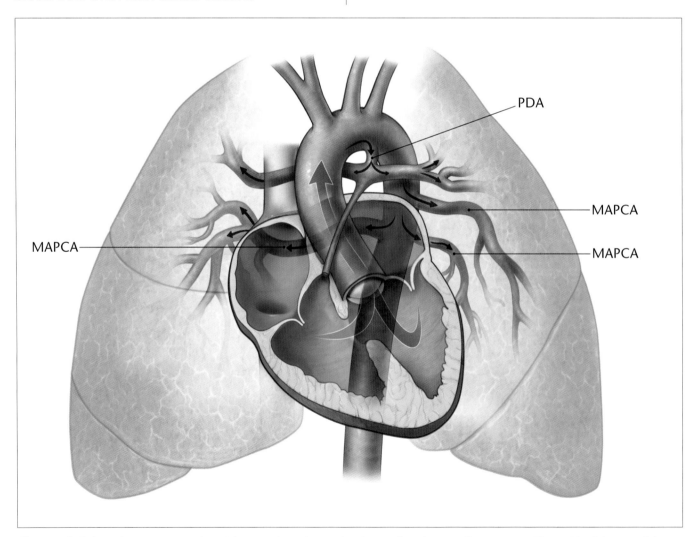

Figure 2.30. Pulmonary atresia with MAPCAs that arise from the descending aorta. The MAPCAs provide pulmonary blood flow. A PDA is also shown.

Murmur

If a heart murmur is present, it will be secondary to a PDA or aortopulmonary collaterals.

Chest X-Ray*

Heart Size

- The heart size is usually normal or slightly enlarged.

- A right aortic arch is present in 25 to 30% of cases. A right aortic arch is strongly associated with 22q11.2DS.

*X-ray not shown

Heart Shape

- As with TOF, the heart shape may be boot shaped.

Pulmonary Vasculature

- Decreased pulmonary vascular markings are seen when pulmonary blood flow is decreased.

- Pulmonary vascular markings are variable and depend upon the size and number of MAPCAs and/or presence of a large PDA.

Initial Stabilization

PA-VSD and No MAPCAs

Treatment is aimed at ensuring pulmonary blood flow and reversing the effects of severe hypoxemia and acidosis. The approach to cyanotic neonates with suspected CHD remains the same as discussed previously:

1. Begin an infusion of PGE to re-establish and maintain ductal patency.

2. Begin oxygen to improve systemic oxygenation and decrease PVR.

3. Maintain O_2 saturation > 75%.

4. If there is a right aortic arch, evaluate for 22q11.2DS; monitor for and treat hypocalcemia.

PA-VSD and MAPCAs

Blood flow through MAPCAs is not dependent upon PGE. However, PGE is often initiated until the sources of pulmonary blood flow have been accurately defined. Flow into the native pulmonary arteries, if present, is important so that these vessels can be preserved and ultimately used in the definitive repair.

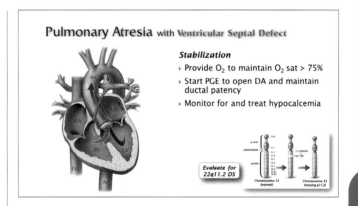

Pulmonary Atresia with Ventricular Septal Defect

Stabilization
- Provide O_2 to maintain O_2 sat > 75%
- Start PGE to open DA and maintain ductal patency
- Monitor for and treat hypocalcemia

Evaluate for 22q11.2 DS

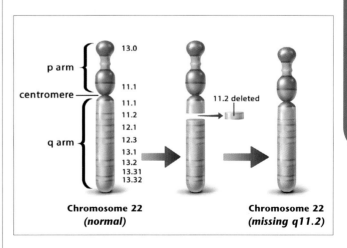

Oftentimes, PGE is continued until another palliative procedure, such as placement of a central shunt, can be performed.

Transposition of the Great Arteries (TGA)[73,170,186,203,219,226,227]

TGA affects approximately 5% of all infants with CHD. The male to female ratio is 2 to 1. As the name suggests, the great arteries are transposed relative to the ventricle. The aorta arises from the right ventricle and ejects deoxygenated blood through the aortic valve to the body. The pulmonary artery arises from the left ventricle and recirculates oxygenated blood back to the lungs. This pattern of blood flow is in *parallel* rather than in *series*, meaning the majority of blood ejected from a ventricle is recirculated back to that same ventricle.

For oxygenated blood to reach the systemic circulation, mixing of the pulmonary and systemic venous return *must* occur at an ASD and/or VSD. A VSD is present in approximately 30 to 40% of patients with TGA (see page 138). In addition to a VSD, associated defects may include left ventricular outflow tract obstruction (COA, IAA) and pulmonary stenosis.

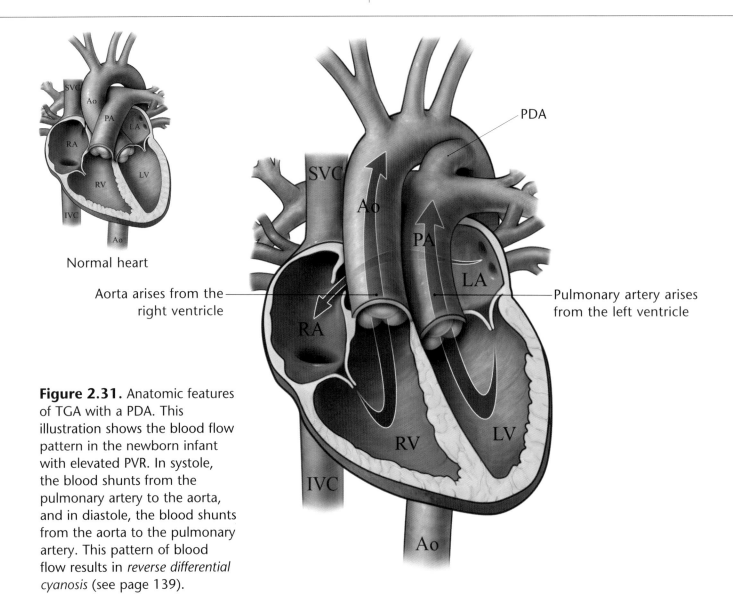

Normal heart

Aorta arises from the right ventricle

Pulmonary artery arises from the left ventricle

Figure 2.31. Anatomic features of TGA with a PDA. This illustration shows the blood flow pattern in the newborn infant with elevated PVR. In systole, the blood shunts from the pulmonary artery to the aorta, and in diastole, the blood shunts from the aorta to the pulmonary artery. This pattern of blood flow results in *reverse differential cyanosis* (see page 139).

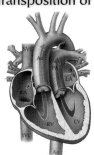

Transposition of the Great Arteries

Anatomic Features

› Parallel circulation
› Aorta arises from RV
  ▪ **Deoxygenated** venous blood → RA → RV → aorta → body
› Pulmonary artery originates from LV
  ▪ **Oxygenated** pulmonary venous blood → LA → LV → PA → lungs
› In the absence of a VSD, adequate mixing at the atrial level is essential for survival

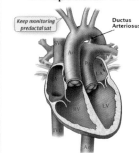

Transposition of the Great Arteries

Keep monitoring preductal sat

Ductus Arteriosus

Video demonstrates

1) Closed ductus arteriosus
2) PGE started to re-open the ductus arteriosus Prostaglandin E₁
3) PDA slowly opens
4) Intercirculatory mixing improves

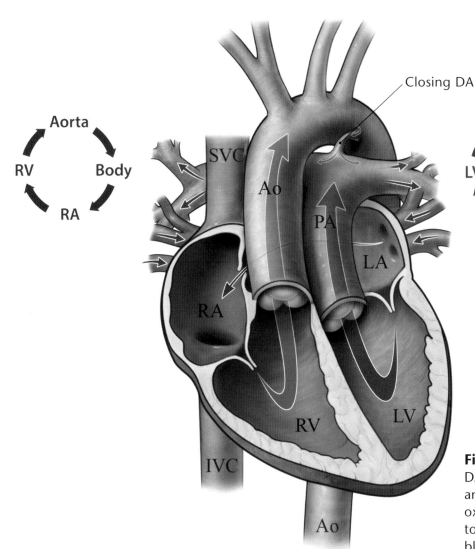

Figure 2.32. TGA with a closing DA. In the absence of a VSD and/or adequate atrial mixing, oxygenated blood will recirculate to the lungs, and deoxygenated blood will circulate systemically. In this setting, cyanosis is severe.

Cyanotic CHD
Ductal Dependent

Transposition of the Great Arteries (TGA)

Clinical Presentation

Cyanosis

TGA with IVS

The size of the ASD influences the degree of mixing between the pulmonary and systemic circulations and thus, the severity of the cyanosis. If the ASD is small, moderate to severe cyanosis is noted at birth or soon after birth. The arterial PO_2 may be as low as 15 to 25 mmHg (2 to 3.3 kPa). Although tachypneic and cyanotic, the baby may initially have unlabored respiratory effort. With ongoing severe hypoxemia and development of metabolic acidosis, work of breathing increases. This observation is important for differentiating between pulmonary and cardiac disease. Infants with pulmonary disease and severe hypoxemia to the same degree as infants with TGA usually present initially with more pronounced respiratory distress, characterized by tachypnea, retractions, and dyspnea.

TGA with VSD

Infants with TGA and VSD have higher arterial saturations than infants with TGA and IVS. As the PVR drops in the first few weeks of age, the infant may develop pulmonary overcirculation and CHF. Signs include tachypnea, retractions, and hepatomegaly. Depending upon institutional preference, surgical repair may be delayed beyond the neonatal period.

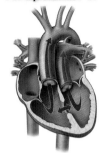

Transposition of the Great Arteries with VSD

Clinical Presentation

- Variable cyanosis → depends on mixing between ventricles
- Tachypnea with easy effort
- May or may not have a murmur
- As pulmonary vascular resistance decreases in first few weeks, pulmonary blood flow ↑ → *pulmonary overcirculation / congestive heart failure*

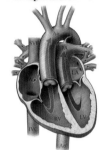

Transposition of the Great Arteries with IVS

Clinical Presentation

- May initially have "comfortable" tachypnea
- With ductal closure → moderate to severe **cyanosis**
- ↑ Work of breathing as hypoxemia worsens
- Often no murmur unless VSD or associated pulmonary stenosis
- Loud single S2

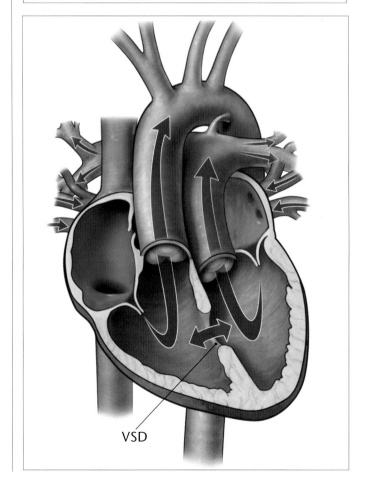

VSD

Reverse Differential Cyanosis

Reverse differential cyanosis (lower O_2 saturation in the right hand, higher O_2 saturation in the foot) may be observed in the initial newborn period when PVR is elevated, or in the setting of TGA with critical coarctation/interrupted aortic arch. This pattern is the opposite of the saturation pattern seen in PPHN and is therefore an important observation.

As PVR declines in the hours and days after birth, the pre and postductal saturations may equalize, with both being low. Continuous assessment of preductal O_2 saturation is critically important because the O_2 saturation in the right hand is the same O_2 saturation as the blood perfusing the brain.

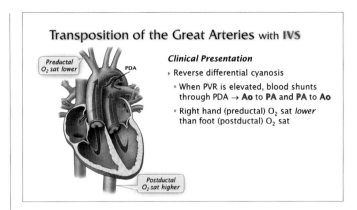

Transposition of the Great Arteries with IVS

Preductal O_2 sat lower

PDA

Clinical Presentation

▸ Reverse differential cyanosis
- When PVR is elevated, blood shunts through PDA → **Ao** to **PA** and **PA** to **Ao**
- Right hand (preductal) O_2 sat *lower* than foot (postductal) O_2 sat

Postductal O_2 sat higher

Heart Sounds

The S2 is single and loud.

Murmur

If the ventricular septum is intact, there is often no murmur. A systolic murmur may be heard in neonates with a VSD and/or associated pulmonary stenosis.

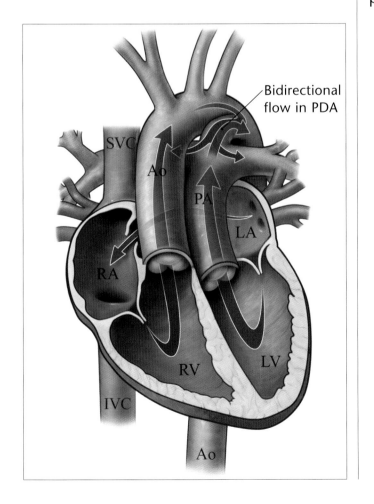

Bidirectional flow in PDA

SVC

Ao

PA

LA

RA

RV

LV

IVC

Ao

Transposition of the Great Arteries (TGA)

Chest X-Ray

Heart Size and Pulmonary Vasculature

TGA with IVS

Normal heart size initially with later development of cardiac enlargement. Pulmonary vascular markings are usually increased secondary to increased pulmonary blood flow.

TGA with VSD

Cardiomegaly and increased pulmonary vascular markings.

Heart Shape

A characteristic oval or egg-shaped appearance ("egg on a string") of the heart is due to a narrow mediastinum, caused by a small thymus and alignment of the great vessels in an anterior-posterior relationship.

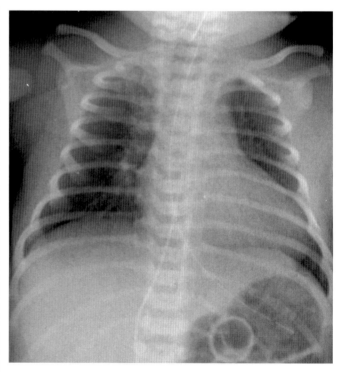

Transposition of the Great Arteries

Chest X-ray
- Normal size or mild cardiomegaly
- Characteristic oval or egg-shaped appearance of heart
  - *"Egg on a string"*
- Narrow mediastinum secondary to alignment of great vessels over each other
- ↑ Pulmonary blood flow → ↑ pulmonary vascular markings

2-hour old term neonate with TGA. The heart size is normal and "egg" on a string configuration.

3-day old term neonate with TGA. The heart is "egg" or oval shaped and there are increased pulmonary vascular markings. The UVC is malpositioned in the right atrium.

TGA with IVS

Treatment is aimed at establishing ductal patency, and if indicated, improving mixing at the atrial level.

1. Start PGE to help increase left atrial pressure by increasing blood flow to the lungs as follows:

- In diastole, the blood will shunt from the aorta through the PDA to the pulmonary arteries. The benefit of increasing pulmonary blood flow is that the increased pulmonary venous return will increase the pressure in the left atrium to help force blood across the PFO or ASD to the right atrium.

- The size of the ASD influences the degree of mixing between the pulmonary and systemic circulations and thus, the severity of the hypoxemia. If the ASD is small, even if the PDA is large, the infant will have moderate to severe cyanosis at birth or soon after birth.

- While PVR is elevated or in the setting of left outflow tract obstruction, in systole, the blood will also shunt from the pulmonary artery to the aorta, thus increasing the amount of oxygenated blood entering the aorta.

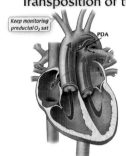

Transposition of the Great Arteries

Keep monitoring preductal O₂ sat

PDA

Initial Stabilization
- Provide O₂
- Maintain preductal O₂ sat > 75%
- *Facilitate intercirculatory mixing*
  - Begin PGE infusion
  - ↑ Pulmonary blood flow → ↑ pulmonary venous return → ↑ L-to-R atrial level shunt
  - Respiratory support → if intubation required, conventional ventilation may facilitate mixing

2. Provide supplemental oxygen.

- Monitor the O₂ saturation in the right hand (preductal) and either foot (postductal). The goal saturation in the right hand is > 75%.

3. Intubation and conventional ventilation may be required to provide respiratory support and to treat apnea that may occur with infusion of PGE.

- Conventional ventilation may be more effective than high frequency oscillatory ventilation (HFOV) in promoting intercirculatory mixing due to the larger changes in intrathoracic pressure.

(Continued on next page)

Cyanotic CHD
Ductal Dependent

Transposition of the Great Arteries (TGA)

TGA with IVS (Initial Stabilization continued)

4. Adequacy of the intra-atrial shunt is essential for survival. If hypoxemia is not sufficiently relieved with administration of PGE, mixing at the atrial level can be improved by performing a balloon atrial septostomy (also called a Rashkind procedure, Figure 2.33 on page 143). Balloon atrial septostomy can be performed at the bedside with transthoracic echocardiographic guidance, or in the cardiac catheterization laboratory. A positive outcome of this procedure is an improvement in systemic O_2 saturation. It may be possible to discontinue the PGE following balloon atrial septostomy.

Transposition of the Great Arteries

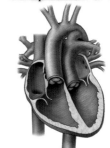

Rashkind – Balloon Atrial Septostomy
- Indications
  - Persistent, severe hypoxemia after opening ductus
  - Persistent acidosis
- Effect
  - Saturation should improve significantly
  - Acidosis should resolve

Transposition of the Great Arteries

Rashkind – Balloon Atrial Septostomy

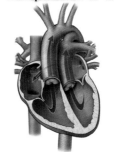
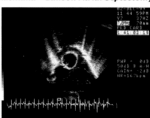

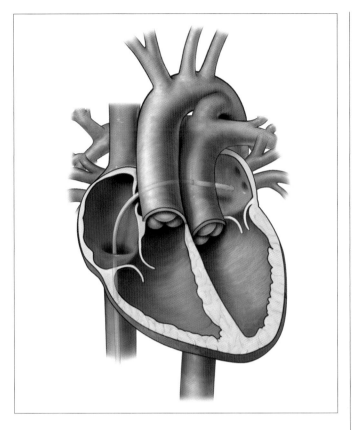

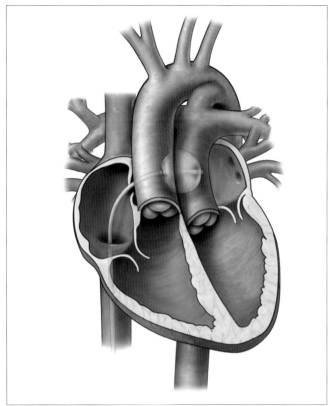

Figure 2.33. Balloon atrial septostomy. A balloon-tipped catheter is inserted via the femoral or umbilical vein into the left atrium and through the PFO (upper left). The balloon is inflated with saline or contrast (upper right) and then is rapidly pulled back into the right atrium. The illustration on the right shows the enlarged atrial septal defect and increased flow of oxygenated blood from the left atrium to the right atrium.

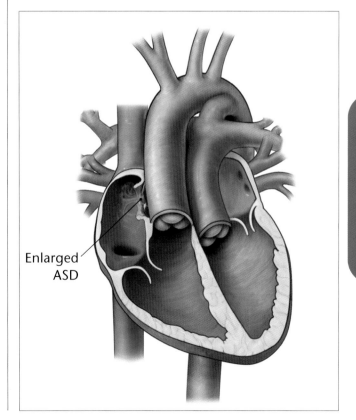

Enlarged
ASD

What does it mean?
What is the difference between D-TGA and L-TGA?[192,226,228,229]

Under normal circumstances, during the 3rd and early 4th weeks of gestation, the straight heart tube bends and loops to the right (dextro or d-looping). This results in the right ventricle being positioned to the right and anterior to the left ventricle. Ventricular *inversion* results when the heart tube bends and loops to the left rather than to the right (levo or l-looping). This also causes the right atrium to drain into the morphologic left ventricle and the left atrium to drain into the morphologic right ventricle, also called *atrioventricular discordance*. Note that the terms *left and right ventricles* refer to ventricular morphology rather than the left or right position of the ventricle in the heart and chest.

In addition to ventricular looping, it is important to consider the relationship between the ventricles and great arteries. There are two basic types of transposition, D-TGA and L-TGA. In D-TGA, the aorta is located anteriorly and rightward and arises from the right-sided right ventricle. In L-TGA, the aorta is located anteriorly and leftward and arises from the left-sided morphologic right ventricle.

Associated lesions with L-TGA are common and include VSD, an abnormal left-sided tricuspid valve (dysplastic and may be Ebstein-like), and left ventricular outflow tract obstruction (i.e., the tract supplying blood to the lungs). The atrioventricular conduction system is also commonly abnormal.

As shown in Figure 2.34, the anatomy and pattern of blood flow in L-TGA is as follows:

- The left ventricle and mitral valve are located on the *right* side of the heart. Deoxygenated systemic venous return enters the right

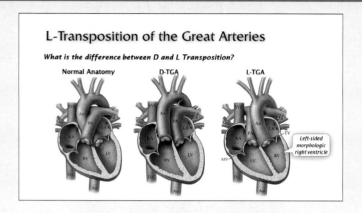

L-Transposition of the Great Arteries

What is the difference between D and L Transposition?

Normal Anatomy | D-TGA | L-TGA

Left-sided morphologic right ventricle

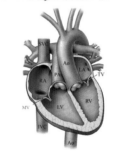

L-Transposition of the Great Arteries

Clinical Presentation
- Also known as congenitally corrected transposition
- May be or symptomatic or asymptomatic secondary to valve regurgitation +/or associated lesions (Ebstein anomaly, coarctation, VSD)

atrium, then passes through the mitral valve to the left ventricle. The deoxygenated blood is then ejected into the transposed pulmonary artery to the lungs.

- The right ventricle and tricuspid valve are located on the *left* side of the heart. Oxygenated pulmonary venous return enters the left atrium, then passes through the tricuspid valve to the right ventricle. Oxygenated blood is then ejected into the transposed aorta to supply the heart, brain, and body.

The combination of ventricular inversion and transposition of the great vessels allows for correct flow of deoxygenated and oxygenated blood to the lungs and body. For this reason, L-transposition is often referred to as "congenitally corrected" transposition of the great arteries.

With D-TGA, deoxygenated systemic venous return enters the right atrium, then passes through the tricuspid valve to the right ventricle. The deoxygenated blood is then ejected into the transposed aorta to supply the heart, brain, and body. Oxygenated pulmonary venous return enters the left atrium, then passes through the mitral valve to the left ventricle. Oxygenated blood is then ejected into the transposed pulmonary artery and back into the lungs.

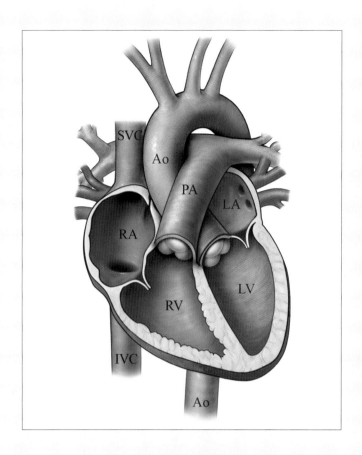

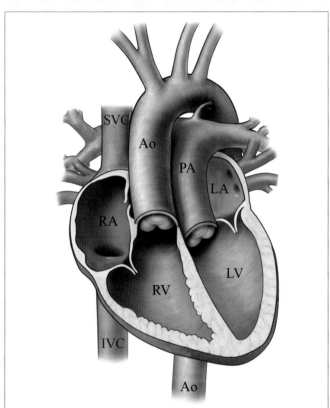

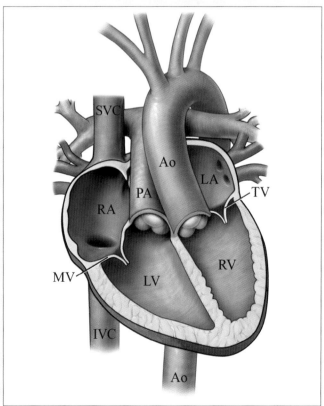

Figure 2.34. Normal heart anatomy (top), D-TGA (bottom left), L-TGA (bottom right). In L-TGA, the terms left and right ventricle refer to ventricular morphology rather than the left or right position of the ventricle in the heart and chest. MV = mitral valve TV = tricuspid valve

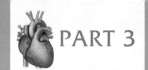

PART 3 | S. T. A. B. L. E. – Cardiac Module

Sugar, Temperature, Airway, Blood Pressure, Lab Work, and Emotional Support

Introduction

Healthcare professionals involved with neonatal and emergency care will occasionally encounter neonates who are ill with cardiac conditions. Prompt, effective, and appropriate care can reduce secondary organ damage, improve short- and long-term outcomes, and reduce morbidity and mortality. This section will briefly discuss the six S.T.A.B.L.E. assessment components (Sugar, Temperature, Airway, Blood pressure, Lab work, and Emotional support) and any modifications specific to neonates with suspected or confirmed CHD.[230]

Care must be provided based on the neonate's condition at presentation. If the infant is in shock, attention must first be devoted to reducing the work of breathing and identifying and treating primary causes of acid-base disturbances. Supportive and resuscitative measures include assisting ventilation and improving oxygenation, improving blood pressure and perfusion, establishing intravenous (IV) and arterial access, administering medications, and maintaining a normal body temperature.

Sugar and Safe Care Module

Sick infants often do not tolerate enteral (oral or gavage) feedings, and if the infant experienced shock, then intestinal perfusion may have been impaired. In the presence of ductal dependent lesions, as the DA closes, infants will display signs of increased distress that include disinterest in feedings, a weak suck, and development of intestinal ileus and vomiting. When an infant has suspected CHD, the safest approach is to withhold feedings and establish IV access as soon as possible to ensure an IV line is available for medications and fluid

resuscitation. In addition, placement of an IV will allow the infusion of appropriate glucose-containing solutions to support the infants' increased energy demands.

Sugar and Safe Care

› Sick infants often do not tolerate enteral feedings
  ▪ Respiratory distress interferes with coordination of suck, swallow, breathing → ↑ Risk of aspiration
  ▪ Disinterest in feedings, easily fatigued, weak suck
› With ductal closure in left heart obstructive lesions
  ▪ Intestinal ileus, vomiting
  ▪ ↑ Risk of intestinal ischemia
› Withhold feedings and establish IV access
  ▪ Provide glucose-containing solutions

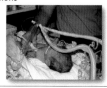

Glucose Production and Utilization Rate[231-235]

Glucose is the primary fuel used by the brain; therefore, adequate blood glucose levels are essential for normal brain function. In healthy term neonates, the liver glycogen breakdown and glucose production rate are approximately 4 to 6 mg/kg/minute. Sick infants are at increased risk for hypoglycemia because of an increased glucose utilization rate that may exceed their glucose production or availability rate. Neonates with CHD may also have concurrent illnesses that place them at higher risk for hypoglycemia, including chromosomal or genetic conditions, hyperinsulinemia, intrauterine growth restriction, and prematurity.

Initial IV Fluid Rate and Target Glucose Levels[230,232,233,235-242]

The S.T.A.B.L.E. Program defines hypoglycemia as "glucose delivery or availability that is inadequate to meet glucose demand." The exact blood glucose value that defines hypoglycemia remains controversial. In addition, glucose values tolerated by individual infants may vary because of their specific diagnoses and medical problems. When the blood sugar is low, action should be taken to restore the blood sugar to an euglycemic, or normal blood glucose concentration.[243,244]

Once IV access is established, administer $D_{10}W$ at 80 mL/kg/day to provide a glucose infusion rate of 5.5 mg/kg/minute. Infants with hyperinsulinemia and/or accelerated glucose utilization may need a higher dextrose concentration than $D_{10}W$. In the first 2 days of age, the goal blood sugar is 50 to 110 mg/dL (2.8 to 6.1 mmol/L) and after 48 hours, the goal blood sugar is 60 to 110 mg/dL (3.3 to 5.1 mmol/L). The addition of electrolytes, calcium, and magnesium should be considered once the infant is greater than 48 hours old.

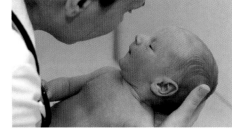

Aerobic and Anaerobic Metabolism

Video created and narrated by the Program Author, Dr. Kris Karlsen

Click to play (3:40 min)

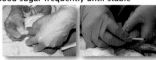

Sugar and Safe Care

Monitor Blood Glucose and Maintain > 50 mg/dL (2.8 mmol/L)

› ↑ Risk for hypoglycemia secondary to:
  ▪ Anaerobic metabolism and ↑ glucose utilization rate
  ▪ Associated chromosomal or genetic conditions, hyperinsulinemia, intrauterine growth restriction, prematurity
› Monitor blood sugar frequently until stable

A neonate who develops cardiogenic shock or obstructive shock related to ductal closure is at increased risk for acute renal failure and oliguria. Hyponatremia, the appearance of edema, and development of CHF are associated with an imbalance between intake and output. If shock has occurred and the patient is normoglycemic, consider decreasing the baseline fluid rate to 60 mL/kg/day. If the infusion rate is decreased, monitor the blood sugar regularly to ensure it remains consistently >50 mg/dL (<48 hours of age), or >60 mg/dL (>48 hours of age).

If the blood sugar is lower than desired, administer a 2 mL/kg $D_{10}W$ glucose bolus, which equals 200 mg/kg of glucose, at a rate of 1 mL per minute. More than one glucose bolus may be required to stabilize the blood sugar. To prevent hyperglycemia and rebound hypoglycemia, do not give $D_{25}W$ or $D_{50}W$ dextrose concentrations. If the blood sugar remains persistently below the desired target range, increase the maintenance IV fluid dextrose concentration to $D_{12.5}W$, $D_{15}W$, or higher. When glucose concentrations exceed $D_{12.5}W$, it is customary to infuse fluids via an umbilical venous catheter (UVC) or a peripherally inserted central catheter (PICC).

IV Access and Central Lines[176,245-259]

Several options for establishing IV access include placing two peripheral IV lines and/or placing a double-lumen UVC or double-lumen PICC. Having a minimum of two IV access ports will allow simultaneous infusion of a glucose-containing solution and medications, such as PGE.

Sugar and Safe Care

Intravenous (IV) Access

▸ $D_{10}W$ at 80 mL/kg/day (5.5 mg/kg/minute glucose infusion rate)

▸ Place 2 IV lines if possible

  ▪ Double lumen central venous catheter and peripheral IV *or* 2 peripheral IVs

▸ Emergency IV access

  ▪ Umbilical vein catheterization

  ▪ Intraosseous route if other IV cannot be established

 In a life-threatening emergency, if not able to rapidly establish reliable venous access, an intraosseous (IO) needle can be inserted into the medial aspect of the tibial bone, just below the tibial tuberosity.[259-261] It should be remembered that the infant who is conscious or who regains consciousness requires numbing of the IO space with lidocaine prior to infusion of medications or fluids.[262]

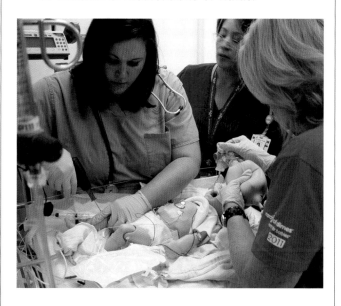

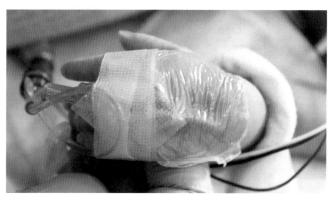

Peripheral IV secured with clear transparent dressing

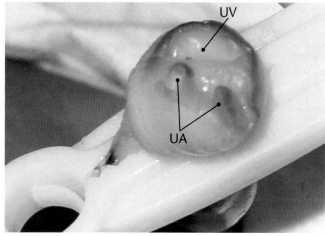

UV = umbilical vein   UA = umbilical artery

Umbilical Vein Catheter (UVC)

The UVC tip should be positioned at the inferior vena cava/right atrial (IVC/RA) junction (also called the cavoatrial junction).

Figures 3.1 and 3.2 demonstrate good position of the UVC at the IVC/RA junction. Figures 3.3 and 3.4 demonstrate malpositioned UVCs.

A UVC tip malpositioned in the heart increases the risk for:

- Arrhythmias
- Intracardiac thrombus formation
- Myocardial perforation
- Pericardial effusion
- Cardiac tamponade
- Pulmonary and systemic emboli (infected emboli will result in abscess formation)
- Endocarditis
- Pulmonary infarction
- Pulmonary hemorrhage

A UVC tip malpositioned in the liver or portal venous system increases the risk for:

- Hepatic necrosis following thrombus formation or infusion of hypertonic or vasoactive solutions into the liver
- Portal hypertension
- Peritoneal perforation
- Intestinal ischemia
- Hepatic vessel perforation and hematoma formation; followed by calcification formation when the hematoma resolves
- Intravascular thrombus formation
- Emboli released into the liver

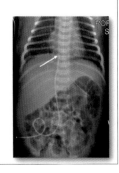

Sugar and Safe Care

Umbilical Venous Catheter (UVC)
- Location
  - Inferior vena cava / right atrial junction
- Administer IV fluids and medications
  - If tip properly positioned, may use for vasopressors
  - Can be used to monitor central venous pressure

Sugar and Safe Care

Umbilical Venous Catheter (UVC) – Safety
- Extra precaution if there is a R-to-L atrial or ventricular shunt → risk of emboli to brain and systemic circulation

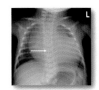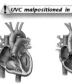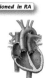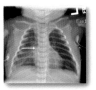

UVC malpositioned in RA

Many infants with severe forms of CHD have right-to-left shunts at the atrial or ventricular level. Therefore, use extra caution to prevent any emboli from entering the central line or any other intravascular catheter.

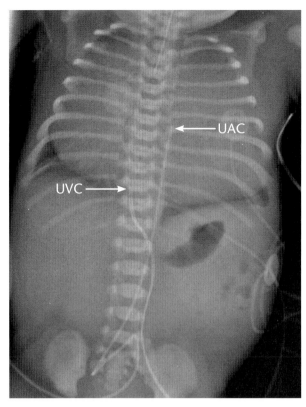

Figure 3.1. Term infant with Ebstein anomaly and massive cardiomegaly. The UVC is in good position at the IVC/RA junction and the UAC is in good position at thoracic vertebrae 7 (T7).

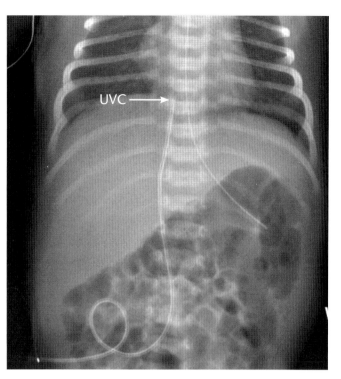

Figure 3.2. Late preterm infant with suspected cyanotic CHD. The UVC is in good position at the IVC/RA junction. The enteric tube tip is in the stomach.

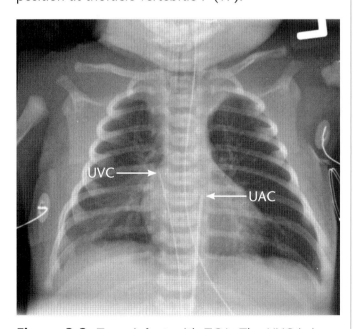

Figure 3.3. Term infant with TGA. The UVC is in the high RA near the SVC and should be retracted approximately 3.5 centimeters. The UAC is in good position at T7. The endotracheal tube projects over the upper intrathoracic area. The enteric tube enters the stomach with the tip not imaged.

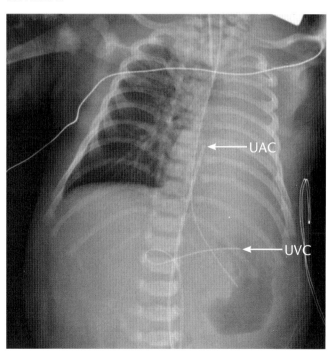

Figure 3.4. Term infant with TGA. The UVC is malpositioned in the portal venous system. The UAC is in good position between T6 and T7. The endotracheal tube tip is in the mid-trachea. The left lung is atelectatic. The enteric tube enters the stomach and could be advanced slightly.

Umbilical Artery Catheter (UAC) and Peripheral Arterial Line (PAL)

UAC insertion is indicated when continuous BP monitoring and/or arterial blood gas assessment is required. The UAC tip should be positioned between thoracic vertebrae 6 and 9 (T6 and T9). If this location cannot be achieved, then the UAC tip may be positioned low at the level of lumbar vertebrae 3 and 4 (L3 and L4). When the UAC tip is in a low location, complications that lead to removal are more common. Figures 3.5 through 3.8 demonstrate umbilical catheters in both good and poor positions.

If unable to insert a UAC, additional options include cannulation of the radial or posterior tibial arteries. Vasopressors, including dopamine and epinephrine, should *never* be administered in any arterial line.

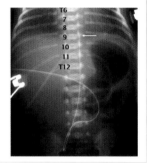

Sugar and Safe Care

Umbilical Arterial Catheter (UAC) - Indications
› Monitor arterial blood pressure
› Monitor arterial blood gases

Sugar and Safe Care

UAC – Tip location
› High line
  ▪ Tip located between T6 and T9
› Low line
  ▪ Tip located between L3 and L4
› Confirm placement with x-ray

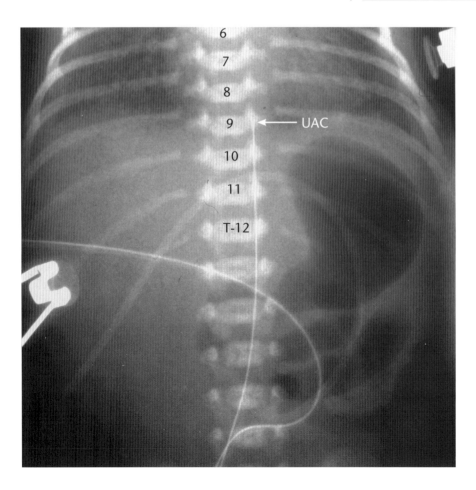

Figure 3.5. Abdominal x-ray showing the UAC tip in good position at T9.

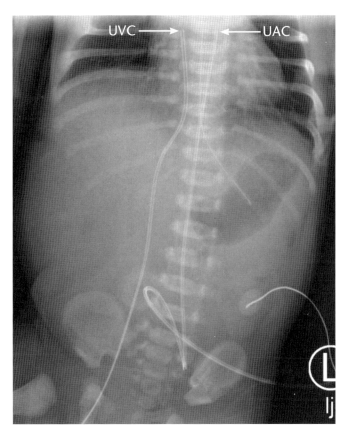

Figure 3.6. Term infant with transposition of the great arteries. The UVC is in the high right atrium near the SVC. The UAC tip is at the inferior aspect of T5 (slightly high). The enteric tube overlies the stomach.

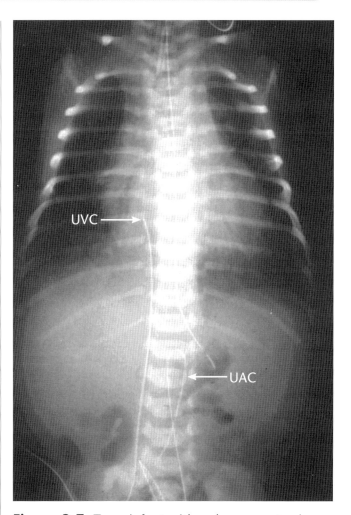

Figure 3.7. Term infant with pulmonary atresia. The UVC is malpositioned in the right atrium and the UAC is coiled back upon itself in the aorta. The enteric tube overlies the stomach.

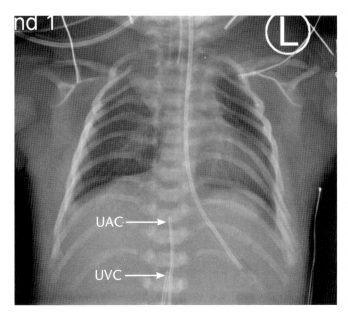

Figure 3.8. Term infant with TAPVC. The UVC tip is malpositioned in the liver and the UAC tip is at T10. The UAC could be pulled to a low line to relocate the tip between L3 and L4. The UVC should be removed and not left in the liver.

S.T.A.B.L.E. Modules

UMBILICAL CATHETER SAFETY

- *Use sterile technique when placing lines.*

- *Once the sterile field is disassembled or the line has been secured, do not advance the UVC or UAC into the vein or artery.*

- *The UAC or PAL should be attached to a transducer. A dampened or flattened arterial waveform may indicate presence of an air bubble in the system, disconnection, development of a thrombus in or around the catheter tip, hypotension, or changes in ductal patency.*

- *Use caution when connecting IV fluids or medications to the central line or when drawing labs to avoid contaminating the sterile line.*

- *If the UVC or UAC is repositioned, a chest or abdominal x-ray should be repeated to confirm correct placement of the catheter tip.*

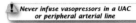

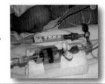

Sugar and Safe Care

UAC – Safety
- Maintain sterile technique and air-tight system
- Rapid and life-threatening blood loss with disconnection
  - Use of transducer assists with detection of disconnection
- Confirm placement with chest x-ray
  - Repeat x-ray if catheter repositioned
- Monitor for catheter complications
  - Blanching or discoloration of toes, legs, groin, buttocks, abdomen

Never infuse vasopressors in a UAC or peripheral arterial line

- *Maintain an air-tight system. Do not allow air bubbles to infuse into the body.*

- *Check connections to be sure they are tight. Rapid, life-threatening blood loss can occur with inadvertent disconnection of the tubing.*

EXAM TIP:

Arterial spasm or development of emboli from small blood clots that form on the tip or in the circulation adjacent to the tip of the catheter may occur when a UAC or other arterial line is in use. The area distal to the spasm or clot may show signs of impaired skin perfusion. Therefore, monitor the infant frequently for white, blue, or black discoloration of the skin on the back,

buttocks, groin, abdomen, legs, feet, or toes. If the arterial line is in a peripheral site, observe the hand and fingers (radial artery) or foot and toes (posterior tibial artery) for altered perfusion, discoloration of the skin, and decreased skin temperature. If concerned, the line will most likely need to be removed.

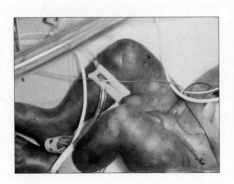
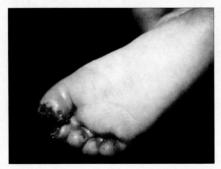
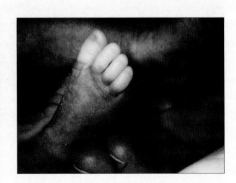

Peripherally Inserted Central Catheter (PICC)

A PICC may be placed in upper or lower extremities. An upper extremity PICC is in a central location when the tip is located in the superior vena cava (SVC), but not deeper than the junction of the SVC and RA (Figure 3.9). After initial insertion, periodic x-ray or imaging surveillance is important to monitor for tip migration to an undesirable location.

If the infant's cardiac defect will lead to single ventricle palliation or a 1.5 ventricle repair, the PICC should not be placed in an upper extremity because patency of the SVC for a future Glenn procedure is essential. For upper and lower extremity PICCs, malposition of the tip in the heart raises the risk for cardiac perforation, pericardial effusion, cardiac tamponade, and arrhythmia. Figure 3.10 shows a large right-sided pleural effusion following PICC malposition.

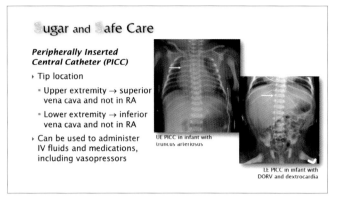

Sugar and **S**afe Care

Peripherally Inserted Central Catheter (PICC)

▸ Tip location
  - Upper extremity → superior vena cava and not in RA
  - Lower extremity → inferior vena cava and not in RA

▸ Can be used to administer IV fluids and medications, including vasopressors

UE PICC in infant with truncus arteriosus

LE PICC in infant with DORV and dextrocardia

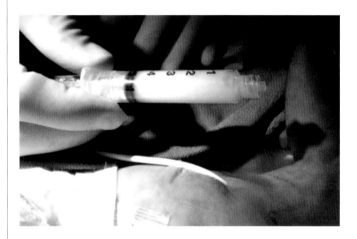

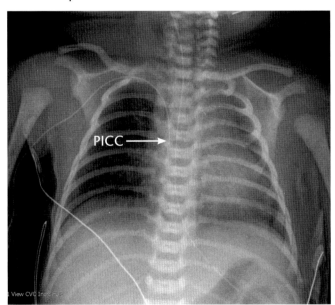

Figure 3.9. Chest x-ray showing an upper extremity PICC correctly positioned in the SVC.

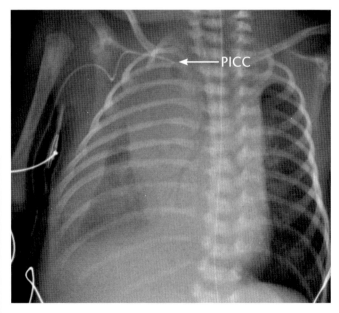

PICC

Figure 3.10. Upper extremity PICC in a noncentral position. The infant developed respiratory distress and the chest x-ray revealed a large right-sided pleural effusion secondary to the PICC eroding through the vein. A chest tube was placed and hyperalimentation solution was aspirated (see photo above). The PICC was removed.

S.T.A.B.L.E. Modules

155

A lower extremity PICC is in a central location when the tip is located in the inferior vena cava (IVC) below the right atrium. When the PICC is initially placed, both anterior-posterior and lateral abdominal x-rays are recommended to ensure the catheter tip is located in the IVC and not in unintended locations, such as lumbar, epigastric, spermatic, kidney, or liver vessels. Periodic abdominal x-ray or imaging surveillance should also occur to monitor for tip migration to an undesirable location. Figures 3.11 and 3.12 show x-rays of infants with lower extremity PICCs. Note: there is controversy regarding acceptable lower extremity PICC tip positions. Consult additional resources as necessary.

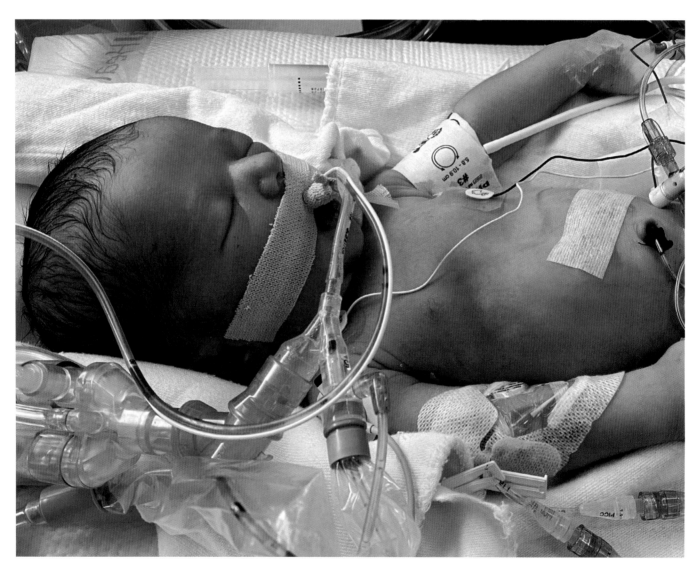

Term infant with critical COA, hypoplastic aortic arch, and congenital diaphragmatic hernia (postoperative). A right arm PICC and umbilical catheter are present.

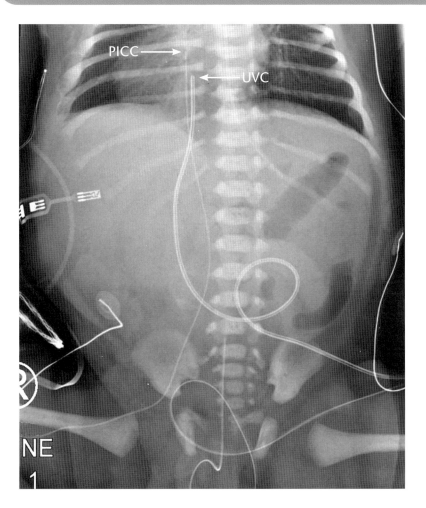

Figure 3.11. Abdominal x-ray of an infant with DORV and dextrocardia. The right lower extremity PICC tip is malpositioned in the high right atrium, 2.5 cm above the diaphragm. The UVC tip is in the lower right atrium, 1.5 cm above the diaphragm. An enteric tube projects over the stomach. A bladder catheter is present.

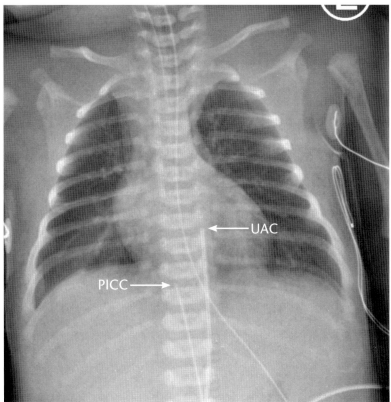

Figure 3.12. Chest x-ray of an infant with TGA. The lower extremity PICC is at T10 and the UAC is at T8. The endotracheal tube is in the mid-trachea and the enteric tube overlies the stomach.

Temperature Module[264,265]

Temperature regulation is controlled by the hypothalamus. When peripheral and core temperature sensors detect cold stress, they send signals to the hypothalamus. The hypothalamus, in turn, activates norepinephrine release. The effects of norepinephrine throughout the body are numerous, including peripheral and pulmonary vasoconstriction, stimulation of brown fat metabolism, and an increase in metabolic rate with increased O_2 and glucose consumption.

Neonates require constant thermal support to prevent hypothermia. When infants are acutely sick, normal care procedures are replaced with activities aimed at resuscitation and stabilization. Infants are usually left undressed and placed on open radiant warming beds (if available) to permit observation and performance of intensive care procedures. During resuscitation and stabilization, the risk of cold stress and hypothermia dramatically increases; therefore, extra care should be directed at preventing hypothermia.

Temperature

> Sick infants are vulnerable to becoming hypothermic
> Provide thermal support at all times
  - Emergency department, labor / delivery, nursery, transport, neonatal intensive care, pediatric intensive care, cardiac cath lab
> Use radiant heat source on servo control
> Chemical thermal mattress (preterm infants), warm blankets, hat

  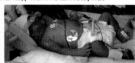

As an example, consider the 2-day-old baby who is rushed to the hospital because of shock secondary to a ductal dependent, left-heart obstructive lesion. The infant is undressed, examined, provided respiratory support, and subjected to x-rays, lab draws, and placement of IVs and lines. During this dramatic resuscitation, the infant's body temperature will drop and will continue to drop until caregivers turn their attention to reversing the decline. Unfortunately, thermoregulation may be far down the list of priorities when faced with such an emergency. As a reminder, all infants are entirely dependent on their caregivers to prevent hypothermia.

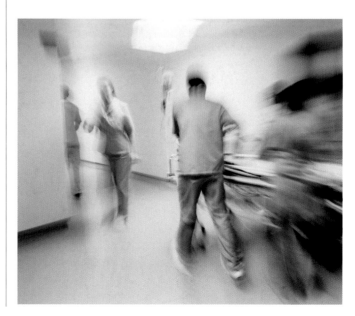

Airway Module[266-270]

Neonates with cardiac disease require varied levels of respiratory support – from nasal cannula O_2 supplementation to more intense therapies, such as high-flow nasal cannula, continuous positive airway pressure, nasal intermittent positive pressure ventilation, and endotracheal intubation with assisted ventilation. Neonates with CHD often have normal lung compliance unless there is concurrent respiratory disease or CHF; therefore, ventilatory support should be adjusted to prevent excessive levels of support.

Hypoxemia is the term used to describe a low arterial blood oxygen content.

Hypoxia is the term used to describe an inadequate level of O_2 in the tissues that is below physiologic levels required for normal cell functioning. In the setting of significant hypoxia and acidosis, there is a significantly increased risk that organs, including the brain, may be damaged, and if severe enough, the infant could die. Tissue hypoxia can result from many causes. Factors that interfere with oxygenation and O_2 delivery to the tissues include:

- Lung disease that can lead to failure to oxygenate pulmonary capillary blood

- Intracardiac mixing that can alter arterial PO_2

- Heart failure that can interfere with pumping blood to the tissues and can lead to pulmonary edema

- Severe anemia with subsequent lower O_2 content of the blood

Airway

Ventilatory Support

› Neonates with CHD usually have normal lung compliance unless there is concurrent respiratory disease

  ▪ Most do not need high inspiratory pressure or rapid ventilation rates

› Left heart obstructive lesions → avoid hyperoxia and hypocarbia

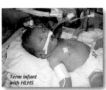
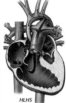

Airway

Hypoxemia

› Low level of oxygen in the arterial blood

Hypoxia

› Insufficient delivery of oxygen to the tissues → below physiologic requirements of the cells

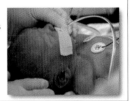

Airway – Causes of Tissue Hypoxia

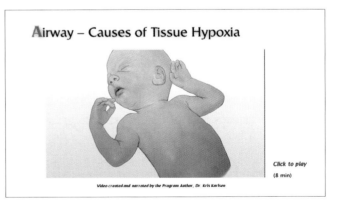

Click to play
(8 min)

Video created and narrated by the Program Author, Dr. Kris Karlsen

O₂ Saturation, Hemoglobin, and CHD

Infants with cyanotic CHD can usually tolerate an O_2 saturation between 75 and 85%. The reason lies in the ability of Hb to release adequate amounts of O_2 to the tissues, providing there is adequate cardiac output and tissue perfusion, a normal body temperature, a normal pH and carbon dioxide level, and an adequate amount of Hb. To ensure adequate amounts of Hb are available to carry O_2, optimizing the Hb level may warrant transfusion of packed red blood cells (PRBCs). The target Hb level is individualized based on the infant's condition, underlying cardiac anomaly, and O_2 saturation goal. The usual volume for PRBC transfusions is between 10 and 20 mL/kg. Consultation with a pediatric cardiologist or neonatologist will help identify cardiac patients who may benefit from transfusion therapy to maximize O_2 carrying capacity.

O₂ Content

At 37° Celsius, 1 gram of Hb binds with a maximum of 1.34 mL of O_2. When Hb is 100% saturated with O_2, the total O_2 content of the blood at varying Hb concentrations is displayed in Figure 3.13. Under normal conditions, a negligible amount of O_2 is also dissolved in plasma and is not included in the calculation of O_2 content. For support of normal metabolism, the tissues require approximately 5 mL of O_2 for every 100 mL of blood perfusing them.

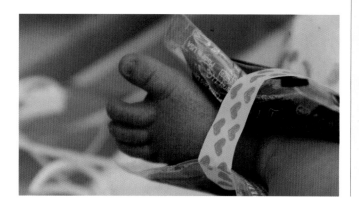

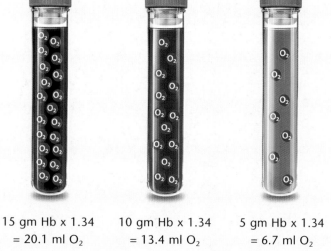

Airway – Causes of Tissue Hypoxia

- Anemia may contribute to tissue hypoxia → low O_2 content
- Cyanotic CHD patients may require a higher target hemoglobin level
- 1 gram of Hgb carries 1.34 mL of O_2
  - Hgb (in grams) x 1.34 mL O_2 = O_2 content/100 mL blood

To support metabolism, tissues require approximately 5 mL of O_2 per 100 mL of blood perfusing them

Consult with cardiologist for optimal hemoglobin level

It is important to understand that infants with cyanotic CHD need sufficient Hb to ensure adequate O_2 content. For example, an infant with a Hb of 15 gm/dL and an O_2 saturation of 100% has a total O_2 content of 20 mL of O_2 per 100 mL of blood. An infant with cyanotic CHD and an O_2 saturation of 75% and the same amount of Hb (15 gm/dL) has an O_2 content that is 75% of normal or 15 mL of O_2 per 100 mL of blood. For this reason, it is important to avoid anemia in infants with cyanotic CHD.

At 37°C, 1 gm Hb x 1.34 ml O_2 = O_2 content/100 mL whole blood

15 gm Hb x 1.34 = 20.1 ml O_2 10 gm Hb x 1.34 = 13.4 ml O_2 5 gm Hb x 1.34 = 6.7 ml O_2

Figure 3.13. Effects of varying Hb levels on O_2 content.

Near infrared reflective spectroscopy (NIRS) monitoring is a noninvasive technology that provides measurement of regional O_2 saturation (rSO_2) of Hb in the tissue bed beneath the sensor. In neonates, two sites are typically monitored (cerebral and somatic – kidney) beds, although mesenteric rSO_2 has also been studied.

Pulse oximetry evaluates the percentage of Hb that is saturated with O_2 to infer the arterial O_2 saturation (SpO_2). Thus, SpO_2 reflects the precapillary amount of O_2 that will be delivered to the tissues. NIRS evaluates an average of the arterial, venous, and capillary beds that are in the light path beneath the sensor. The venous portion is the largest at 75%. Thus, NIRS monitoring closely reflects the *postcapillary* tissue O_2 saturation after the O_2 has been extracted.

NIRS monitoring can help detect changes in perfusion that can lead to tissue hypoxia so that targeted interventions can be employed to improve O_2 delivery to the tissues and organs. NIRS is used to monitor the hemodynamic status in critically ill patients, including:

- Neonates on PGE because of left or right heart obstructive lesions

- Neonates undergoing therapeutic hypothermia for hypoxic ischemic encephalopathy

- Patients (of all ages) who are receiving ECMO

- Following heart surgery

- Other critical illnesses

One example of how NIRS can be used is for the infant with HLHS and who is on PGE to maintain ductal patency. A high SpO_2 reading (reflecting arterial oxygenation) but a low somatic NIRS reading (reflecting O_2 saturation at the tissue level) can inform the clinician of a

Airway

Near Infrared Reflective Spectroscopy (NIRS) Monitoring

- Noninvasive technology – usually monitor cerebral and somatic (kidney) beds
- Measures *regional* O_2 saturation (rSO_2) of Hb in tissue bed beneath sensor
- Evaluates average of arterial, venous, and capillary beds → venous portion (75%)
- NIRS reflects the *postcapillary* tissue O_2 saturation after O_2 is extracted

Infant with complex CHD and cerebral NIRS monitoring

potential imbalance related to pulmonary versus systemic blood flow. PVR declines when there is a higher PO_2. Blood leaving the heart will follow the pathway of least resistance, which in the setting of hyperoxia, will be left-to-right from the aorta through the PDA to the lungs (and to the detriment of blood flow to the systemic circulation). The SpO_2 and somatic NIRS readings will reflect this imbalance of pulmonary to systemic blood flow that may increase the risk for somatic tissue hypoxia, including to the intestines and kidneys.

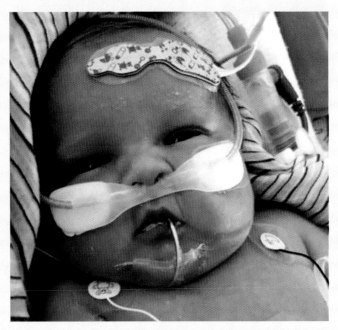

Cerebral NIRS monitoring in an infant with complex CHD.

Pulse Oximetry Screening (POS) for Critical Congenital Heart Disease (CCHD)

In 2012, the U.S. Secretary of Health and Human Services recommended that POS for CCHD be added to the recommended universal newborn screening panel (RUSP).[278] The RUSP is a list of disorders that can be identified through newborn screening and that if detected, can support an overall net health benefit to infants.[279] Since 2018, all U.S. states and the District of Columbia have implemented CCHD screening policies.[280] Worldwide, many hospitals also perform CCHD screening prior to discharging an infant to home.[112-116,281-283] A study conducted in the Netherlands evaluated POS for CCHD in the setting of a high number of home births (18%) and early postnatal discharges within 5 hours of birth, and concluded that CCHD screening was likely to be cost effective. In addition, the opportunity to detect noncardiac pathology, such as respiratory or infectious illnesses, could reduce morbidity and mortality in neonates.[284]

Purpose of POS

The purpose of POS is to detect lower than normal O_2 saturation values secondary to previously undiagnosed CCHD. The goal is to screen healthy-appearing infants prior to discharge to home, since there is significant risk of morbidity or even mortality if the infant is home when the ductus arteriosus (DA) begins to close and symptoms develop.[7,117] For hospitalized neonates, POS screening is recommended in the absence of a postnatal echocardiogram and once the infant is no longer on supplemental O_2.[116,285] Most POS studies were conducted at or near sea level; therefore, the effect of altitude on lowering the O_2 saturation must be considered when interpreting results.[286,287]

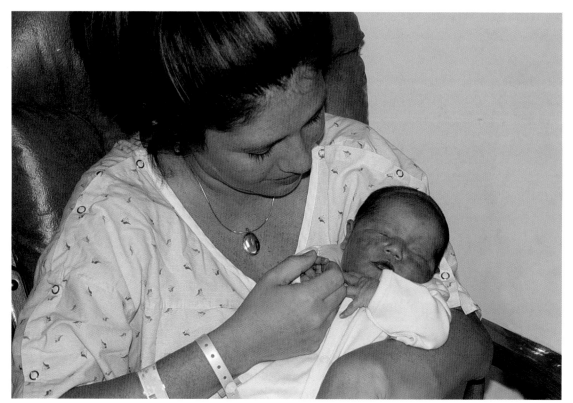

24-hour old, healthy term infant

When is CCHD Screening Done?

After birth, transition from fetal to neonatal circulation involves closure of fetal shunts (foramen ovale and DA) and stabilization of O_2 saturation levels. To prevent false positive results (meaning it is determined there is a CCHD when in fact, there is not), it is best to wait until the infant is at least 24 hours old to perform POS. If the infant is being discharged to home prior to 24 hours, the screening can be done earlier.

The 7 primary heart lesions that may be detected by CCHD screening include:[116,288,289]

- Hypoplastic left heart syndrome
- Pulmonary atresia
- Tetralogy of Fallot
- Total anomalous pulmonary venous connection
- Transposition of the great arteries
- Tricuspid atresia
- Truncus arteriosus

> ### Airway
>
> ***Pulse Oximetry Screening for Critical Congenital Heart Disease (CCHD)***
>
> › Purpose → detect lower than normal O_2 saturation values to identify undiagnosed CCHD
>
> › **7 primary heart lesions**
>   - Hypoplastic left heart syndrome
>   - Pulmonary atresia
>   - Tetralogy of Fallot
>   - Total anomalous pulmonary venous connection
>   - Transposition of the great arteries
>   - Tricuspid atresia
>   - Truncus arteriosus
>
> › **5 secondary targets**
>   - Coarctation of the aorta
>   - Double-outlet right ventricle
>   - Ebstein anomaly
>   - Interrupted aortic arch
>   - Single ventricle CH

The 5 secondary targets that may be detected by CCHD screening include:[285,289,290]

- Coarctation of the aorta
- Double-outlet right ventricle
- Ebstein anomaly
- Interrupted aortic arch
- Various forms of single ventricle CHD

Pulse oximetry screening also reveals infants who have a lower O_2 saturation secondary to:[281,285,291,292]

- Noncritical CHD
- Noncardiac problems such as infections, PPHN, pulmonary diseases, hypothermia, and hemoglobinopathies

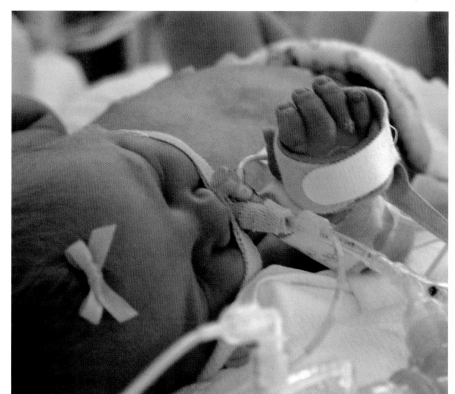

CCHD Screening Protocols
American Academy of Pediatrics

One CCHD screening protocol recommended by the American Academy of Pediatrics (AAP) since 2011 involves measuring and comparing O_2 saturations in both the right hand (preductal) and either foot (postductal).[116] If the O_2 saturation is > 95% in the right hand or foot and the difference between the right hand and foot is < 3 percentage points, the infant passes the screen. If the initial or any subsequent O_2 saturations are < 90%, the infant fails the screen. If the O_2 saturation is between 90% and 94% or there is a preductal to postductal difference of >3%, the test is repeated at one hour intervals up to two times. The test is failed if the O_2 saturation remains less than 95% or the preductal to postductal difference is > 3 percentage points. The AAP's CCHD screening algorithm can be found[293] at

https://www.cdc.gov/ncbddd/heartdefects/hcp.html and the AAP website.[288]

Alternative, Simplified Screening Protocol

In 2018, an expert panel with representatives from 14 organizations, plus state public health officials and CCHD parent advocates, was convened to evaluate evidence obtained following 7 years of CCHD screening. This panel recommended a modification (Figure 3.14)[294] to the AAP's algorithm in order to simplify the algorithm without increasing the false-positive rate by an unacceptable level. The primary differences between this newer algorithm and the AAP's algorithm are as follows:

- A pass is assigned if the O_2 saturation is > 95% in both the upper and lower extremities (instead of either the upper or lower extremity).

- Requiring only 1 repeat screen (instead of 2) for infants who do not initially pass nor fail.

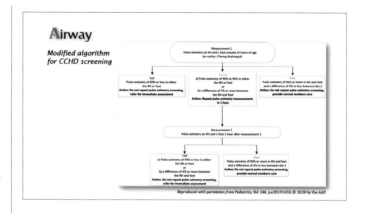

The advantages of simplifying the algorithm include reducing human error associated with interpreting results or in carrying out the repeat screening that occurs when there is not a pass or a fail. Eliminating a second screen may also help to more rapidly identify neonates with CHD or other illnesses that present with hypoxemia.

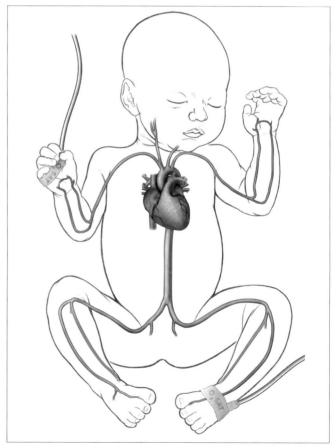

Right hand (preductal) and either foot (postductal) O_2 saturation measurement.

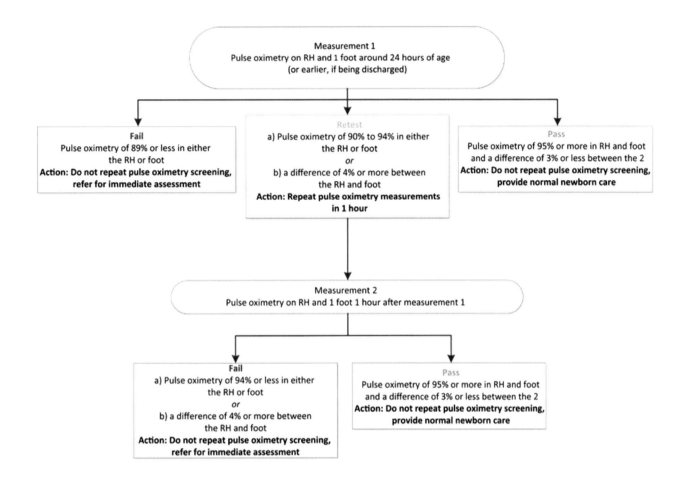

Figure 3.14. Revised CCHD screening algorithm.[294]

Reproduced with permission from Pediatrics, Vol. 146, p.e20191650, © 2020 by the AAP.

Notes:

1. When the infant fails CCHD screening, additional follow-up, including a thorough physical exam and possibly an echocardiogram, is indicated.

2. Infants who pass CCHD screening may still have CHD. For example, coarctation of the aorta does not typically present with abnormal O_2 saturations.

3. Staff should be properly trained in how to perform pulse oximetry screening so that both false negative and false positive results are avoided.

4. At times, the results of oximetry screening will lead to a delay in discharge or possibly a neonatal transport to another facility if additional diagnostic testing is required. This creates a financial and emotional burden since neonatal transport is expensive, and it results in separation of the infant from the family.

5. In the United States, state laws vary regarding newborn CCHD pulse oximetry screening; individual institution algorithms may reflect their individual state Department of Health rules and regulations.

Blood Pressure Module[125,130-133,135,260]

A neonate with severe CHD, poor cardiac output, and/or severe hypoxemia is at risk for developing shock. Delayed or insufficient treatment may lead to permanent tissue injury, organ damage, and death. Rapid, effective treatment of shock may include the following:

- Respiratory support to increase tissue oxygenation, assist with CO_2 removal, and decrease work of breathing.

- Volume resuscitation to increase preload and cardiac output.

- Administration of medications to improve heart function and systemic and pulmonary blood flow (including PGE, as applicable).

- Normalizing energy (glucose), electrolytes (sodium, potassium, and chloride), or mineral imbalances (magnesium and calcium), that reduce heart contractility when abnormal.

- Treatment of arrhythmias (too fast or too slow) that impair cardiac output.

- Relief of noncardiac causes of obstructive shock that may be secondary to cardiac tamponade, air leak, or hyperinflation.

- Obstructive shock secondary to left outflow tract obstructive lesions is treated with PGE.

Methods for Measuring BP[138,295]
Arterial

Common sites for arterial, invasive BP monitoring in neonates include the umbilical, radial, and posterior tibial arteries. When the transducer is located at the level of the heart, the catheter and transducer are free of air bubbles, and the waveform is not dampened by clots or other obstructions, arterial BP is the most accurate method for assessing BP.

Blood Pressure

- Neonates with severe forms of CHD → at risk to develop shock
- Treatment for shock includes:
  - Respiratory support
  - Volume resuscitation to ↑ preload and cardiac output
  - Medication administration
  - Normalizing energy, electrolyte, mineral imbalances
  - Treatment of arrhythmias
  - Treatment of various causes of obstructive shock

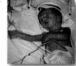

Blood Pressure

Methods for Measuring
- Arterial
  - Umbilical artery, radial, posterior tibialis

Increasing Accuracy of Oscillometric BP Measurement
- Take BP when infant is calm
- Use correct cuff size
- Keep limb at same height as heart
- Gently hold arm or leg in straight position
- Ensare arterial arrow lined up over the artery

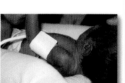

Oscillometric Measurement

Noninvasive blood pressure (NIBP) monitoring allows for the determination of systolic, diastolic, and mean arterial BP. Practitioners should be aware of circumstances in which NIBP monitoring may yield inaccurate results compared to results obtained by invasive BP (IBP) monitoring. Poor correlation between NIBP and IBP measurements is observed in infants with lower gestational ages and weights, lower postmenstrual age, ill preterm and term infants, and infants receiving mechanical ventilation.[147,295-297] The direction of inaccuracy is toward false elevations of mean, systolic, and diastolic BPs when compared to IBP measurements.[147,297] Thus, it is essential that thorough patient assessment accompanies interpretation of NIBP measurements since results obtained may overestimate the actual BP. Figure 3.15 provides information about how oscillometric BP is determined and guidelines about how to improve accuracy when taking a cuff BP.

Oscillometric Measurement – How Does it Work?[137,147,148,295,298-304] and personal communication

Bruce Friedman D.Eng., Principal Engineer Analytics, GE Healthcare Technologies, June 9, 2020

The cuff inflates to a level above systolic BP. As the cuff slowly deflates, arterial blood flow increases, and pulsatile signals or oscillations are detected in the arterial wall. The oscillations increase in intensity; when they reach their peak, the mean arterial BP is determined first. The cuff further deflates and when blood flows smoothly through the artery without further detection of oscillations, systolic and diastolic BPs are calculated.

Information obtained during cuff deflation is sensed by a pressure transducer located in the NIBP monitor. The monitor analyzes data via a proprietary algorithm, resulting in display of a systolic, diastolic, and mean arterial BP.

The cuff may be placed on the arm, thigh, or calf. To enable comparison of results, it is helpful to take the BP on the same limb (right upper arm, if possible). Abnormal BP results should be repeated and always correlate findings with patient assessment.

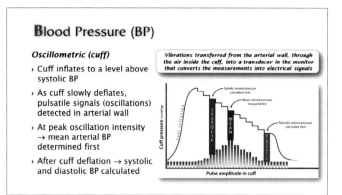

The following items help improve accuracy of oscillometric BP measurement:

- Take the BP when the infant is in a calm state because movement interferes with accuracy of the reading.

- Use the correct cuff size. Calf and arm BPs correlate closely, providing the proper cuff size is selected based on the circumference of the midarm or calf. Too small of a cuff overestimates BP, whereas too large of a cuff underestimates BP.

- Keep the arm or leg at the level of the heart. Gently hold the extremity in a straight position distal to the cuff placement.

- Line up the arterial arrow that is on the cuff with the brachial artery (for an arm BP) or the popliteal artery (for a leg BP). The bladder of the cuff underlies where the tubing is located, and it is the bladder that is detecting the oscillations in the artery.

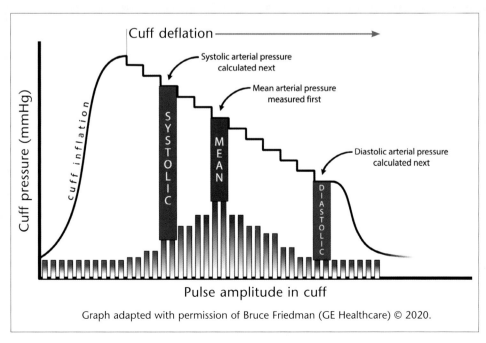

Graph adapted with permission of Bruce Friedman (GE Healthcare) © 2020.

Figure 3.15. Noninvasive oscillometric blood pressure (BP) measurement in neonates.

Lab Work Module

A variety of laboratory tests are useful to evaluate the health and condition of an infant with suspected or confirmed CHD.

Blood Sugar

As discussed in the Sugar module section, neonates with CHD are at increased risk for hypoglycemia. Recognizing this risk, it is important to prevent hypoglycemia by promptly initiating IV therapy and administering dextrose-containing solutions. Signs of hypoglycemia may be subtle and nonspecific. Neurologic signs of hypoglycemia include lethargy, hypotonia, tremors, jitteriness, irritability, abnormal or weak cry, disinterest in feedings, weak suck, hypothermia, and in severe cases, seizures. Cardiorespiratory signs of hypoglycemia include tachypnea, cyanosis, and apnea.

Blood Gas[260,266]

- This test is especially important if the infant is experiencing respiratory distress or there is a history of shock.

- Arterial samples are the gold standard to assess oxygenation, ventilation, and acid/base status.

- Capillary samples obtained from a well-warmed heel (arterialized capillary sample) provide an estimation of ventilation and acid/base status. Oxygenation should be evaluated by pulse oximetry.

- If a venous blood gas is obtained, the pH value will be lower and the PCO_2 level will be higher than an arterial sample. Venous blood pH values are usually 0.02 to 0.04 lower and PCO_2 4 to 8 mmHg higher than arterial results.[36,305] For venous samples, oxygenation should be evaluated by pulse oximetry.

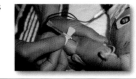

Lab Work

- Blood sugar
- Blood gas
- Lactate
- Electrolytes and renal function tests
- Calcium, magnesium
- Liver function tests, coagulation studies
- Complete blood count with differential
- Cardiac enzymes → B-type natriuretic peptide (BNP) and Troponin I

Lactic Acid/Lactate[36,109,306,307]

- Lactic acid exists as L-lactate and D-lactate. The only form produced in human metabolism is L-lactate and therefore, is the commonly measured level. Cells require adequate amounts of O_2 for survival. When tissue perfusion and O_2 delivery to the cells is inadequate, cells rely on anaerobic metabolism to produce energy. Lactic acid is produced as a by-product of anaerobic metabolism, and as lactic acid accumulates, pH declines (acidosis/acidemia).

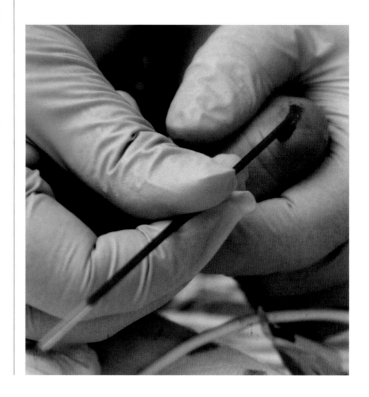

- A normal blood lactate concentration is between 0.5 and 1 mmol/L. A persistently elevated lactate or lactic acid level > 2 mmol/L is concerning. In combination with metabolic acidosis, the higher the number, the more dire the situation. Lactate levels may also be elevated secondary to other causes; thus, evaluating a blood gas helps identify when tissue hypoxia is the cause.

- Sampling error can account for some causes of a falsely elevated lactate level. In particular, the test should be drawn from a free-flowing sample that is promptly analyzed. In neonates, if the feet are cool or poorly perfused, a capillary lactic acid or lactate level may be more elevated than a sample drawn from a vein or artery.

Electrolytes and Renal Function Tests[308-310]

These tests are useful to evaluate renal function and to detect abnormalities that may negatively affect heart function, including hypo- or hyperkalemia and hyponatremia. Infants with acute kidney injury (AKI) secondary to perinatal asphyxia or shock often have oliguria, elevated creatinine levels (reflecting changes in kidney function), and electrolyte abnormalities.

Blood Urea Nitrogen (BUN) and Creatinine

Urea is a waste product of protein breakdown and is cleared from the bloodstream by the kidneys. An elevated BUN may be observed when there is acute kidney injury, heart failure, dehydration, or a diet high in protein.

In the first few days after birth, the serum creatinine level reflects maternal values. After a hypoxic insult, serum creatinine may not rise for 48 to 72 hours, therefore, trending this test will help to evaluate improving or declining renal function.

Sodium and Potassium

Hyponatremia may occur for various reasons, but in infants with CHD, the reason may be related to retention of free water before kidney function normalizes. Treatment involves restricting free water administration until kidney function improves. Hyponatremia may also occur with administration of loop diuretics.

Hypokalemia may occur because of diuretic administration, renal dysfunction, diarrhea, or gastric losses. ECG signs of hypokalemia include flattened T waves, prolongation of the QT interval, or appearance of U waves. Hypokalemia should be avoided in infants receiving digoxin or in infants with prolonged QT syndrome.

Hyperkalemia can cause a life-threatening cardiac arrhythmia. ECG signs of hyperkalemia include peaked T waves, a widened QRS, bradycardia or tachycardia, supraventricular tachycardia, and ventricular tachycardia or fibrillation. An infant with acidosis may have acutely rising potassium levels. Treatment of symptomatic hyperkalemia centers around stabilizing cardiac membranes by administering one or more of the following medications: calcium gluconate, insulin/glucose, inhaled albuterol, sodium bicarbonate, and Lasix.

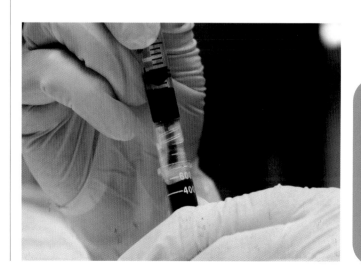

Ionized Calcium[271,311-314]

The most abundant mineral in the body is calcium, with the majority of calcium accumulating during the last trimester. Ionized calcium is the measure of 'free calcium' and is the physiologically active fraction of calcium in the blood. By 24 to 36 hours of age, ionized calcium stabilizes at approximately 1.2 mmol/L (4.9 mg/dL). Table 3.1 summarizes the normal serum concentrations of total and ionized calcium in term infants. By 1 week of age, in healthy, term infants, the serum calcium concentration rises to levels found throughout childhood.

Calcium plays an important part in the excitation-contraction coupling and generation of impulses in myocardial cells and is also a major factor in vascular smooth muscle tone. An adequate ionized calcium concentration optimizes myocardial contractility. Therefore, if the infant with CHD is hypocalcemic, an infusion of calcium gluconate may be necessary to improve the inotropic function of the heart.

Hypocalcemia and 22q11.2 Deletion Syndrome (22q11.2DS)

Calcium regulation is maintained through interaction between parathyroid hormone, calcitonin, and vitamin D. Therefore, infants with 22q11.2DS may be prone to persistent hypocalcemia because of impaired parathyroid function.

Magnesium[119,271,314,315]

Magnesium is an essential mineral that has many important roles in physiologic functions. Magnesium is the second most abundant intracellular cation, influencing membrane integrity, neuromuscular excitability, nervous tissue conduction, protein synthesis, muscle contractility, and hormone secretion.

Causes of hypomagnesemia (usually considered < 1.6 mg/dL) may include the following:

- Insulin-dependent and gestational maternal diabetes
- Intrauterine growth restriction
- Neonatal hypoparathyroidism
- Maternal hyperparathyroidism
- Defect of intestinal magnesium transport – primary hypomagnesemia with hypocalcemia
- Infantile isolated renal magnesium wasting
- Hypomagnesemia with hypercalciuria and nephrocalcinosis

Signs of hypomagnesemia are similar to signs of hypocalcemia – tremors, irritability, and seizures. When hypocalcemia is present, then assessment for hypomagnesemia should follow since the two are closely associated.

Maintenance of a normal serum magnesium is an important goal when a patient is prone to arrhythmias, including long QT syndrome. In particular, hypomagnesemia can aggravate

Term Infant, Age	Serum Concentration		
	Total Calcium	Ionized Calcium	
	mg/dL	mg/dL	mmol/L
Birth (cord blood)	10.2 (9.0-11.4)	5.82 (5.22-6.42)	1.45 (1.3-1.6)
2 hours old	9.7 (8.5-10.9)	5.34 (4.84-5.84)	1.33 (1.21-1.46)
24 hours old	9.0 (7.8-10.2)	4.92 (4.40-5.44)	1.23 (1.1-1.36)

Table 3.1. Normal serum concentrations of total and ionized calcium from birth through 24 hours, term infants. Adapted from Loughead (1988)[312] and Namgung (2020).[313]

a potentially fatal arrhythmia, Torsades de Pointes (a polymorphic ventricular tachycardia). Treatment of Torsades de Pointes includes a magnesium infusion and synchronized cardioversion, or defibrillation, as indicated.

Liver Function Tests (LFTs)[316-319]

LFTs are useful to assess and monitor the degree of liver damage that may have occurred during periods of shock or injury to the liver from other etiologies, such as hepatitis. Infants with left-sided obstructive lesions (i.e., COA, IAA, critical aortic valve stenosis, and HLHS), are especially vulnerable to kidney and liver damage if the ductus closed and impaired systemic perfusion.

Liver Enzymes

Elevated levels of enzymes released by liver cells in response to damage or disease include the following:

- Alanine aminotransferase (ALT; also called alanine transaminase)

- Aspartate aminotransferase (AST; also called serum glutamic-oxaloacetic transaminase; SGOT)

- Gamma-glutamyl transpeptidase (GGT)

- Alkaline phosphatase (i.e., liver fraction portion)

In addition to enzymes, liver function testing evaluates levels of proteins made in the liver (albumin and total protein), and bilirubin that is processed in the liver.

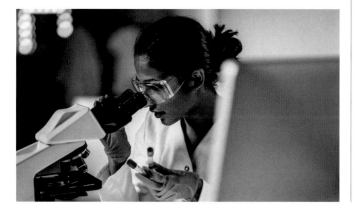

Coagulation Tests

These lab tests are obtained if bleeding is observed, if there is a family history of bleeding disorders, or if there is a history of shock or liver injury.

- **Prothrombin time** (PT). Measures how long it takes for a clot to form after adding thromboplastin to a patient's blood sample. Prothrombin itself is a protein made by the liver which is involved in blood clotting. A prolonged PT may also indicate a vitamin K deficiency.

- **Partial Thromboplastin Time** (PTT). Measures how long it takes for a clot to form after the cellular components are first removed from the blood sample using a centrifuge. Calcium and other substances are then added and the number of seconds it takes for the clot to form is measured. The PTT is commonly monitored when patients are receiving a continuous infusion of heparin to adjust the dose and achieve the desired level of anticoagulation.

- **Internationalized Normalized Ratio** (INR). The INR is simply a method of standardizing the value of a patient's PT. The INR is calculated by dividing the patient's PT by a control PT value obtained using a reference reagent developed by the World Health Organization.

- **Fibrinogen** is a protein made by the liver.

- **Anti-Factor Xa (anti-Xa) Level**. Instead of a continuous infusion of IV heparin, some patients receive once or twice daily subcutaneous injections of low molecular weight heparin (enoxaparin). The anti-Xa is commonly monitored when patients are receiving low molecular weight heparin injections to adjust the dose and achieve the desired level of anticoagulation.

Complete Blood Count [320-331]

A CBC is a set of tests that indicate the counts of white blood cells, red blood cells, and platelets. The CBC also includes information about the amount of Hb and the size of the red blood cells. A *differential* provides the count of each type of white blood cell present in the sample.

Especially important for neonates with CHD is assessment of the red cell count to detect anemia or polycythemia. Infants with cyanotic CHD who have O_2 saturation goals lower than infants without CHD may need periodic blood transfusions or administration of erythropoiesis-stimulating agents (ESAs) to maintain an adequate Hb level. The target Hb level is individualized based on the infant's condition, underlying cardiac anomaly, and O_2 saturation goal.

Infants with CHD may also have concurrent infection; thus, evaluation of the white blood cells, including presence of immature forms that may indicate infection, is helpful to guide treatment decisions and response to therapy.

White blood cells are involved in protection against infective organisms and foreign substances and are produced in the bone marrow along with red blood cells and platelets. There are five main types of WBCs: neutrophils, eosinophils, basophils, lymphocytes, and monocytes. Neutrophils are WBCs primarily responsible for killing and digesting bacteria. In neonates and especially in preterm neonates, neutrophil chemotaxis (movement) is immature; in the face of serious bacterial infection, the neutrophils may not be capable of mounting an adequate response. It is important to recognize that neonates with sepsis may have a completely normal CBC in the early phase of illness. The time between the onset of infection and the first change in CBC may be between 4 and 6 hours.

The decision to treat with antibiotics should be based on clinical signs and history, including risk factors for sepsis and timing of presentation – not solely on CBC results.

Platelets (also called thrombocytes) are made in the bone marrow and are cells involved with clot formation to help stop or prevent bleeding. Low platelet counts (thrombocytopenia) may result from either decreased platelet production or increased platelet utilization (or destruction) because of the following various pathological conditions:

- Infectious etiology – bacterial, fungal, or viral (e.g., CMV, HIV, rubella, and herpes)

- Maternal medical conditions (e.g., pregnancy-induced hypertension)

- Maternal auto- or isoimmunization – alloimmune or autoimmune thrombocytopenia (i.e., idiopathic thrombocytopenic purpura, systemic lupus erythematosus)

- Genetic etiologies – chromosomal (trisomy 13, 18, 21, turner syndrome), familial thrombocytopenias, or specific mutations in the genes MPL, RUNX1, or PTPN11

- Other etiologies – necrotizing enterocolitis, hyperviscosity, disseminated intravascular coagulation following perinatal asphyxia, metabolic (i.e., propionic methylmalonic, or isovaleric acidemias)

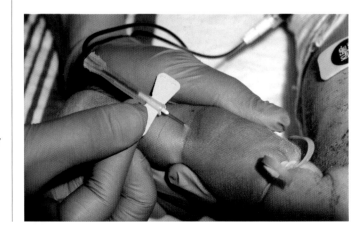

Cardiac Enzymes: B-Type Natriuretic Peptide (BNP)[271,332-341] and Troponin[271,342-346]

In patients with CHD, two cardiac biomarkers, BNP and troponin are useful to evaluate CHF and myocardial dysfunction (BNP) and myocardial cell injury (troponin).

- **BNP** is synthesized and secreted by the ventricular myocardium in response to increased right and left ventricular pressure overload, volume expansion, and myocardial wall stress (i.e., stretching of cardiac myocytes). In neonates, BNP levels are initially elevated, with a rapid decline observed after 3 days through the first weeks of life. In infants with CHD or cardiomyopathy, BNP may begin a progressive rise after 4 days of age. BNP levels are also increased in preterm infants with a hemodynamically significant PDA. Other causes of elevated BNP levels include PPHN, septic shock, and renal failure (because BNP is cleared by the kidneys).

- **Troponin** is an enzyme that is released from cardiac myocytes in response to myocardial injury. Troponin levels may be elevated with sepsis, heart failure, tachyarrhythmias, heart block, cardiomyopathies, myocarditis, pericarditis, chest trauma (cardiac contusion), and severe pulmonary hypertension. Troponin levels are also often elevated after cardiac surgery. If levels fail to decline after surgery, there is a higher risk of poor outcomes.

In neonates, one study measured troponin levels on the 3rd day after birth[344] and found elevated levels in infants delivered by cesarean section compared to those delivered vaginally. The authors suggested troponin may have been released in response to intrauterine stress that may have prompted a cesarean delivery. In another study, troponin levels were measured at approximately 12 hours of age and were significantly elevated in infants who experienced perinatal asphyxia compared to control infants with Apgar scores > 7 at 1 minute and > 8 at 5 minutes.[347]

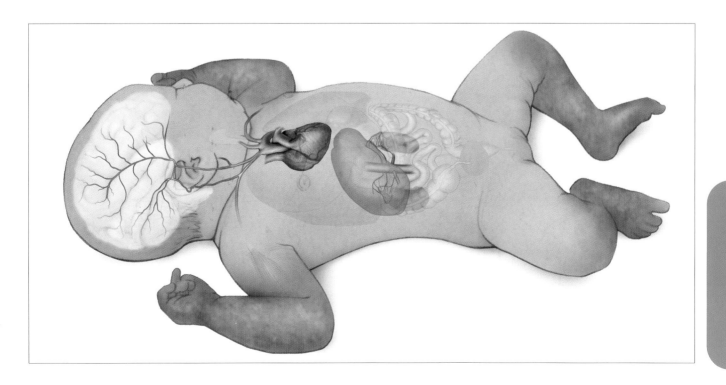

What does it mean? Let's talk about Genetic Testing[348-354]

Cell-Free DNA – Noninvasive Prenatal Testing

Prenatal Cell-Free DNA (cfDNA) testing is a peripheral blood test that determines the amount of fetal DNA that is circulating in maternal blood. This is accomplished by isolating cfDNA, which are small, free-floating fragments of DNA. A small portion of the cfDNA in maternal blood is cell-free fetal DNA (cffDNA) derived from the placenta. These fetal fragments can be detected as early as 10 weeks of gestation and up until the time of delivery. Abnormal quantities of cffDNA are associated with aneuploidy,* in particular, chromosomes 13, 18, and 21 and sex chromosomes. Of note, cfDNA may also identify maternal conditions (i.e. Turner syndrome or malignancy). Multiple gestation, maternal obesity, and early first trimester pregnancy (< 10 weeks) may affect the accuracy of cfDNA results. Prenatal cfDNA testing is expanding to include screening for many common, single-gene disorders and some microdeletion syndromes, but does not screen for all genetic syndromes or congenital defects (i.e., neural tube, heart, and abdominal wall).

If the test result is negative, then the predictive value of the test (i.e., negative predictive value) is high for the common aneuploidies, but may not be as high for the microdeletion or other less common chromosomal conditions. In addition, there may be other chromosomal conditions or genetic disorders present that the cfDNA test does not identify. If the result is positive, then the result is interpreted in the context of the maternal risk for that aneuploidy. At times, the test yields a no-call result (neither negative nor positive) because of a low fraction

of cffDNA in the maternal blood. This can result from normal variations in cfDNA quantity in pregnant individuals; however, several large studies have reported low cffDNA fractions associated with an increased risk of aneuploidy. Therefore, in any situation in which there is a negative, positive, or no-call result, additional testing and fetal evaluation may be indicated. Obstetric counseling should inform the mother of these possibilities and available options for more genetic testing and counseling.

Karyotype

A karyotype (also known as chromosome analysis) is used to analyze an individual's chromosomes and is the first-line test for situations in which balanced translocations or aneuploidy (i.e., trisomy and monosomy conditions) are suspected. The short arm of the chromosome is called *p* and the long arm is called *q*. The centromere is the region of the chromosome that divides the *p* and *q* arms.

Fluorescence In Situ Hybridization (FISH) Process

FISH uses fluorescently tagged DNA probes that are added to the chromosome preparation. If matching DNA material is present, the fluorescent signal is visible under the fluorescent

---

> **Lab Work**
>
> *Genetic Testing*
> ‣ Cell-free DNA (cfDNA) testing → noninvasive prenatal testing
> ‣ Karyotype
> ‣ Fluorescence in situ hybridization (FISH) process
> ‣ Chromosomal microarray analysis (CMA)
> ▪ Also referred to as single nucleotide polymorphism (SNP)
> ‣ Next generation sequencing (NGS)
> ▪ Targeted gene panel, whole exome sequencing (WES), whole genome sequencing (WGS)

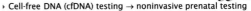

---

*Aneuploidy refers to the presence of an extra chromosome number or a missing chromosome.

microscope. If the matching chromosomal material is deleted, then no fluorescence is seen. FISH is typically used when there is suspicion of a microdeletion syndrome, like 22q11.2DS or William's syndrome.

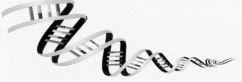

Chromosomal Microarray Analysis[355]

Chromosomal microarray analysis (CMA), also referred to as single nucleotide polymorphism (SNP) microarray is a chromosomal analysis testing option that is used to identify copy number variants (CNVs) with much higher resolution than traditional karyotyping. CMA testing also provides more quantitative and consistent results compared to FISH analysis. CMA can detect microdeletions (including 22q11.2DS) and duplications and can also identify unbalanced translocations. Thus, CMA is the recommended first-line test for an infant with multiple congenital anomalies. It may also be indicated if the phenotype is highly associated with a deletion or duplication syndrome (e.g. conotruncal anomalies and/or arch abnormalities with 22q11.2DS). CMA cannot detect single nucleotide variants; therefore, when a patient has suspected CHARGE syndrome or other single-gene syndromes (e.g., Noonan syndrome), CMA and FISH analysis will not identify these disorders. Rather, gene(s)-specific sequencing analysis is indicated.

Next Generation Sequencing (NGS)[356-358]

NGS involves rapid, large-scale sequencing of deoxyribonucleic acid (DNA). DNA codes for genes that make proteins for the body. During sequencing, DNA variants are detected. A DNA variant is a change in the DNA sequence that is different from what is typically seen in the general population. All humans have thousands of DNA variants; most of these variants are harmless or have an unknown effect. However, some DNA variants may cause disease and typically these are classified as pathogenic variants. These pathogenic variants range from larger-scale chromosomal abnormalities and copy number variations (CNVs) to smaller-scale insertion/deletions (indels) and single nucleotide variants (SNVs) including autosomal and X-linked mutations.

Targeted gene panel (TGP), whole exome sequencing (WES), and whole genome sequencing (WGS) are three NGS methods currently used to help establish genetic diagnosis. A TGP tests a defined number of genes that may have a suspected or known association with a disease. WES refers to the sequencing of all coding regions of a patient's genome, whereas WGS refers to sequencing the entire genome (both coding and noncoding regions). In theory, WES should be sufficient to identify the vast majority of pathogenic variants; however, studies have demonstrated that this method identifies, at best, only 85% of pathogenic variants when compared to WGS.

WES and WGS testing is often done in a trio, with blood obtained from both the patient and parents. While trio testing is not necessary for WES/WGS, it can increase the likelihood of identifying a genetic etiology. Having both parents included in the analysis allows determination of the inheritance of a particular variant of interest. Having this information is valuable to the lab as they can then determine if the variant was new (e.g. de novo; not identified in the parents) or if one or both of the parents also carried the variant. This is particularly important for recessive conditions to ensure that the two variants identified in the patient are indeed on separate chromosomes, (i.e. each parent carries one of the two variants).

Emotional Support Module[359-362]

The birth of a baby is typically a momentous life event. The birth of a sick baby creates immense stress and sense of crisis. Imagine the shock and fear when parents hear the words, "we think there may be something wrong with your baby's heart." Parents must struggle to absorb their infant's complicated medical situation which may have arrived without warning.

Birth of an infant with a cardiac defect is a very disruptive time for the family. Parents will worry not only about their immediate situation and separation from the infant, but also about the future. Their thoughts may include: Will my child be normal? Will he or she be able to play like other children? Will he or she endure pain and need to be in and out of the hospital for the rest of their life? What will this mean for our family, our lifestyle, our finances, and our other children? Parents may not come right out and voice these concerns when you interact with them, but these thoughts and concerns are naturally there.

Each family brings a unique and potentially complicated history, as well as a diverse cultural background, to each childbirth experience. Parental reactions are sometimes hard to interpret and styles of coping vary, as do responses seen from the parents of the same baby. It is important to approach the family in a nonjudgmental manner and to activate support resources as necessary.

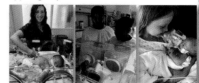
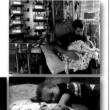

Emotional Support
- Keep parents informed and involved
- Provide illustrations of cardiac lesions
- Expect to repeat explanations
- Refer to appropriate resources and support groups

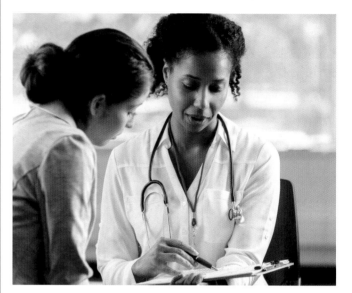

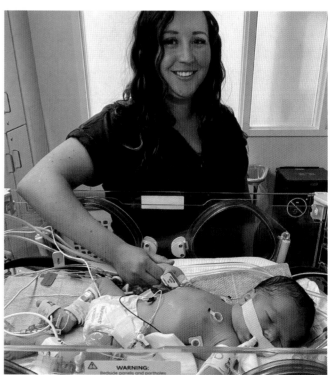

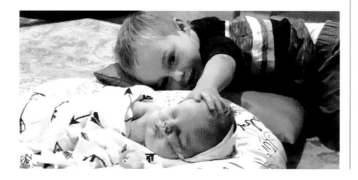

While in your care, remember that adults are accustomed to having control over events in their lives. To a degree, having an infant in the neonatal or cardiac intensive care unit takes parental control away. Depending upon the infant's state of health, the parents may not be able to do many of the normal parenting activities such as hold or feed their infant or change their infant's diaper. Ways to facilitate parenting in neonatal and cardiac intensive care units includes teaching parents how to assist in their infant's care and allowing them to hold their infant as soon as is safe.

Be consistent with explanations regarding the plan of care. Oftentimes, parents complain that "everyone is telling me something different" and "no-one seems to agree with the plan of care". Encourage parents to participate in patient rounds so they hear the discussions that take place and to contribute to decision making. Encourage the family to speak up if they are hearing conflicting or confusing information from the healthcare team.

Finally, explain the infant's condition in understandable, accurate, and honest terms. Use illustrations and written information as needed so that parents may fully comprehend their infant's medical issues. At all times, remain empathetic, supportive, non-judgmental, and culturally sensitive.

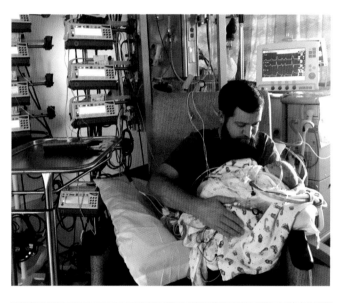

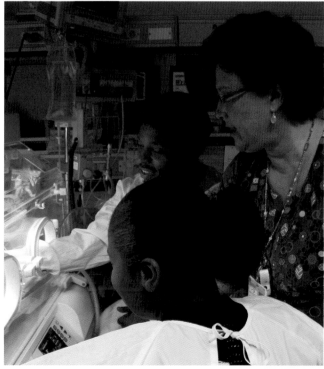

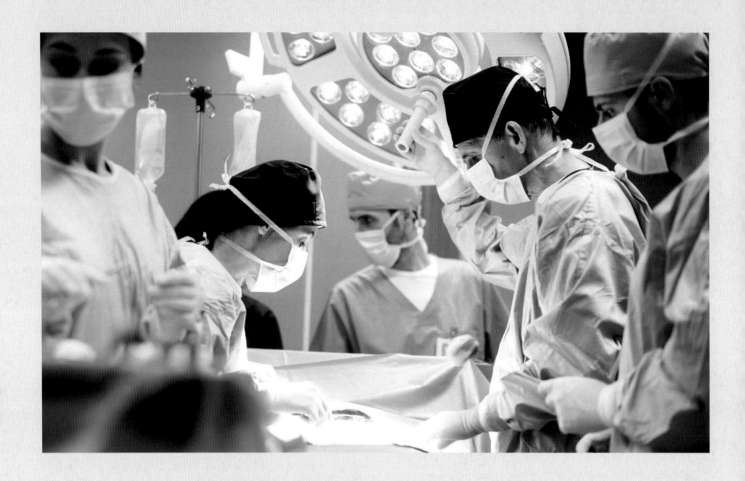

Left-Sided Obstructive Lesions, Ductal Dependent for Systemic Blood Flow............................ **183**

Coarctation of the Aorta 184

Interrupted Aortic Arch 186

Aortic Valve Stenosis 188

Hypoplastic Left Heart Syndrome 190

Cyanotic Congenital Heart Disease, Not Ductal Dependent for Pulmonary Blood Flow........... **197**

Tetralogy of Fallot 198

Tricuspid Atresia 202

Truncus Arteriosus.. 204

Ebstein Anomaly... 206

Cyanotic Congenital Heart Disease, Ductal Dependent for Pulmonary Blood Flow **207**

Pulmonary Atresia with Intact Ventricular Septum (PA-IVS).. 208

Pulmonary Atresia and Ventricular Septal Defect (PA-VSD)... 212

Transposition of the Great Arteries (TGA) 214

Introduction

Complete surgical repair of heart defects is performed when possible. However, some infants may be too small or have co-morbidities or other factors that need to be considered when deciding the best timing and approach. These co-morbidities and factors include the following:

- Prematurity, corrected gestational age, and the infant's weight.

- Concurrent illnesses including lung disease and infection.

- Any organ damage that occurred during the acute phase of illness.

Decisions regarding surgical approach are based upon factors including:

- Institutional approaches based on available resources and expertise of the multidisciplinary specialty teams.

- Availability of extracorporeal membrane oxygenation therapy.

- Whether there is a heart transplant program.

Palliation and Surgical Repair

Co-Morbidities and Factors to Consider

- Gestational age, corrected gestational age, infant's weight
- Concurrent illness
  - Severity of lung disease
  - Infection
  - Organ damage that occurred during acute phase of illness
    - Liver, kidneys, brain, intestine

Palliation and Surgical Repair

Institutional Factors

- Institutional approach to treatment varies based on available resources and expertise of the multidisciplinary specialty team:
  - Extracorporeal membrane oxygenation (ECMO) therapy, heart transplant program
  - Multidisciplinary specialty team includes:
    - Cardiology, cardiac surgery, nursing, neonatology, pediatric critical care, radiology, and anesthesia

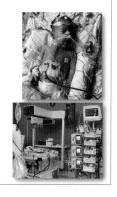

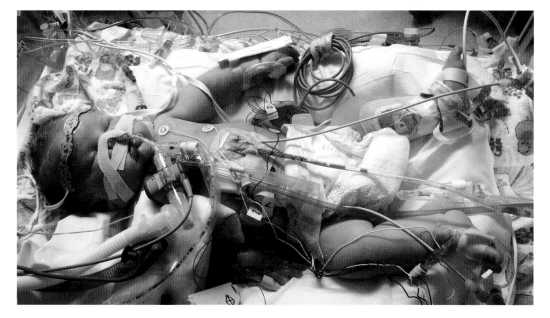

Infant with DORV and dextrocardia following surgical intervention.

*This Appendix of palliative and surgical repair options will follow the order of the lesions presented in Part 2.

Open Heart Surgery

Cardiac surgery is performed with or without cardiopulmonary bypass, which is a mechanical means of providing systemic perfusion and gas exchange independent of the heart.

Outcomes of Heart Surgery

- Complete correction of the heart defect as occurs following repair of a coarctation of the aorta or closure of a ventricular septal defect.

- If initial complete repair is not possible, staged surgical correction or palliation may be utilized. For example, in hypoplastic left heart syndrome, the stage 1 Norwood procedure and subsequent operations are palliative with the goal of these surgeries to result in one functioning ventricle that will provide systemic perfusion.

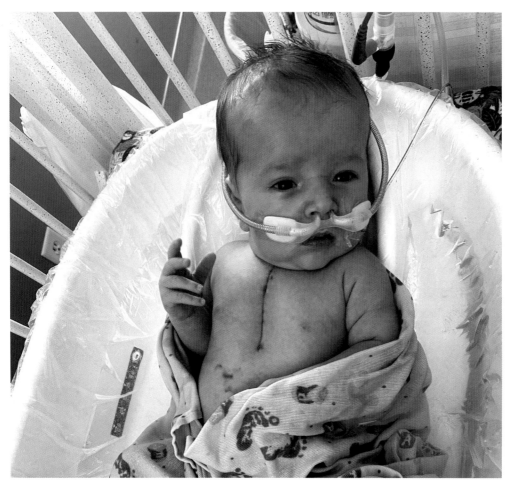

Eight-week old infant, post-operative repair of COA and hypoplastic aortic arch.

What does it mean? Let's talk about a 2 Ventricle Repair, a 1.5 Ventricle Repair, and Single Ventricle Palliation

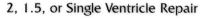

2, 1.5, or Single Ventricle Repair

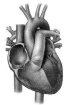 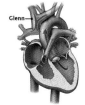 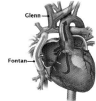

2 Ventricle Repair
› RV pumps blood to lungs and LV pumps blood to body

1.5 Ventricle Repair
› Glenn procedure → to augment pulmonary blood flow and help offload the small RV

Single Ventricle Palliation
› One ventricle becomes systemic pumping chamber → pulmonary blood flow provided by Glenn and Fontan connections

2 ventricle repair

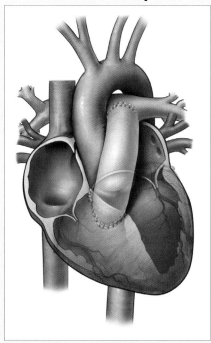

After surgical repair, the RV will pump blood to the lungs and the LV will pump blood to the body.

Truncus Arteriosus post surgical repair

The pulmonary arteries are now connected to the right ventricle and the VSD is closed.

1.5 ventricle repair

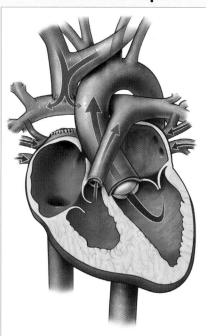

Pulmonary blood flow will be augmented by addition of a Glenn anastomosis.

Pulmonary atresia post balloon valvuloplasty

Glenn procedure performed to augment pulmonary blood flow and help offload the small RV.

Single ventricle palliation

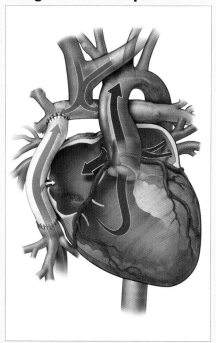

One ventricle (right or left) will provide systemic perfusion. Systemic venous return will flow to the lungs via Glenn and Fontan connections.

Hypoplastic left heart syndrome post Fontan procedure

The right ventricle is responsible for pumping blood systemically. Pulmonary blood flow is provided by Glenn and Fontan connections.

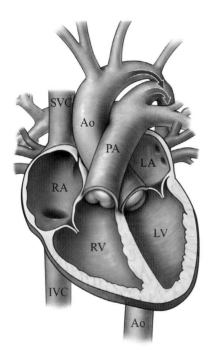

Coarctation of the aorta – page 184

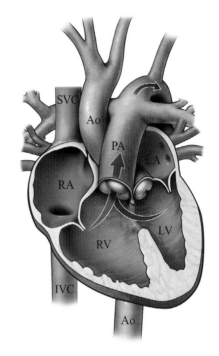

Interrupted aortic arch – page 186

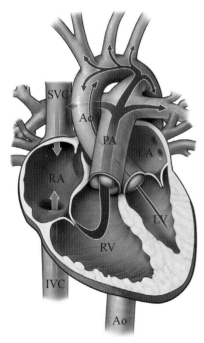

Aortic valve stenosis – page 188

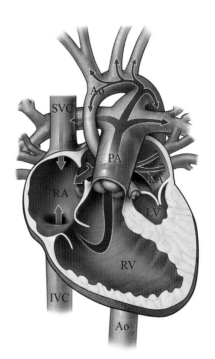

Hypoplastic left heart syndrome – page 190

APPENDIX – Palliative and Surgical Repair Options

Coarctation of the Aorta – Surgical Repair of the Aortic Arch

For more information about COA see page 74.

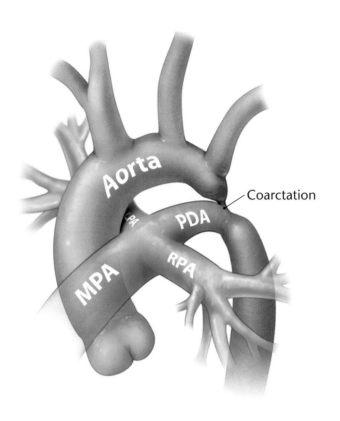

Coarctation

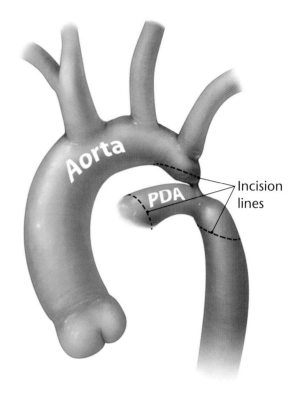

Incision lines

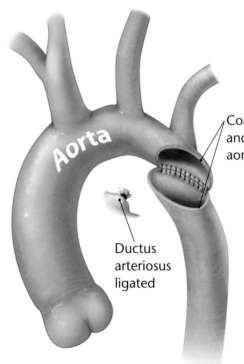

Coarctectomy and back wall of aorta sutured

Ductus arteriosus ligated

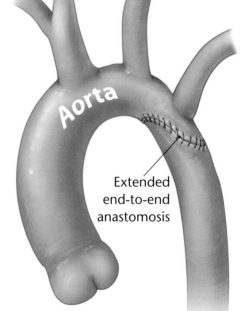

Extended end-to-end anastomosis

Coarctation of the Aorta – Surgical Repair of the Aortic Arch

Surgical morbidity may include:

- Injury to the recurrent laryngeal nerve that may lead to vocal cord dysfunction
- Weak cry, impaired swallow that may increase the risk for aspiration
- Injury to the phrenic nerve
- Chylothorax
- Bleeding
- Infection

- Postoperative paradoxical hypertension
- Spinal cord ischemia / injury
- Recurrent obstruction

  Treatment options include:
  - ◆ Percutaneous balloon angioplasty to widen the narrowed area *(interventional cardiac catheterization procedure)*
  - ◆ Stent insertion (for older patients)

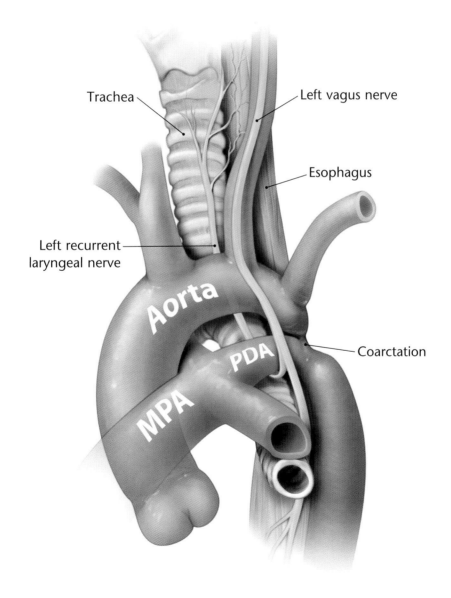

Trachea

Left vagus nerve

Esophagus

Left recurrent laryngeal nerve

Aorta

PDA

MPA

Coarctation

Interrupted Aortic Arch – Surgical Repair

For more information about IAA see page 76.

IAA type B is shown. Possible surgical morbidities are similar to coarctation of the aorta.

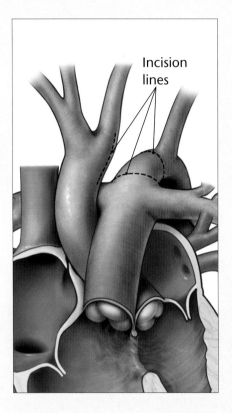

Incision lines

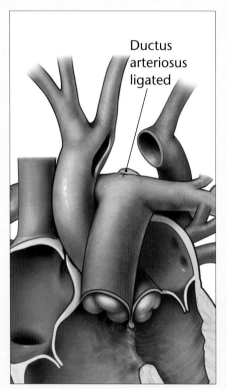

Ductus arteriosus ligated

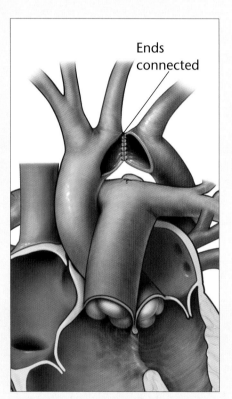

Ends connected

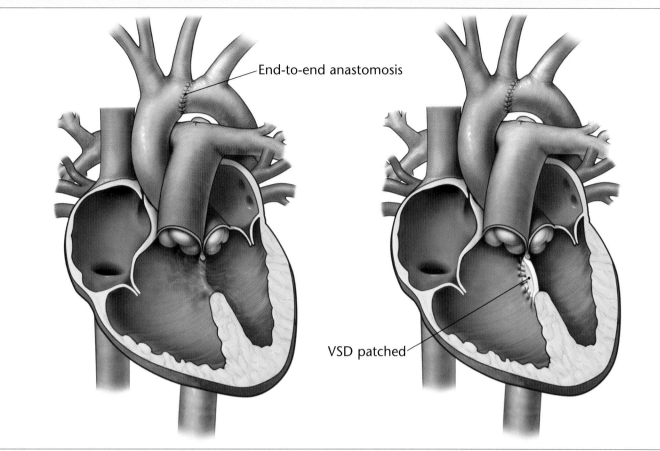

End-to-end anastomosis

VSD patched

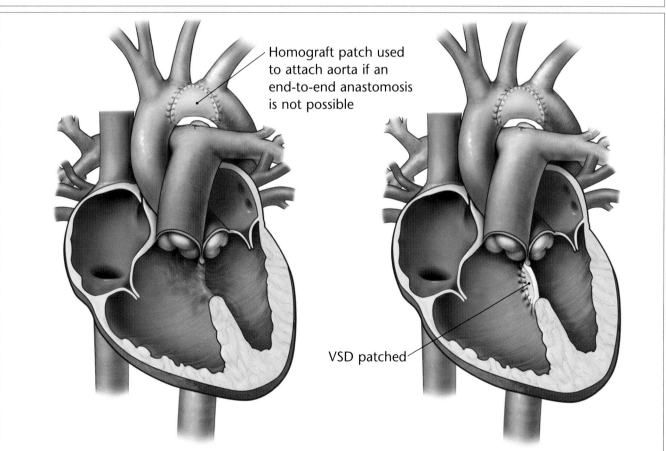

Homograft patch used to attach aorta if an end-to-end anastomosis is not possible

VSD patched

Critical Aortic Valve Stenosis

For more information about critical AV stenosis see page 78.

Balloon Valvuloplasty
(Interventional cardiac catheterization procedure)

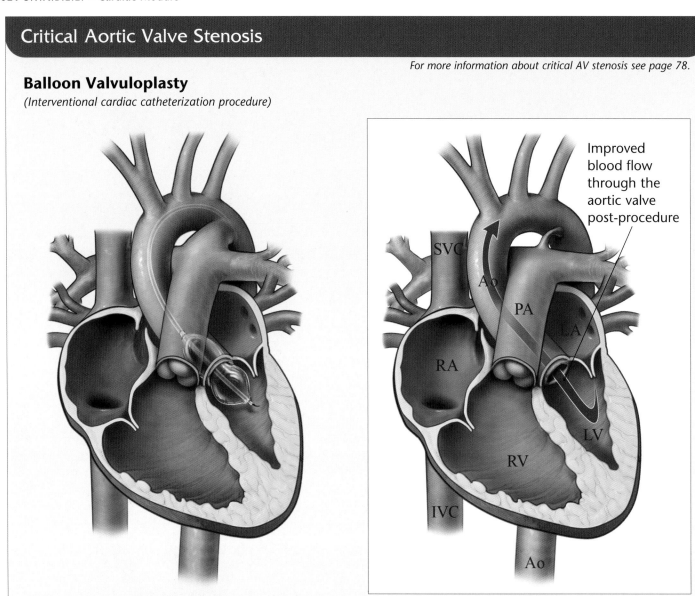

Improved blood flow through the aortic valve post-procedure

Aortic Valvotomy – *a bicuspid aortic valve is shown*

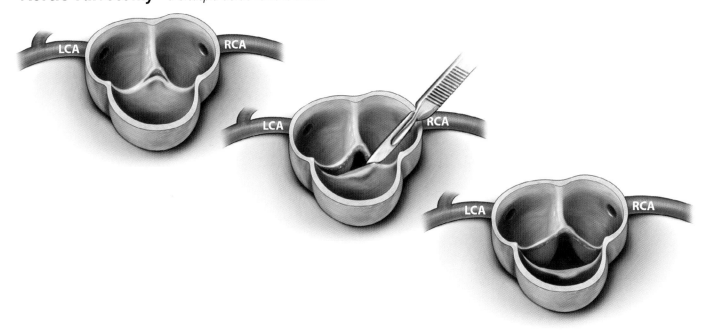

Critical Aortic Valve Stenosis – Ross Procedure (surgical)

Selected if the aortic valve disease is not amenable to balloon valvuloplasty or surgical valvotomy. Future reoperations are usually necessary to replace the pulmonary valve. Complications may include residual or recurrent aortic valve disease, heart block, and pulmonary valve stenosis or regurgitation.

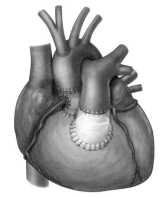

Completed surgery

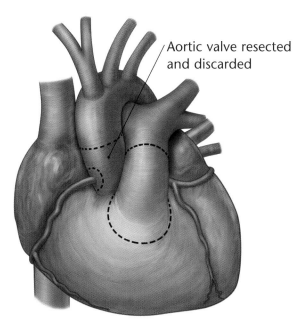

Aortic valve resected and discarded

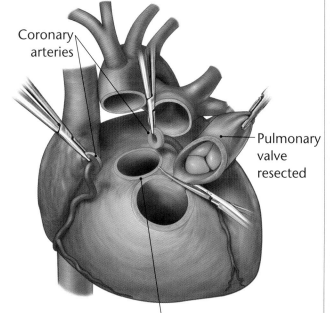

Coronary arteries

Pulmonary valve resected

Aortic annular hypoplasia may require enlargement (called a Konno procedure; not shown)

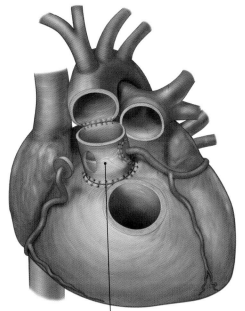

Pulmonary valve moved into aortic position and coronary arteries attached

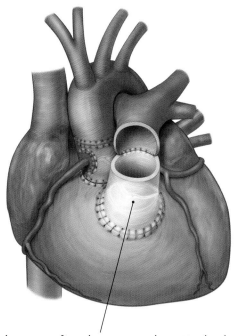

New homograft pulmonary valve attached

Hypoplastic Left Heart Syndrome

For more information about HLHS see page 80.

Palliative, single ventricle surgery for HLHS occurs in 3 separate surgeries:

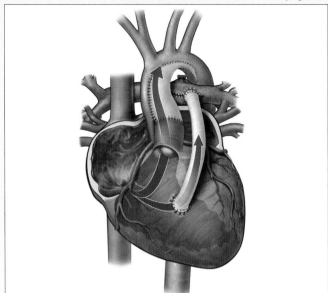

Stage ❶ Operation

The first-stage (Norwood) operation is performed in the neonatal period. If the infant cannot undergo a Norwood procedure, a hybrid procedure may be performed (see page 196).

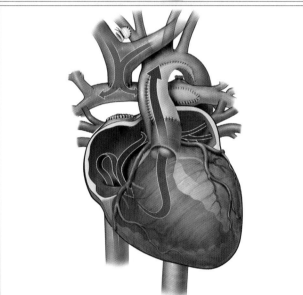

Stage ❷ Operation

The second-stage operation (bidirectional Glenn or the hemi-Fontan procedure) is performed when the infant is approximately 4 to 6 months old. Selection of surgical approach is generally based on institutional preference for the final planned Fontan operation.

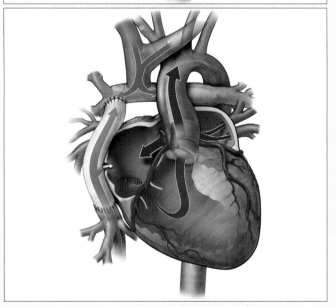

Stage ❸ Operation

The third-stage operation (Fontan) is typically performed between 18 months and 3 years of age. Occasionally, Fontan completion is delayed to an older age.

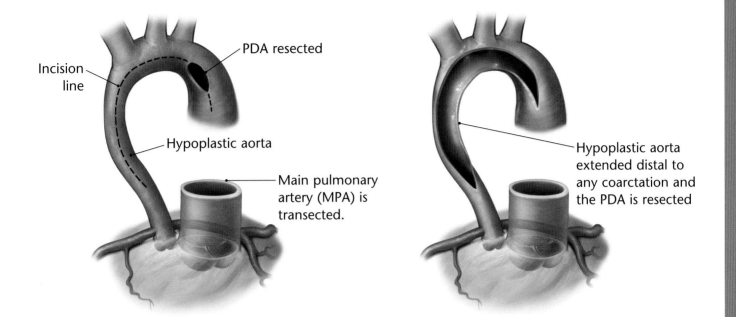

Incision line

Hypoplastic aorta

PDA resected

Main pulmonary artery (MPA) is transected.

Hypoplastic aorta extended distal to any coarctation and the PDA is resected

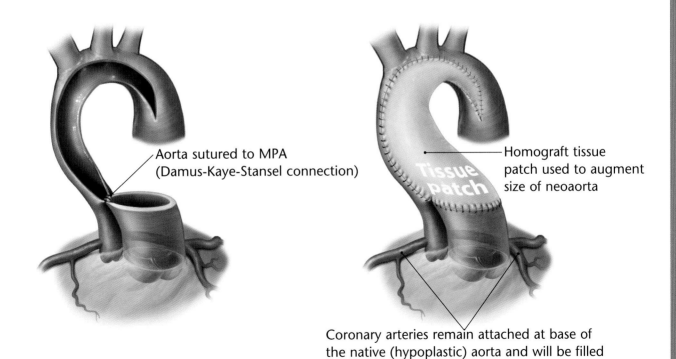

Aorta sutured to MPA (Damus-Kaye-Stansel connection)

Homograft tissue patch used to augment size of neoaorta

Coronary arteries remain attached at base of the native (hypoplastic) aorta and will be filled by retrograde flow through neoaorta

APPENDIX – Palliative and Surgical Repair Options

(Continued next page)

Hypoplastic Left Heart Syndrome - Stage 1 Norwood Operation

At the conclusion of the stage 1 Norwood procedure, the right ventricle pumps blood to the systemic circulation. Pulmonary blood flow is provided by a Sano shunt or BT shunt.

Sano shunt

Right ventricle to pulmonary artery conduit.

Advantage

■ Blood is pumped to the body and lungs with RV contraction and there is no systemic diastolic runoff.

Disadvantage

■ An incision is made into the RV which is the systemic pumping ventricle.

BT shunt

■ Right subclavian artery to pulmonary artery shunt.

■ Blood flows to the pulmonary arteries during systole and diastole.

Disadvantage

■ Systemic diastolic blood pressure is lower as blood flows through the shunt during diastole. As a result, coronary artery perfusion may be compromised secondary to the lower diastolic blood pressure.

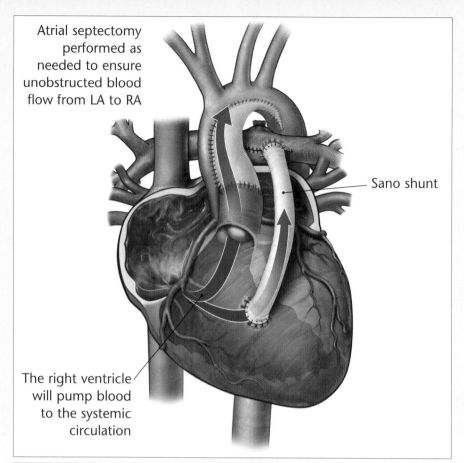

Atrial septectomy performed as needed to ensure unobstructed blood flow from LA to RA

Sano shunt

The right ventricle will pump blood to the systemic circulation

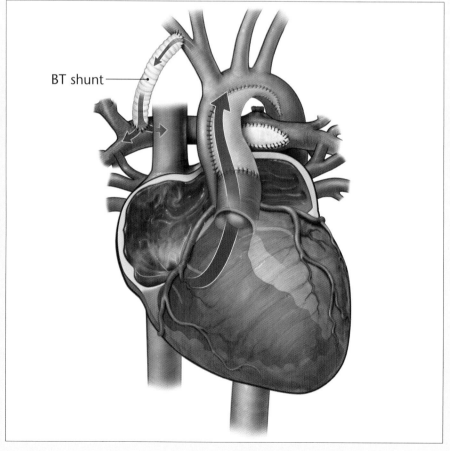

BT shunt

Performed at approximately 4 to 6 months of age. Two surgical options are the Glenn procedure or the hemi-Fontan procedure. A Glenn or hemi-Fontan procedure is also referred to as a superior cavopulmonary anastomosis.

Glenn Procedure

- The Sano or BT shunt is removed (illustration shows BT shunt ligated).
- The SVC is connected directly to the right pulmonary artery (RPA).
- The SVC is oversewn at the entrance to the RA.
- Infant remains desaturated (O_2 saturation ~ 82 to 84%) because the IVC blood goes directly into the systemic circulation.

Hemi-Fontan Operation

Alternative to the Glenn Procedure

- Sano or BT shunt removed (not shown)
- As with the Glenn procedure, the SVC is connected to the RPA, however, the surgical steps are different. The procedural steps to create a hemi-Fontan are shown on page 194.

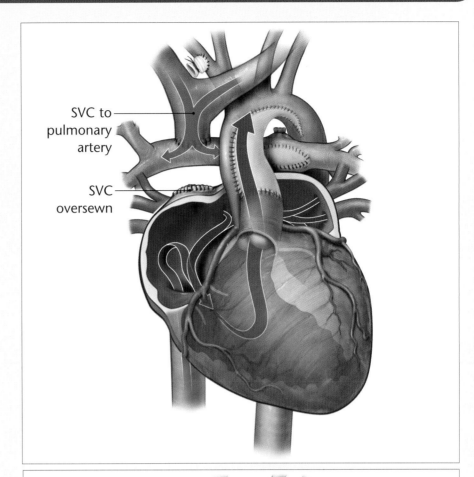

SVC to pulmonary artery

SVC oversewn

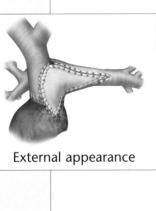

External appearance

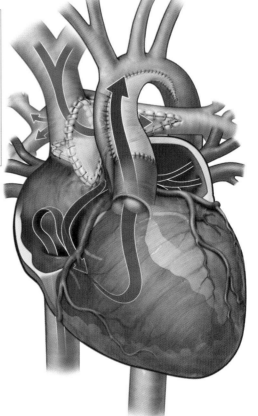

APPENDIX – Palliative and Surgical Repair Options

Hypoplastic Left Heart Syndrome – Procedural Steps – Hemi-Fontan

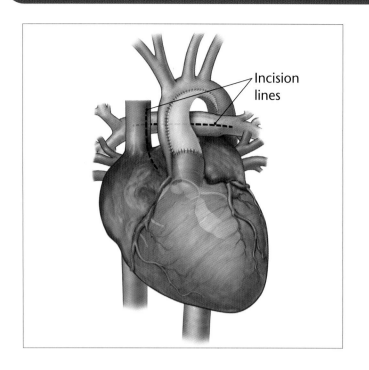

Incision lines

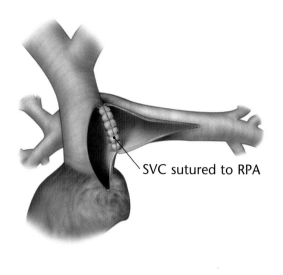

SVC sutured to RPA

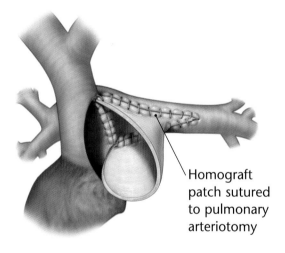

Homograft patch sutured to pulmonary arteriotomy

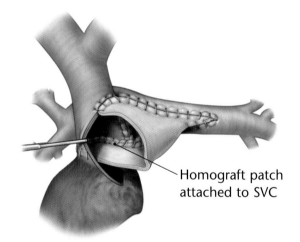

Homograft patch attached to SVC

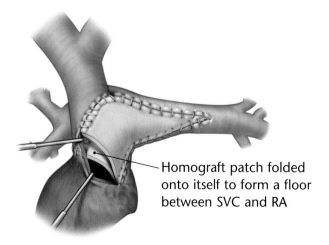

Homograft patch folded onto itself to form a floor between SVC and RA

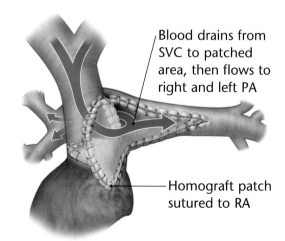

Blood drains from SVC to patched area, then flows to right and left PA

Homograft patch sutured to RA

The Fontan operation is typically performed between 18 months and 3 years of age. Occasionally, Fontan completion is delayed to an older age.

Extracardiac Fontan

(if Glenn was initially performed)

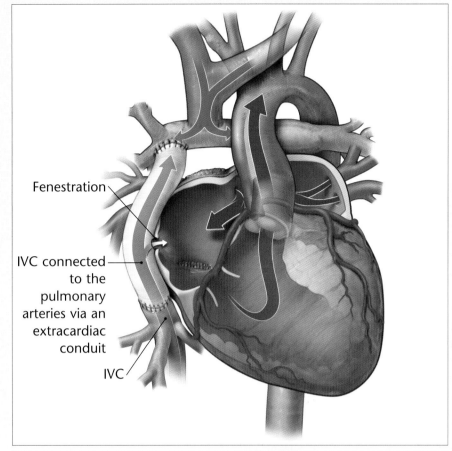

Fenestration

IVC connected to the pulmonary arteries via an extracardiac conduit

IVC

Lateral tunnel Fontan

(if hemi-Fontan was initially performed)

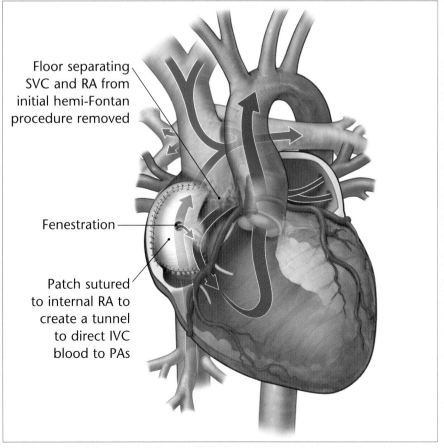

Floor separating SVC and RA from initial hemi-Fontan procedure removed

Fenestration

Patch sutured to internal RA to create a tunnel to direct IVC blood to PAs

Hypoplastic Left Heart Syndrome – Hybrid Approach

1 Neonatal Period

The hybrid approach may be selected based on institutional preference, or other clinical factors that increase the risk of cardiopulmonary bypass. These include prematurity, small size, intracranial hemorrhage, or other organ injury.

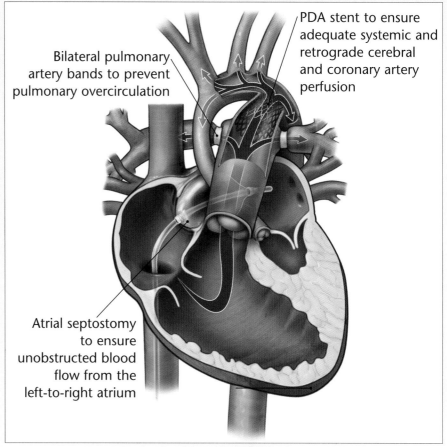

Bilateral pulmonary artery bands to prevent pulmonary overcirculation

PDA stent to ensure adequate systemic and retrograde cerebral and coronary artery perfusion

Atrial septostomy to ensure unobstructed blood flow from the left-to-right atrium

2 Comprehensive Stage 2 Operation – 4 to 6 months of age

- Removal of the pulmonary artery bands and PDA stent
- Pulmonary artery reconstruction
- Damus-Kaye-Stansel aortic arch reconstruction (Norwood procedure)
- Glenn procedure
- Atrial septectomy

Challenges related to this operation include:

- Surgically more complex - stage 1 and stage 2 operations performed together.
- Longer time on cardiopulmonary bypass.

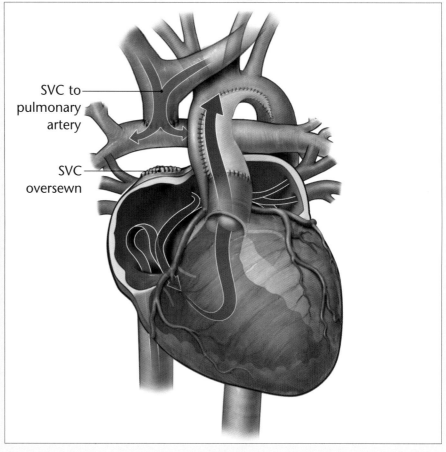

SVC to pulmonary artery

SVC oversewn

3 Fontan Operation (see page 195 for illustration).

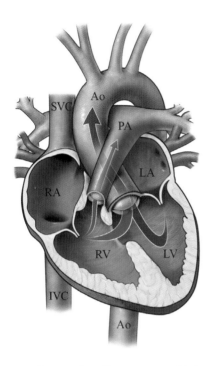

Tetralogy of Fallot – page 198

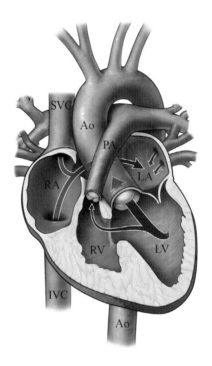

Tricuspid atresia – page 202

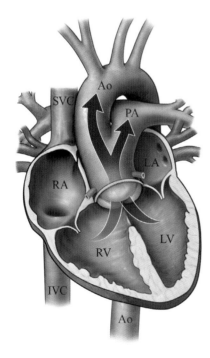

Truncus arteriosus – page 204

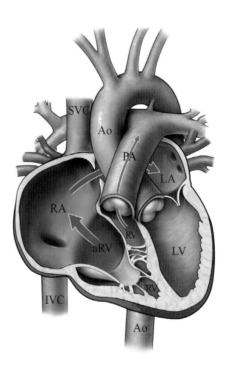

Ebstein anomaly – page 206

Tetralogy of Fallot – Palliative Options

For more information about TOF see page 88.

Prior to definitive surgical repair at approximately 4 to 6 months of age, 4 palliative options are available to address reduced pulmonary blood flow.

Balloon Valvuloplasty

Relieves obstruction at the pulmonary valve.
(Interventional cardiac catheterization procedure)

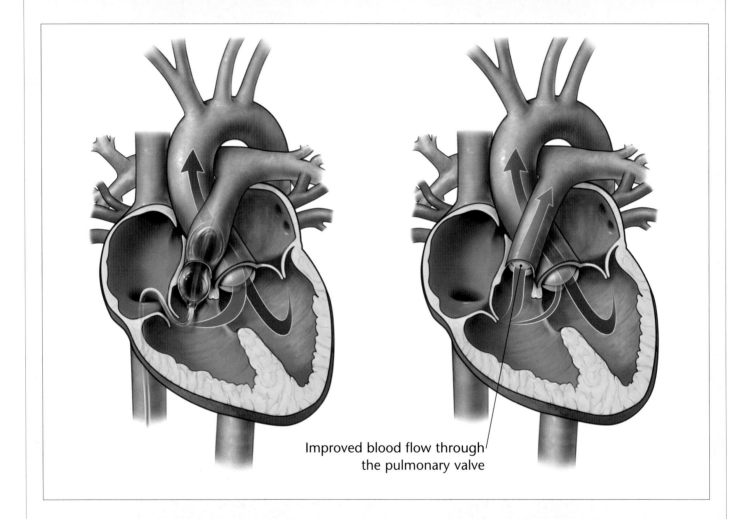

Improved blood flow through the pulmonary valve

Right Ventricular Outflow Tract (RVOT) Stent

Treats muscular RVOT obstruction.

(Interventional cardiac catheterization procedure)

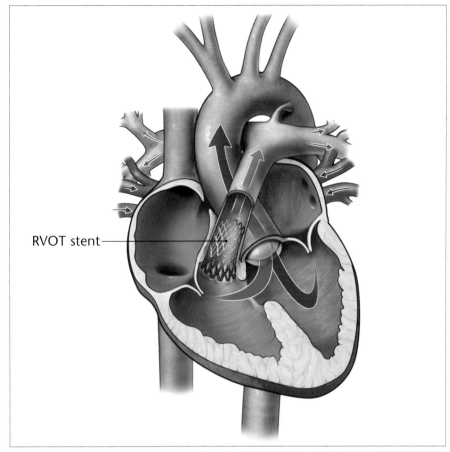

RVOT stent

Stent the Ductus Arteriosus

To provide adequate pulmonary blood flow. The size and location of the DA must be amenable to placement of a stent.

(Interventional cardiac catheterization procedure)

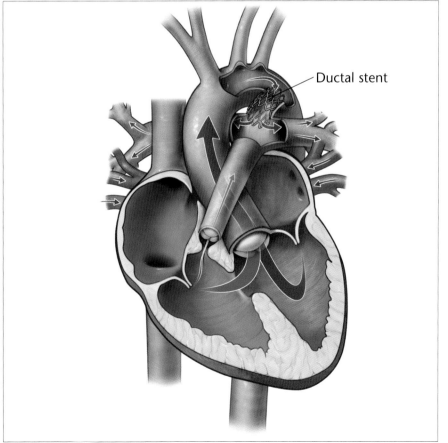

Ductal stent

APPENDIX – Palliative and Surgical Repair Options

Tetralogy of Fallot – Palliative Options

Systemic-pulmonary artery shunt (Blalock-Taussig/ BT shunt)

To provide adequate pulmonary blood flow *(surgical procedure)*.

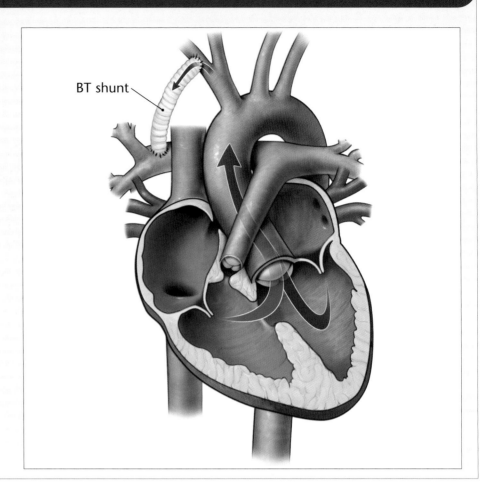

BT shunt

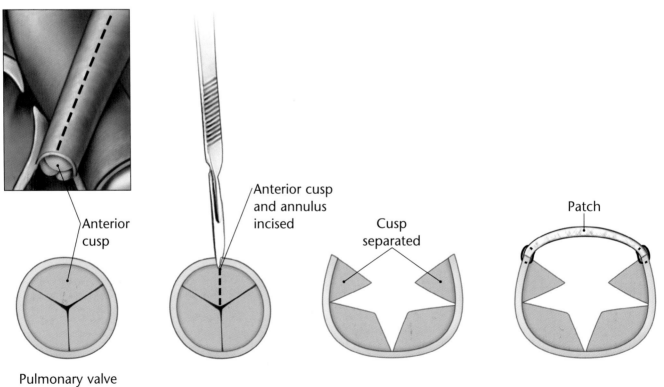

Anterior cusp

Pulmonary valve

Anterior cusp and annulus incised

Cusp separated

Patch

Patient will require future placement of a competent pulmonary valve.

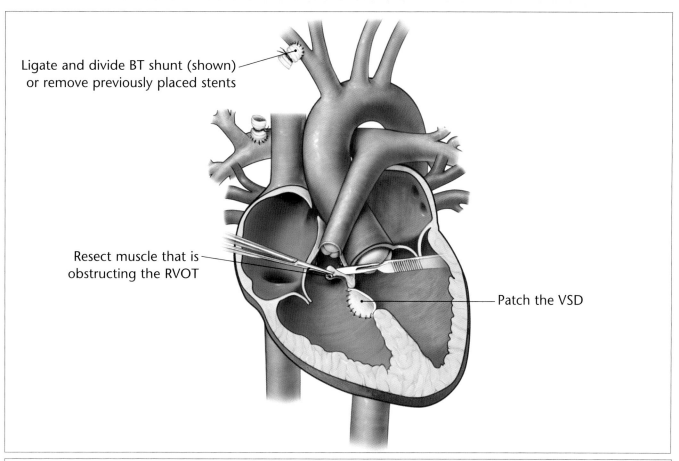

Ligate and divide BT shunt (shown) or remove previously placed stents

Resect muscle that is obstructing the RVOT

Patch the VSD

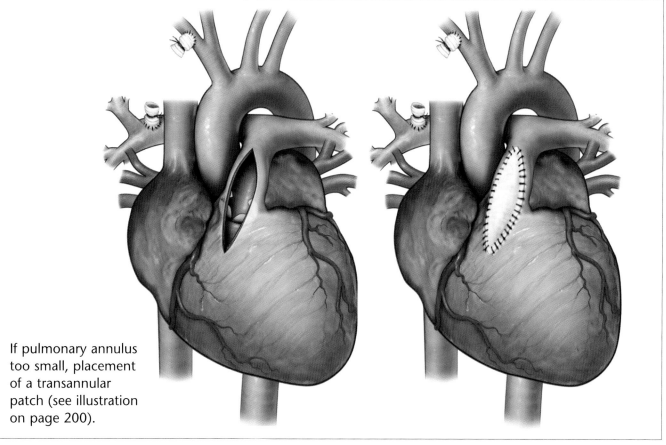

If pulmonary annulus too small, placement of a transannular patch (see illustration on page 200).

Tricuspid Atresia

For more information about tricuspid atresia see page 102.

Single ventricle surgical palliation of tricuspid atresia usually occurs in 3 separate surgeries. The timing of intervention is influenced by the size of the VSD and the degree of pulmonary stenosis. Infants with adequate pulmonary blood flow may not need intervention as a neonate; their first surgery may be the Glenn procedure when they are 4 to 6 months old.

Stage 1 Operation

For inadequate pulmonary blood flow, a BT shunt may be necessary. However, some institutions may elect to stent the ductus arteriosus (see illustration on page 199).

If there is excessive pulmonary blood flow, pulmonary artery banding may be necessary.

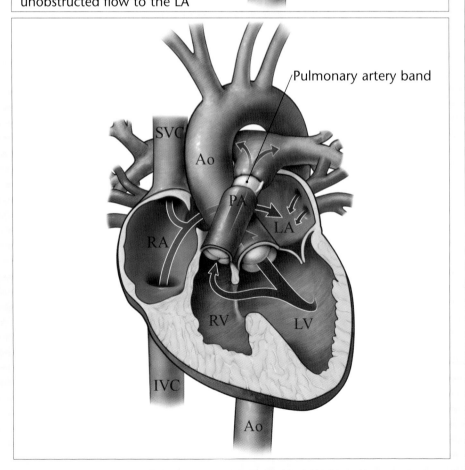

Atrial septectomy to ensure unobstructed flow to the LA

Stage ② Operation

The Glenn procedure is performed when the infant is 4 to 6 months old when the PVR should be low enough to allow passive drainage of venous blood from the head and arms to the pulmonary arteries and lungs. If a BT shunt was previously placed, it is taken down when the Glenn procedure is done. The goal O_2 saturation following this operation is approximately 85%.

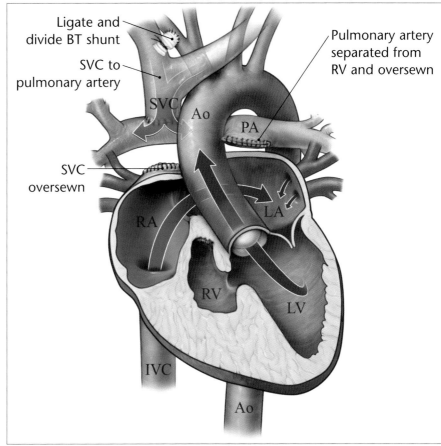

Ligate and divide BT shunt

SVC to pulmonary artery

Pulmonary artery separated from RV and oversewn

SVC oversewn

SVC

Ao

PA

RA

LA

RV

LV

IVC

Ao

Stage ③ Operation

The Fontan operation is typically performed between 18 months and 3 years of age. Occasionally, Fontan completion is delayed to an older age.

The timing varies based on regional preference and patient clinical status. At the conclusion of this surgery, the IVC and SVC blood flows passively to the pulmonary arteries via surgically constructed anastomoses. The pulmonary venous return flows to the left atrium, left ventricle, and then out the aorta. The O_2 saturation following this operation is usually in the 90s.

Some centers utilize a hemi-Fontan and lateral tunnel Fontan approach for stage 2 and 3 surgeries.

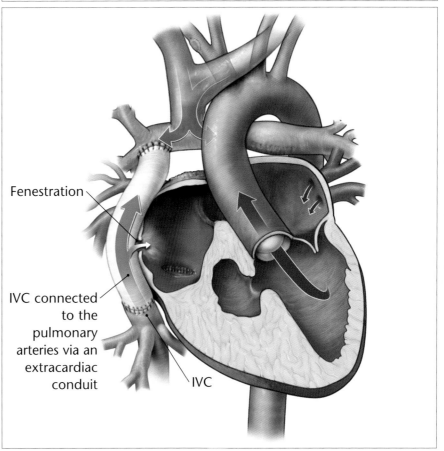

Fenestration

IVC connected to the pulmonary arteries via an extracardiac conduit

IVC

Truncus Arteriosus

Complete 2-ventricle surgical repair occurs in the neonatal period and preferably within the first few weeks after birth. With closure of the VSD, the left ventricle will eject blood across the truncal valve into the aorta and the right ventricle will eject blood through a valved conduit to the lungs. The coronary arteries remain connected to the truncal root (neoaorta). The patient will be monitored regularly for development of truncal valve disorders that may require additional intervention.

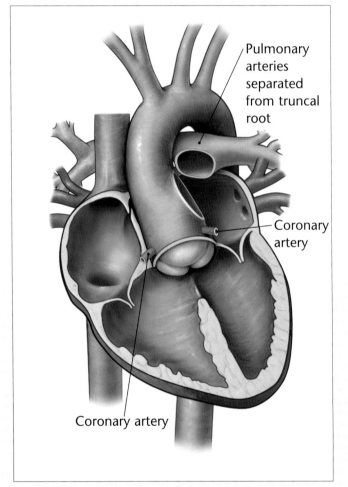

Pulmonary arteries separated from truncal root

Coronary artery

Coronary artery

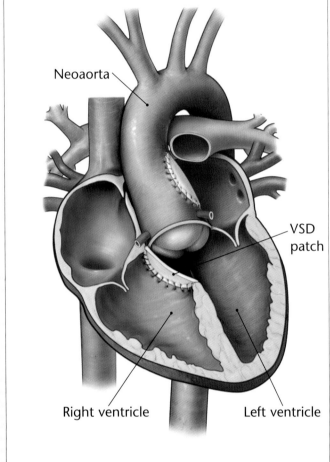

Neoaorta

VSD patch

Right ventricle

Left ventricle

For more information about truncus arteriosus see page 108.

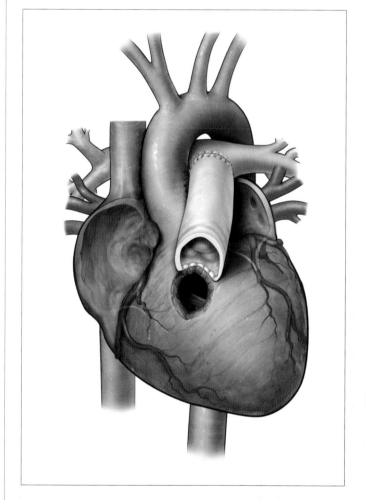

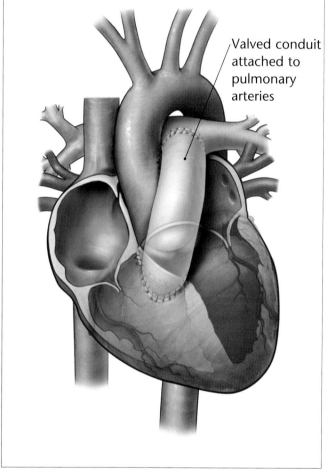

Valved conduit attached to pulmonary arteries

Ebstein Anomaly - Surgical Repair - Cone Procedure

For more information about Ebstein anomaly see page 120.

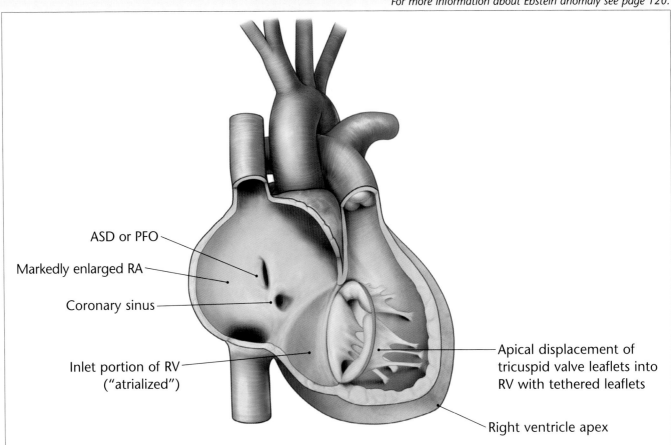

ASD or PFO

Markedly enlarged RA

Coronary sinus

Inlet portion of RV
("atrialized")

Apical displacement of
tricuspid valve leaflets into
RV with tethered leaflets

Right ventricle apex

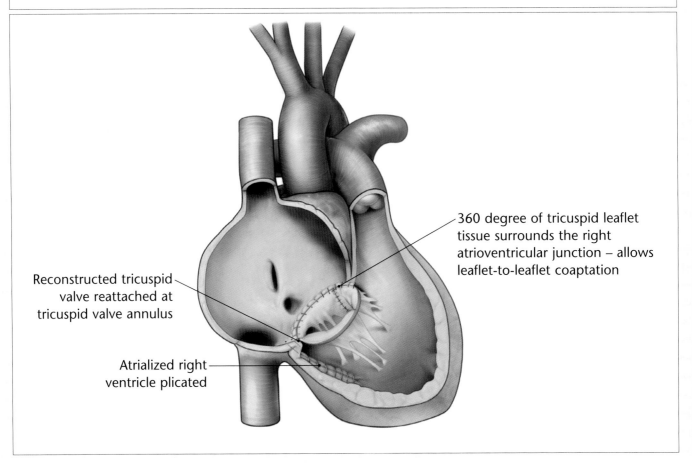

Reconstructed tricuspid
valve reattached at
tricuspid valve annulus

Atrialized right
ventricle plicated

360 degree of tricuspid leaflet
tissue surrounds the right
atrioventricular junction – allows
leaflet-to-leaflet coaptation

Cyanotic Congenital Heart Disease
Ductal Dependent for Pulmonary Blood Flow

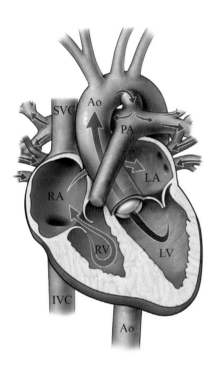

Pulmonary atresia with intact ventricular septum
– page 208

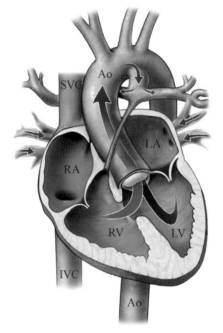

Pulmonary atresia with ventricular septal defect
– page 212

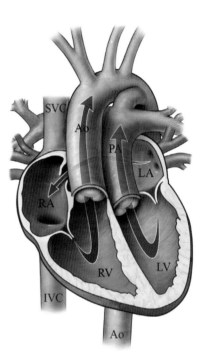

Transposition of the great arteries
– page 214

APPENDIX – Palliative and Surgical Repair Options

Pulmonary Atresia with Intact Ventricular Septum – Surgical and Palliative Options

For more information about PA-IVS see page 126.

Surgical options depend upon the size of the right ventricle (RV), the size, anatomy, and function of the tricuspid valve, and the presence or absence of RV dependent coronary circulation.

2 Ventricle Repair

There is no RV-dependent ventriculocoronary circulation, an adequate sized RV, and a functional tricuspid valve.

Initially, antegrade blood flow from the RV through the atretic pulmonary valve is established via radiofrequency perforation and pulmonary balloon valvuloplasty.
(Interventional cardiac catheterization procedure)

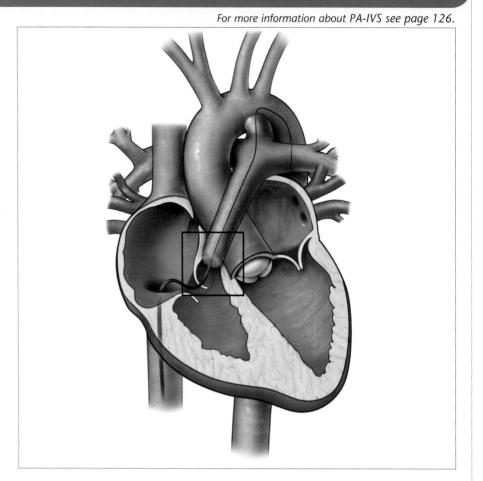

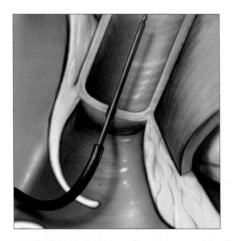 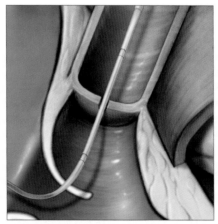 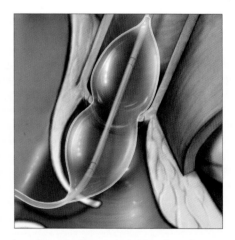

Radiofrequency perforation and balloon dilation of the atretic pulmonary valve (i.e., balloon valvuloplasty).

Until ventricular compliance improves, antegrade blood flow through the pulmonary valve may still be inadequate following balloon valvuloplasty. If unable to discontinue PGE, then options to improve pulmonary blood flow include placement of a ductal stent *(interventional cardiac catherization procedure)*, or a BT shunt *(surgical procedure)*. If there is valvar and subvalvar (muscular or infundibular) obstruction of the RVOT, then a transannular patch may be necessary to widen the RVOT (not shown). When the patient is older, a second-stage operation may be necessary to reconstruct the RVOT and close the ASD.

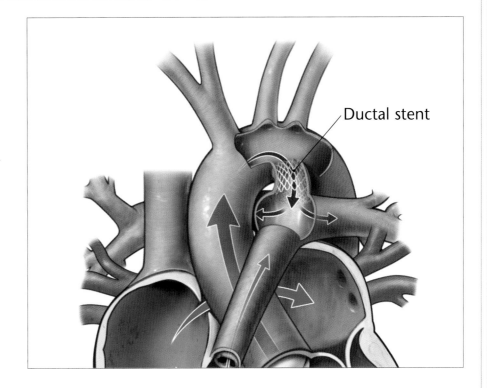

Ductal stent

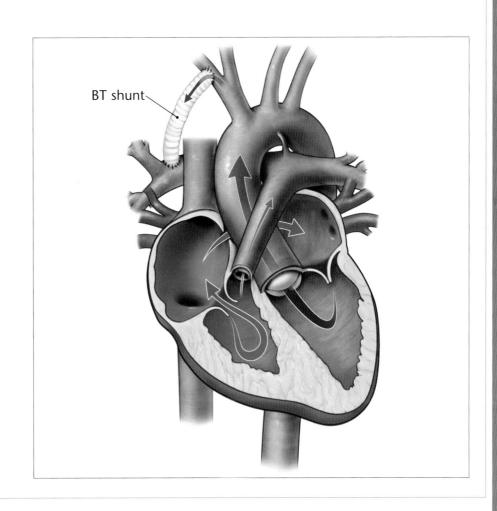

BT shunt

1.5 Ventricle Repair

There is mild to moderate RV hypoplasia.

Forward blood flow from the RV to the pulmonary artery is initially established via radiofrequency perforation and balloon pulmonary valvuloplasty. At around 4 to 6 months of age, a Glenn anastomosis is performed. The smaller RV now only has to pump half the systemic venous return to the lungs since the SVC drains the other half directly to the pulmonary arteries. As the child grows, the RV and tricuspid valve will hopefully grow in size, so that the Fontan operation will not be necessary.

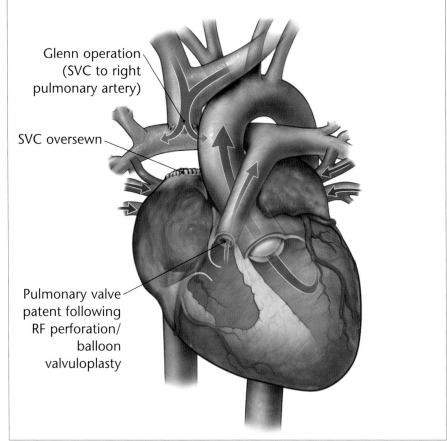

Glenn operation (SVC to right pulmonary artery)

SVC oversewn

Pulmonary valve patent following RF perforation/ balloon valvuloplasty

Single Ventricle Palliation

There is severe RV hypoplasia, a very small tricuspid valve, and/or RV-dependent coronary circulation.

Palliative steps include establishment of reliable pulmonary blood flow via a BT shunt or ductal stent until the infant is old enough to have a Glenn or hemi-Fontan procedure. If there is RV-dependent coronary circulation, decompression of the RV is avoided since there is increased risk for myocardial ischemia.

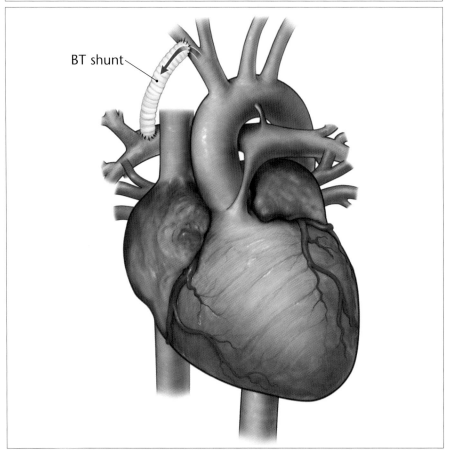

BT shunt

A Glenn procedure is typically performed when the infant is 4 to 6 months old.

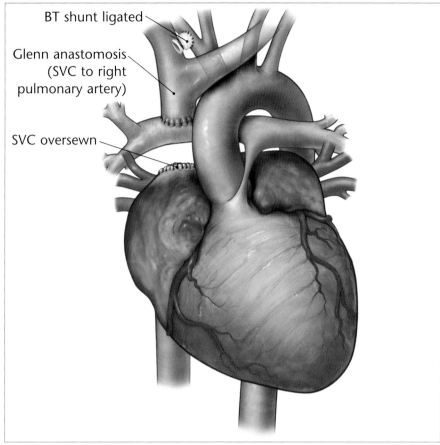

BT shunt ligated

Glenn anastomosis (SVC to right pulmonary artery)

SVC oversewn

The Fontan operation is typically performed between 18 months and 3 years of age. Occasionally, Fontan completion is delayed to an older age. Cardiac transplantation may eventually be necessary.

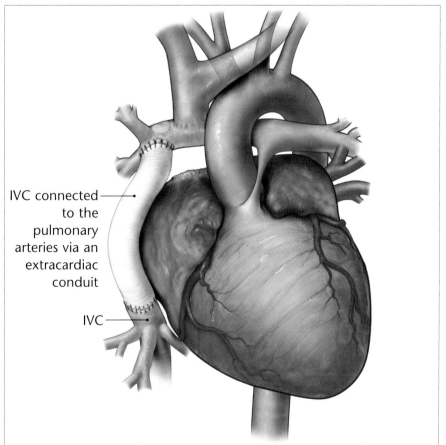

IVC connected to the pulmonary arteries via an extracardiac conduit

IVC

APPENDIX – Palliative and Surgical Repair Options

Pulmonary Atresia with Ventricular Septal Defect

For more information about PA-VSD see page 132.

Placement of a central shunt between the aorta and hypoplastic main pulmonary artery to provide pulmonary blood flow and promote growth of the true pulmonary arteries prior to surgical repair.

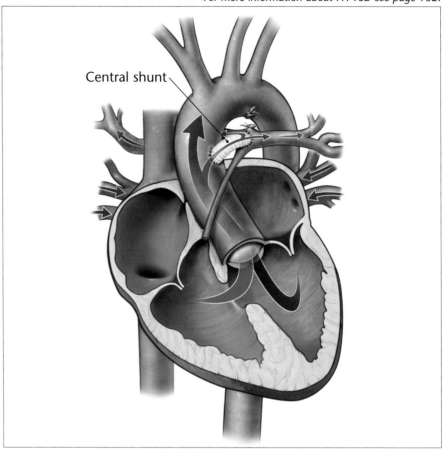

Central shunt

When the patient is older, surgical repair includes patch closure of the VSD and providing pulmonary blood flow via a valved conduit between the RV and pulmonary arteries.

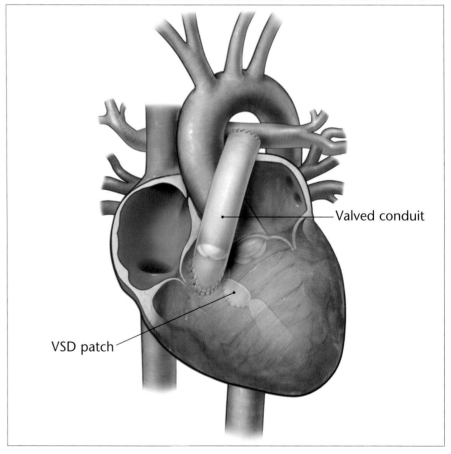

Valved conduit

VSD patch

Placement of a central shunt between the aorta and hypoplastic main pulmonary artery to provide pulmonary blood flow and promote growth of the true pulmonary arteries prior to surgical repair.

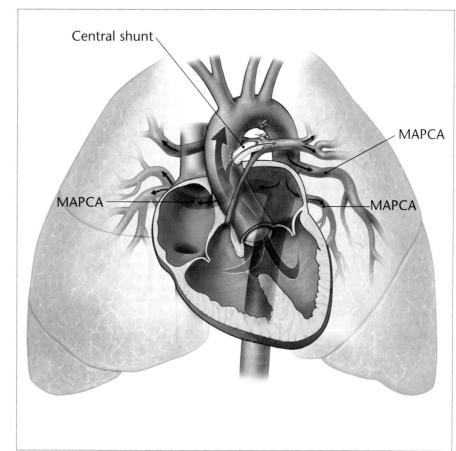

Unifocalization Procedure

The collateral arteries are disconnected from the aorta and connected to the pulmonary arteries. Pulmonary blood flow is provided via a valved (homograft) conduit between the RV and pulmonary arteries.

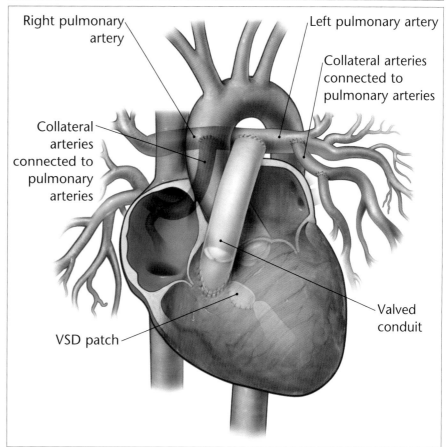

Transposition of the Great Arteries – Arterial Switch Operation

For more information about TGA see page 136.

Most patients undergo surgical repair in the early neonatal period via an arterial switch operation (ASO) to relocate the great arteries. The aorta and coronary arteries are translocated to arise from the left ventricle and the pulmonary artery is translocated to arise from the right ventricle.

If a balloon atrial septostomy was performed, the ASD is closed (not shown). The patient will be followed for development of coronary artery stenosis, supravalvar pulmonary artery stenosis, branch pulmonary stenosis, dilation of the neoaortic root, and supravalvar aortic narrowing

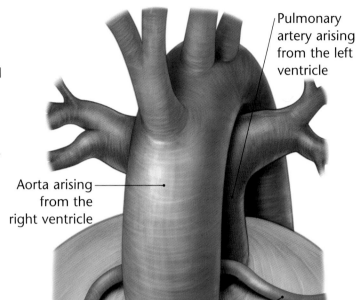

Pulmonary artery arising from the left ventricle

Aorta arising from the right ventricle

Coronary arteries

Before surgery

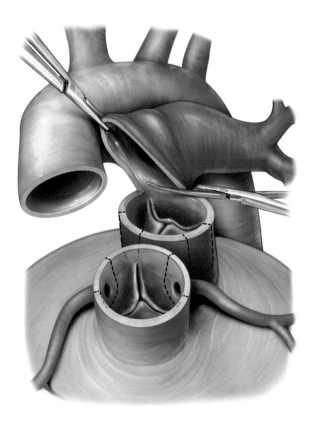

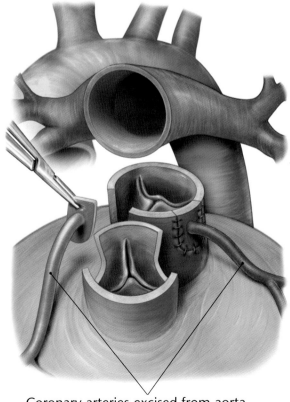

Coronary arteries excised from aorta and translocated to the pulmonary root

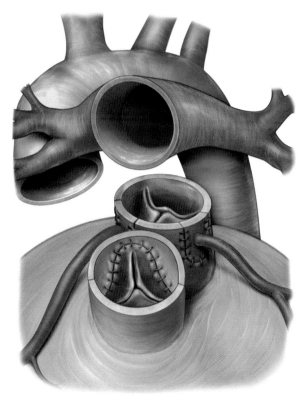

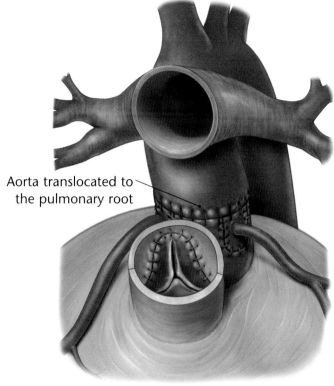

Aorta translocated to the pulmonary root

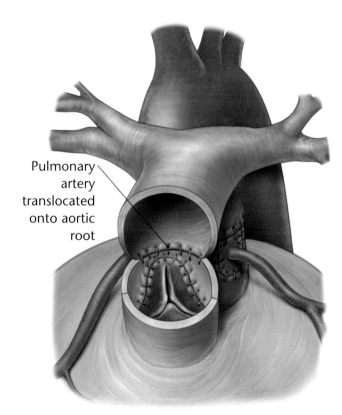

Pulmonary artery translocated onto aortic root

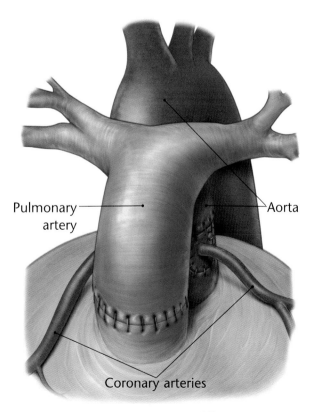

Pulmonary artery

Aorta

Coronary arteries

After surgery

References

1. Botto LD. Epidemiology and Prevention of Congenital Heart Defects. In: Allen HD, Shaddy RE, Penny DJ, Feltes TF, Cetta F, eds. *Moss and Adams' Heart Disease in Infants, Children, and Adolescents.* 9 ed. Philadelphia: Wolters Kluwer; 2016:55-86.

2. Scholz T, Reinking B. Congenital Heart Disease. In: Gleason CA, Juul SE, eds. *Avery's Diseases of the Newborn.* 10 ed. Philadelphia PA: Elsevier; 2018:801-827.

3. van der Linde D, Konings EE, Slager MA, et al. Birth prevalence of congenital heart disease worldwide: a systematic review and meta-analysis. *J Am Coll Cardiol.* 2011;58(21):2241-2247.

4. Martin JA, Hamilton BE, Osterman MJ, Driscoll AK, Mathews TJ. Births: Final Data for 2015. *Natl Vital Stat Rep.* 2017;66(1):1.

5. Oster ME, Lee KA, Honein MA, Riehle-Colarusso T, Shin M, Correa A. Temporal trends in survival among infants with critical congenital heart defects. *Pediatrics.* 2013;131(5):e1502-1508.

6. Hoffman JI, Kaplan S. The incidence of congenital heart disease. *J Am Coll Cardiol.* 2002;39(12):1890-1900.

7. Brown KL, Ridout DA, Hoskote A, Verhulst L, Ricci M, Bull C. Delayed diagnosis of congenital heart disease worsens preoperative condition and outcome of surgery in neonates. *Heart.* 2006;92(9):1298-1302.

8. Costello JM, Almodovar MC. Emergency Care for Infants and Children with Acute Cardiac Disease. *Clinical Pediatric Emergency Medicine.* 2007;8(3):145-155.

9. Guveli BT, Rosti RO, Guzeltas A, et al. Teratogenicity of Antiepileptic Drugs. *Clin Psychopharmacol Neurosci.* 2017;15(1):19-27.

10. Tomson T, Battino D. Teratogenicity of antiepileptic drugs: state of the art. *Curr Opin Neurol.* 2005;18(2):135-140.

11. Vajda FJ, Graham J, Roten A, Lander CM, O'Brien TJ, Eadie M. Teratogenicity of the newer antiepileptic drugs--the Australian experience. *J Clin Neurosci.* 2012;19(1):57-59.

12. Vajda FJ, O'Brien TJ, Lander CM, Graham J, Eadie MJ. The teratogenicity of the newer antiepileptic drugs - an update. *Acta Neurol Scand.* 2014;130(4):234-238.

13. Granzotti JA, Amaral FT, Sassamoto CA, Nunes MA, Grellet MA. [Congenital rubella syndrome and the occurrence of congenital heart disease]. *J Pediatr (Rio J).* 1996;72(4):242-244.

14. Basu M, Zhu JY, LaHaye S, et al. Epigenetic mechanisms underlying maternal diabetes-associated risk of congenital heart disease. *JCI Insight.* 2017;2(20):1-20.

15. Hoang TT, Marengo LK, Mitchell LE, Canfield MA, Agopian AJ. Original Findings and Updated Meta-Analysis for the Association Between Maternal Diabetes and Risk for Congenital Heart Disease Phenotypes. *Am J Epidemiol.* 2017;186(1):118-128.

16. Oyen N, Diaz LJ, Leirgul E, et al. Prepregnancy Diabetes and Offspring Risk of Congenital Heart Disease: A Nationwide Cohort Study. *Circulation.* 2016;133(23):2243-2253.

17. Nassr AA, El-Nashar SA, Shazly SA, White WM, Brost BC. Expected probability of congenital heart disease and clinical utility of fetal echocardiography in pregnancies with pre-gestational diabetes. *Eur J Obstet Gynecol Reprod Biol.* 2016;201:121-125.

18. History Taking. In: Park MK, Salamat M, eds. *Park's Pediatric Cardiology for Practitioners.* 7 ed. Philadelphia: Elsevier; 2021:2-5.

19. Mitchell AL, Snyder CS. Genetic and Environmental Contributions to Congenital Heart Disease. In: Martin RJ, Fanaroff AA, Walsh MC, eds. *Fanaroff and Martin's Neonatal-Perinatal Medicine: Diseases of the Fetus and Infant.* 10 ed. Philadelphia: Elsevier Saunders; 2015:1210-1214.

20. Singh Y, Chee Y-H, Gahlaut R. Evaluation of suspected congenital heart disease. *Paediatrics and Child Health.* 2015;25(1):7-12.

21. Baley JE, Gonzalez BE. Perinatal Viral Infections. In: Martin RJ, Fanaroff AA, Walsh MC, eds. *Fanaroff and Martin's Neonatal-Perinatal Medicine: Diseases of the Fetus and Infant.* 10 ed. Philadelphia: Elsevier Saunders; 2015:782-833.

22. Wren C, Birrell G, Hawthorne G. Cardiovascular malformations in infants of diabetic mothers. *Heart.* 2003;89(10):1217-1220.

23. Brite J, Laughon SK, Troendle J, Mills J. Maternal overweight and obesity and risk of congenital heart defects in offspring. *Int J Obes (Lond).* 2014;38(6):878-882.

24. Mills JL, Troendle J, Conley MR, Carter T, Druschel CM. Maternal obesity and congenital heart defects: a population-based study. *Am J Clin Nutr.* 2010;91(6):1543-1549.

25. Watanabe M, Wikenheiser J. Cardiac Embryology. In: Martin RJ, Fanaroff AA, Walsh MC, eds. *Fanaroff and Martin's Neonatal-Perinatal Medicine: Diseases of the Fetus and Infant.* 10 ed. Philadelphia: Elsevier Saunders; 2015:1188-1191.

26. Gill HK, Splitt M, Sharland GK, Simpson JM. Patterns of recurrence of congenital heart disease: An analysis of 6,640 consecutive pregnancies evaluated by detailed fetal echocardiography. *Journal of the American College of Cardiology.* 2003;42(5):923-929.

27. Loffredo CA, Chokkalingam A, Sill AM, et al. Prevalence of congenital cardiovascular malformations among relatives of infants with hypoplastic left heart, coarctation of the aorta, and d-transposition of the great arteries. *Am J Med Genet A.* 2004;124A(3):225-230.

28. Hinton RB, Martin LJ, Tabangin ME, Mazwi ML, Cripe LH, Benson DW. Hypoplastic Left Heart Syndrome Is Heritable. *Journal of the American College of Cardiology.* 2007;50(16):1590-1595.

29. Calcagni G, Digilio MC, Sarkozy A, Dallapiccola B, Marino B. Familial recurrence of congenital heart disease: an overview and review of the literature. *Eur J Pediatr.* 2007;166(2):111-116.

30. Patel A, Costello JM, Backer CL, et al. Prevalence of Noncardiac and Genetic Abnormalities in Neonates Undergoing Cardiac Operations: Analysis of The Society of Thoracic Surgeons Congenital Heart Surgery Database. *Ann Thorac Surg.* 2016;102(5):1607-1614.

31. Bailliard F, Anderson RH. Tetralogy of Fallot. *Orphanet J Rare Dis.* 2009;4:2. doi: 10.1186/1750-1172-4-2.

32. Loffredo CA, Wilson PD, Ferencz C. Maternal diabetes: an independent risk factor for major cardiovascular malformations with increased mortality of affected infants. *Teratology.* 2001;64(2):98-106.

33. Goldmuntz E, Crenshaw ML. Genetic Aspects of Congenital Heart Defects. In: Allen HD, Shaddy RE, Penny DJ, Feltes TF, Cetta F, eds. *Moss and Adams' Heart Disease in Infants, Children, and Adolescents.* 9 ed. Philadelphia: Wolters Kluwer; 2016:87-115.

34. Orofino DHG, Passos SRL, de Oliveira RVC, et al. Cardiac findings in infants with in utero exposure to Zika virus- a cross sectional study. *PLoS Negl Trop Dis.* 2018;12(3):e0006362.

35. Anders JF, Schneider KA. The Sick Neonate With Cardiac Disease. *Clinical Pediatric Emergency Medicine*.12(4):301-312.

36. AHA. Part 3: Systematic Approach to the Seriously Ill or Injured Child. In: Samson RA, Schexnayder SM, Hazinski MF, Meeks R, Knight LJ, eds. *Pediatric Advanced Life Support Provider Manual*. Dallas: American Heart Association; 2016:29-67.

37. Townsend SF. The Large-for-Gestational-Age and the Small-for-Gestational-age Infant. In: Thureen PJ, Deacon J, Hernandez JA, Hall DM, eds. *Assessment and care of the well newborn*. 2nd ed. St. Louis: Elsevier; 2005:267-278.

38. Nodine PM, Arruda J, Hastings-Tolsma M. Prenatal Environment: Effect on Neonatal Outcome. In: Gardner SL, Carter BS, Enzman-Hines M, Hernandez JA, eds. *Merenstein & Gardner's Handbook of Neonatal Intensive Care*. 7th ed. St. Louis: Mosby Elsevier; 2011:13-38.

39. Simmons R. Abnormalities of Fetal Growth. In: Gleason CA, Devaskar SU, eds. *Avery's Diseases of the Newborn*. 9th ed. Philadelphia: Elsevier Saunders; 2012:51-59.

40. Vora N, Bianchi DW. Genetic considerations in the prenatal diagnosis of overgrowth syndromes. *Prenat Diagn*. 2009;29(10):923-929.

41. Metzger BE, Lowe LP, Dyer AR, et al. Hyperglycemia and Adverse Pregnancy Outcome (HAPO) Study: associations with neonatal anthropometrics. *Diabetes*. 2009;58(2):453-459.

42. Eriksson UJ. Congenital anomalies in diabetic pregnancy. *Seminars in fetal & neonatal medicine*. 2009;14(2):85-93.

43. Correa A, Gilboa SM, Besser LM, et al. Diabetes mellitus and birth defects. *Am J Obstet Gynecol*. 2008;199(3):237 e231-239.

44. Correa A, Gilboa SM, Botto LD, et al. Lack of periconceptional vitamins or supplements that contain folic acid and diabetes mellitus-associated birth defects. *Am J Obstet Gynecol*. 2012;206(3):218 e211-213.

45. Madsen NL, Schwartz SM, Lewin MB, Mueller BA. Prepregnancy body mass index and congenital heart defects among offspring: a population-based study. *Congenit Heart Dis*. 2013;8(2):131-141.

46. Cai GJ, Sun XX, Zhang L, Hong Q. Association between maternal body mass index and congenital heart defects in offspring: a systematic review. *Am J Obstet Gynecol*. 2014;211(2):91-117.

47. Gilboa SM, Correa A, Botto LD, et al. Association between prepregnancy body mass index and congenital heart defects. *Am J Obstet Gynecol*. 2010;202(1):51.e1-51.e10.

48. Hoffman TM, Welty SE. Physiology of the Preterm and Term Infant. In: Allen HD, Shaddy RE, Penny DJ, Feltes TF, Cetta F, eds. *Moss and Adams' Heart Disease in Infants, Children, and Adolescents*. 9 ed. Philadelphia: Wolters Kluwer; 2016:655-664.

49. Ullmo S, Vial Y, Di Bernardo S, et al. Pathologic ventricular hypertrophy in the offspring of diabetic mothers: a retrospective study. *Eur Heart J*. 2007;28(11):1319-1325.

50. Blickstein I, Perlman S, Hazan Y, Topf-Olivestone C, Shinwell ES. Diabetes Mellitus During Pregnancy. In: Martin RJ, Fanaroff AA, Walsh MC, eds. *Fanaroff and Martin's Neonatal-Perinatal Medicine: Diseases of the Fetus and Infant*. 10 ed. Philadelphia: Elsevier Saunders; 2015:265-270.

51. Yeh J, Berger S. Cardiac findings in infants of diabetic mothers. *NeoReviews*. 2015;16(11):e624-e630.

52. Primary Myocardial Disease. In: Park MK, Salamat M, eds. *Park's Pediatric Cardiology for Practitioners*. 7 ed. Philadelphia PA: Elsevier; 2021:248-263.

53. Mehta A, Hussain K. Transient hyperinsulinism associated with macrosomia, hypertrophic obstructive cardiomyopathy, hepatomegaly, and nephromegaly. *Arch Dis Child*. 2003;88(9):822-824.

54. ADA. Diagnosis and classification of diabetes mellitus. *Diabetes Care*. 2010;33 Suppl 1:S62-69.

55. Gabbe SG, Landon MB, Warren-Boulton E, Fradkin J. Promoting health after gestational diabetes: a National Diabetes Education Program call to action. *Obstet Gynecol*. 2012;119(1):171-176.

56. ADA. Standards of medical care in diabetes--2011. *Diabetes Care*. 2011;34 Suppl 1:S11-61.

57. Cheung NW. The management of gestational diabetes. *Vasc Health Risk Manag*. 2009;5(1):153-164.

58. Heideman WH, Middelkoop BJ, Nierkens V, et al. Changing the odds. What do we learn from prevention studies targeted at people with a positive family history of type 2 diabetes? *Prim Care Diabetes*. 2011;5(4):215-221.

59. Brown Z, Chang J. Maternal Diabetes. In: Gleason CA, Juul SE, eds. *Avery's Diseases of the Newborn*. 10 ed. Philadelphia PA: Elsevier; 2018:90-103.

60. Simmons R. Abnormalities of Fetal Growth. In: Gleason CA, Devaskar SU, eds. *Avery's Diseases of the Newborn*. 9 ed. Philadelphia PA: Elsevier/Saunders; 2012:51-59.

61. Wallenstein MB, Harper LM, Odibo AO, et al. Fetal congenital heart disease and intrauterine growth restriction: a retrospective cohort study. *J Matern Fetal Neonatal Med*. 2012;25(6):662-665.

62. Morris SA, Maskatia SA, Altman CA, Ayres NA. Fetal and Perinatal Cardiology. In: Martin RJ, Fanaroff AA, Walsh MC, eds. *Fanaroff and Martin's Neonatal-Perinatal Medicine: Diseases of the Fetus and Infant*. 10 ed: Elsevier Health Sciences; 2015:137-180.

63. Haldeman-Englert CR, Saitta SC, Zackai EH. Specific Chromosome Disorders in Newborns. In: Gleason CA, Devaskar SU, eds. *Avery's Diseases of the Newborn*. 9 ed. Philadelphia, PA: Elsevier/Saunders; 2012:196-208.

64. Korlimarla A, Hart SJ, Spiridigliozzi GA, Kishnani PS. Down Syndrome. In: Carey JC, Battaglia A, Viskochil D, Cassidy SB, eds. *Cassidy and Allanson's Management of Genetic Syndromes*. 4 ed. Hoboken NJ: John Wiley & Sons; 2021:355-387.

65. Left-to-Right Shunt Lesions. In: Park MK, Salamat M, eds. *Park's Pediatric Cardiology for Practitioners*. 7 ed. Philadelphia PA: Elsevier; 2021:120-142.

66. Kleinman CS, Seri I. Syndromic Congenital Heart Disease. In: Polin RA, ed. *Hemodynamics and Cardiology: Neonatology Questions and Controversies E-Book*. 2 ed: Elsevier Saunders; 2012:368-376.

67. Jones KL, Jones MC, Del Campo M. Chromosomal Abnormality Syndromes Identifiable on Routine Karyotype. *Smith's Recognizable Patterns of Human Malformation*. 7 ed. Philadelphia, PA: Elsevier Saunders; 2013:7-83.

68. Pathophysiology of Left-to-Right Shunt Lesions. In: Park MK, Salamat M, eds. *Park's Pediatric Cardiology for Practitioners*. 7 ed. Philadelphia PA: Elsevier; 2021:96-101.

69. Dees E, Baldwin HS. Developmental Biology of the Heart. In: Gleason CA, Juul SE, eds. *Avery's Diseases of the Newborn*. 10 ed. Philadelphia PA: Elsevier; 2018:724-740.

70. Cetta F, Truong D, Minich LL, et al. Atrioventricular Septal Defects. In: Allen HD, Shaddy RE, Penny DJ, Feltes TF, Cetta F, eds. *Moss and Adams' Heart Disease in Infants, Children, and Adolescents*. 9 ed. Philadelphia: Wolters Kluwer; 2016:757-781.

References

71. Everett AD, Lim DS. Chapter 2. Congenital Heart Defects. In: Everett AD, Lim DS, eds. *Illustrated Field Guide to Congenital Heart Disease and Repair*. 3 ed. Charlottesville, VA: Scientific Software Solutions, Inc.; 2010:31-119.

72. Cohen MS, Lopez L. Ventricular Septal Defects. In: Allen HD, Shaddy RE, Penny DJ, Feltes TF, Cetta F, eds. *Moss and Adams' Heart Disease in Infants, Children, and Adolescents*. 9 ed. Philadelphia: Wolters Kluwer; 2016:783-802.

73. Prapa M, Pepper, J. & Gatzoulis, M.A. . Abnormalities of the Aortic Root. In: Allen HD, Shaddy RE, Penny DJ, Feltes TF, Cetta F, eds. *Moss and Adams' Heart Disease in Infants, Children, and Adolescents*. 9 ed. Philadelphia: Wolters Kluwer; 2016:871-880.

74. Sachdeva R. Atrial Septal Defects. In: Allen HD, Shaddy RE, Penny DJ, Feltes TF, Cetta F, eds. *Moss and Adams' Heart Disease in Infants, Children, and Adolescents*. 9 ed. Philadelphia: Wolters Kluwer; 2016:739-756.

75. Carey JC. Trisomy 18 and Trisomy 13 Syndromes. In: Carey JC, Battaglia A, Viskochil D, Cassidy SB, eds. *Cassidy and Allanson's Management of Genetic Syndromes*. 4 ed. Hoboken NJ: John Wiley & Sons; 2021:937-956.

76. Van Praagh S, Truman T, Firpo A, et al. Cardiac malformations in trisomy-18: a study of 41 postmortem cases. *J Am Coll Cardiol*. 1989;13(7):1586-1597.

77. Musewe NN, Alexander DJ, Teshima I, Smallhorn JF, Freedom RM. Echocardiographic evaluation of the spectrum of cardiac anomalies associated with trisomy 13 and trisomy 18. *J Am Coll Cardiol*. 1990;15(3):673-677.

78. Balderston SM, Shaffer EM, Washington RL, Sondheimer HM. Congenital polyvalvular disease in trisomy 18: echocardiographic diagnosis. *Pediatr Cardiol*. 1990;11(3):138-142.

79. Meyer RE, Liu G, Gilboa SM, et al. Survival of children with trisomy 13 and trisomy 18: A multi-state population-based study. *Am J Med Genet A*. 2016;170A(4):825-837.

80. Nelson KE, Rosella LC, Mahant S, Guttmann A. Survival and Surgical Interventions for Children With Trisomy 13 and 18. *Jama*. 2016;316(4):420-428.

81. Lantos JD. Trisomy 13 and 18--Treatment Decisions in a Stable Gray Zone. *Jama*. 2016;316(4):396-398.

82. Benitz WE. Patent Ductus Arteriosus. In: Martin RJ, Fanaroff AA, Walsh MC, eds. *Fanaroff and Martin's Neonatal-Perinatal Medicine: Diseases of the Fetus and Infant*. 10 ed. Philadelphia: Elsevier Saunders; 2015:1223-1229.

83. Clyman RI. Mechanisms Regulating Closure of the Ductus Arteriosus. In: Polin RA, Fox WW, Abman SH, eds. *Fetal and Neonatal Physiology*. 4 ed. Philadelphia: Elsevier Saunders; 2011:821-825.

84. Zaidi AN, Daniels CJ. The Adolescent and Adult with Congenital Heart Disease. In: Allen HD, Shaddy RE, Penny DJ, Feltes TF, Cetta F, eds. *Moss and Adams' Heart Disease in Infants, Children, and Adolescents*. 9 ed. Philadelphia: Wolters Kluwer; 2016:1559-1599.

85. Davenport ML. Turner Syndrome. In: Cassidy SB, Allanson JE, eds. *Management of Genetic Syndromes*. 3 ed. Hoboken NJ: John Wiley & Sons; 2010:847-869.

86. Ravenswaaij-Arts CM, Hefner M, Blake K, Martin DM. GeneReviews. *CHD7 Disorder* 2006-2020; https://www.ncbi.nlm.nih.gov/books/NBK1117/. Accessed 02/21/2021.

87. Wong MT, Scholvinck EH, Lambeck AJ, van Ravenswaaij-Arts CM. CHARGE syndrome: a review of the immunological aspects. *Eur J Hum Genet*. 2015;23(11):1451-1459.

88. Jyonouchi S, McDonald-McGinn DM, Bale S, Zackai EH, Sullivan KE. CHARGE (coloboma, heart defect, atresia choanae, retarded growth and development, genital hypoplasia, ear anomalies/deafness) syndrome and chromosome 22q11.2 deletion syndrome: a comparison of immunologic and nonimmunologic phenotypic features. *Pediatrics*. 2009;123(5):e871-877.

89. Janssen N, Bergman JE, Swertz MA, et al. Mutation update on the CHD7 gene involved in CHARGE syndrome. *Hum Mutat*. 2012;33(8):1149-1160.

90. Corsten-Janssen N, Kerstjens-Frederikse WS, du Marchie Sarvaas GJ, et al. The cardiac phenotype in patients with a CHD7 mutation. *Circ Cardiovasc Genet*. 2013;6(3):248-254.

91. Corsten-Janssen N, Scambler PJ. Clinical and molecular effects of CHD7 in the heart. *Am J Med Genet C Semin Med Genet*. 2017;175(4):487-495

92. Blake KD, Hudson AS. Gastrointestinal and feeding difficulties in CHARGE syndrome: A review from head-to-toe. *Am J Med Genet C Semin Med Genet*. 2017;175C:496–506.

93. Martin DM, Oley CA, Van Ravenswaaij-Arts CM. Charge Syndrome. In: Carey JC, Battaglia A, Viskochil D, Cassidy SB, eds. *Cassidy and Allanson's Management of Genetic Syndromes*. Hoboken, NJ: John Wiley & Sons; 2021:157-170.

94. Jones KL, Jones MC, Del Campo M. Miscellaneous Associations. *Smith's Recognizable Patterns of Human Malformation*. 7 ed. Philadelphia, PA: Elsevier Saunders; 2013:850-855.

95. Solomon BD, Pineda-Alvarez DE, Raam MS, Cummings DA. Evidence for inheritance in patients with VACTERL association. *Hum Genet*. 2010;127(6):731-733.

96. England RJ, Eradi B, Murthi GV, Sutcliffe J. Improving the rigour of VACTERL screening for neonates with anorectal malformations. *Pediatr Surg Int*. 2017;33(7):747-754.

97. Solomon BD, Baker LA, Bear KA, et al. An approach to the identification of anomalies and etiologies in neonates with identified or suspected VACTERL (vertebral defects, anal atresia, tracheo-esophageal fistula with esophageal atresia, cardiac anomalies, renal anomalies, and limb anomalies) association. *J Pediatr*. 2014;164(3):451-457.

98. Hall BD. Vater/Vacterl Association. In: Cassidy SB, Allanson JE, eds. *Management of Genetic Syndromes*. 3 ed. Hoboken NJ: John Wiley & Sons; 2010:871-879.

99. Solomon BD. VACTERL/VATER Association. *Orphanet J Rare Dis*. 2011;6:56.

100. Jones KL, Jones MC, Del Campo M. Facial-Limb Defects as Major Feature. *Smith's Recognizable Patterns of Human Malformation*. 7 ed. Philadelphia, PA: Elsevier Saunders; 2013:342-396.

101. Gardner RM, Sutherland GR, Shaffer LG. Structural Rearrangements. *Chromosome Abnormalities and Genetic Counseling*. 4 ed. New York, NY: Oxford University Press; 2012:295-332.

102. Botto LD, May K, Fernhoff PM, et al. A population-based study of the 22q11.2 deletion: phenotype, incidence, and contribution to major birth defects in the population. *Pediatrics*. 2003;112(1 Pt 1):101-107.

103. McDonald McGinn DM, Kohut T, H ZE. Deletion 22q11.2 (Velo-cardio-facial syndrome/DiGeorge syndrome). In: Cassidy SB, Allanson JE, eds. *Management of Genetic Syndromes*. 3 ed. Hoboken NJ: John Wiley & Sons, Inc.; 2010:263-284.

104. Swillen A, McDonald-McGinn D. Developmental trajectories in 22q11.2 deletion. *Am J Med Genet C Semin Med Genet*. 2015;169(2):172-181.

105. Lacour-Gayet F, Bove EL, Hraska V, Morell VO, Spray TL. *Surgery of Conotruncal Anomalies.* Switzerland: Springer; 2016.

106. Sadler TW. Head and Neck. *Langman's Medical Embryology.* 13 ed. Philadelphia: Wolters Kluwer; 2015:278-305.

107. Physical Examination. In: Park MK, Salamat M, eds. *Park's Pediatric Cardiology for Practitioners.* 7 ed. Philadelphia: Elsevier; 2021:6-30.

108. Cassidy S, Allen H, Phillips J, Kyle W. History and Physical Examination. In: Allen HD, Shaddy RE, Penny DJ, Feltes TF, Cetta F, eds. *Moss and Adams' Heart Disease in Infants, Children, and Adolescents.* 9 ed. Philadelphia: Wolters Kluwer; 2016:249-259.

109. Keszler M, Abubakar MK. Physiologic Principles. In: Goldsmith JP, Karotkin EH, Siede BL, eds. *Assisted Ventilation of the Neonate.* 5 ed. St. Louis: Elsevier Saunders; 2011:19-46.

110. Steinhorn RH, Abman SH. Persistent Pulmonary Hypertension. In: Gleason CA, Juul SE, eds. *Avery's Diseases of the Newborn.* 10 ed. Philadelphia PA: Elsevier; 2018:768-778.

111. Ewer AK, Middleton LJ, Furmston AT, et al. Pulse oximetry screening for congenital heart defects in newborn infants (PulseOx): a test accuracy study. *Lancet.* 2011;378(9793): 785-794.

112. Smith AE, Vedder TG, Hunter PK, Carr MR, Studer MA. The use of newborn screening pulse oximetry to detect cyanotic congenital heart disease: a survey of current practice at Army, Navy, and Air Force hospitals. *Mil Med.* 2011;176(3):343-346.

113. de-Wahl Granelli A, Wennergren M, Sandberg K, et al. Impact of pulse oximetry screening on the detection of duct dependent congenital heart disease: a Swedish prospective screening study in 39,821 newborns. *BMJ.* 2009;338:a3037.

114. Mellander M, Sunnegardh J. Failure to diagnose critical heart malformations in newborns before discharge--an increasing problem? *Acta Paediatr.* 2006;95(4):407-413.

115. Riede FT, Worner C, Dahnert I, Mockel A, Kostelka M, Schneider P. Effectiveness of neonatal pulse oximetry screening for detection of critical congenital heart disease in daily clinical routine--results from a prospective multicenter study. *Eur J Pediatr.* 2010;169(8):975-981.

116. Kemper AR, Mahle WT, Martin GR, et al. Strategies for implementing screening for critical congenital heart disease. *Pediatrics.* 2011;128(5):e1259-1267.

117. Mahle WT, Newburger JW, Matherne GP, et al. Role of pulse oximetry in examining newborns for congenital heart disease: a scientific statement from the American Heart Association and American Academy of Pediatrics. *Circulation.* 2009;120(5): 447-458.

118. Congestive Heart Failure. In: Park MK, Salamat M, eds. *Park's Pediatric Cardiology for Practitioners.* 7 ed. Philadelphia PA: Elsevier; 2021:346-356.

119. Cannon B, Snyder C. Disorders of Cardiac Rhythm and Conduction. In: Allen HD, Shaddy RE, Penny DJ, Feltes TF, Cetta F, eds. *Moss and Adams' Heart Disease in Infants, Children, and Adolescents.* 9 ed. Philadelphia: Wolters Kluwer; 2016:623-654.

120. Bernstein D. History and Physical Examination. In: Kliegman R, Stanton B, St. Geme III J, Schor N, Behrman R, eds. *Nelson Textbook of Pediatrics.* 19 ed. Philadelphia: Elsevier Saunders; 2011:1529-1536.

121. Disturbances of Atrioventricular Conduction. In: Park MK, Salamat M, eds. *Park's Pediatric Cardiology for Practitioners.* 7 ed. Philadelphia PA: Elsevier; 2021:335-337.

122. Blickstein I, Hershkovich-Shporen C. Fetal Effects of Autoimmune Disease. In: Martin RJ, Fanaroff AA, Walsh MC, eds. *Fanaroff and Martin's Neonatal-Perinatal Medicine: Diseases of the Fetus and Infant.* 11 ed. Philadelphia: Elsevier; 2020:346-354.

123. Simmons PM, Magann EF. Immune and Nonimmune Hydrops Fetalis. In: Martin RJ, Fanaroff AA, Walsh MC, eds. *Fanaroff and Martin's Neonatal-Perinatal Medicine: Diseases of the Fetus and Infant.* 11 ed. Philadelphia: Elsevier; 2020:371-385.

124. Cannon B, Snyder C. Disorders of Cardiac Rhythm and Conduction in Newborns. In: Martin RJ, Fanaroff AA, Walsh MC, eds. *Fanaroff and Martin's Neonatal-Perinatal Medicine: Diseases of the Fetus and Infant.* 11 ed. Philadelphia: Elsevier; 2020: 1375-1392.

125. AHA. Part 8: Recognition of Shock. In: Samson RA, Schexnayder SM, Hazinski MF, et al., eds. *Pediatric Advanced Life Support Provider Manual.* Dallas: American Heart Association; 2016: 171-195.

126. AHA. Part 11 Management of Arrhythmias. In: Samson RA, Schexnayder SM, Hazinski MF, Meeks R, Knight LJ, eds. *Pediatric Advanced Life Support Provider Manual.* Dallas: American Heart Association; 2016:253-275.

127. Morelli J. Diseases of Subcutaneous Tissue. In: Kliegman R, Stanton B, St. Geme III J, Schor N, Behrman R, eds. *Nelson Textbook of Pediatrics.* 19 ed. Philadelphia: Elsevier Saunders; 2011:2282-2284.

128. Craig JE, Scholz TA, Vanderhooft SL, Etheridge SP. Fat necrosis after ice application for supraventricular tachycardia termination. *J Pediatr.* 1998;133(6):727.

129. APA. *American Pharmacists Association Lexicomp Pediatric & Neonatal Dosage Handbook with International Trade Names Index.* 24 ed. Philadelphia: Wolters Kluwer; 2018.

130. Seri I, Markovitz B. Cardiovascular Compromise in the Newborn Infant. In: Gleason CA, Devaskar SU, eds. *Avery's Diseases of the Newborn.* 9th ed. Philadelphia: Elsevier Saunders; 2012:714-731.

131. Agrawal PB. Shock. In: Cloherty JP, Eichenwald EC, Hansen AR, Stark AR, eds. *Manual of Neonatal Care.* 7th ed. Philadelphia: Lippincott, Williams & Wilkins; 2012:463-468.

132. Turner DA, Cheifetz IM. Shock. In: Kliegman RM, Stanton BF, St. Geme JW, Schor NF, Behrman RE, eds. *Nelson Textbook of Pediatrics.* 19th ed. Philadelphia: Elsevier Saunders; 2011: 305-314.

133. Noori S, Friedlich PS, Seri I. Pathophysiology of Shock in the Fetus and Neonate. In: Polin RA, Fox WW, Abman SH, eds. *Fetal and Neonatal Physiology.* 4 ed. Philadelphia: Elsevier Saunders; 2011:853-863.

134. Carcillo JA, Kuch BA, Han YY, et al. Mortality and functional morbidity after use of PALS/APLS by community physicians. *Pediatrics.* 2009;124(2):500-508.

135. Engle WD. Definition of Normal Blood Pressure Range: The Elusive Target. In: Kleinman CS, Seri I, Polin RA, eds. *Hemodynamics and Cardiology: Neonatology Questions and Controversies.* 2 ed. Philadelphia: Elsevier Saunders; 2012:49-77.

136. Vargo L. Cardiovascular Assessment. In: Tappero EP, Honeyfield ME, eds. *Physical Assessment of the Newborn.* 5 ed: NICU Ink; 2015:93-110.

137. Dionne JM, Bremner SA, Baygani SK, et al. Method of Blood Pressure Measurement in Neonates and Infants: A Systematic Review and Analysis. *J Pediatr.* 2020;221:23-31.e5.

References

138. Dionne JM, Abitbol CL, Flynn JT. Hypertension in infancy: diagnosis, management and outcome. *Pediatr Nephrol.* 2012;27(1):17-32.

139. Zubrow AB, Hulman S, Kushner H, Falkner B. Determinants of blood pressure in infants admitted to neonatal intensive care units: a prospective multicenter study. Philadelphia Neonatal Blood Pressure Study Group. *J Perinatol.* 1995;15(6):470-479.

140. Versmold HT, Kitterman JA, Phibbs RH, Gregory GA, Tooley WH. Aortic blood pressure during the first 12 hours of life in infants with birth weight 610 to 4,220 grams. *Pediatrics.* 1981;67(5):607-613.

141. Kitterman JA, Phibbs RH, Tooley WH. Aortic blood pressure in normal newborn infants during the first 12 hours of life. *Pediatrics.* 1969;44(6):959-968.

142. Johnson GL. Clinical Examination. In: Long WA, Tooley WH, McNamara DG, eds. *Fetal and Neonatal Cardiology.* Philadelphia: W.B. Saunders Company; 1990:223-235.

143. Bernstein D. Acyanotic Congenital Heart Disease: The Left-to-Right Shunt Lesions. In: Kliegman RM, Stanton BF, St. Geme JW, Schor NF, Behrman RE, eds. *Nelson Textbook of Pediatrics.* 19th ed. Philadelphia: Elsevier Saunders; 2011:1551-1561.

144. Johnson WH. Diagnostic Methods. In: Johnson WH, Moller JH, eds. *Pediatric Cardiology.* Philadelphia: Lippincott, Williams, & Wilkins; 2001:1-55.

145. Lennox EG. Cardiology. In: Tschudy MM, Arcara KM, eds. *The Harriet Lane Handbook.* 19 ed. Philadelphia: Elsevier Mosby; 2012:154-200.

146. Lissauer T. Physical Examination of the Newborn. In: Martin RJ, Fanaroff AA, Walsh MC, eds. *Fanaroff and Martin's Neonatal-Perinatal Medicine: Diseases of the Fetus and Infant.* 10 ed. Philadelphia: Elsevier Saunders; 2015:391-406.

147. Dasnadi S, Aliaga S, Laughon M, Warner DD, Price WA. Factors Influencing the Accuracy of Noninvasive Blood Pressure Measurements in NICU Infants. *Am J Perinatol.* 2015;32(7):639-644.

148. Chock VY, Wong RJ, Hintz SR, Stevenson DK. Biomedical Engineering Aspects of Neonatal Monitoring. In: Martin RJ, Fanaroff AA, Walsh MC, eds. *Fanaroff and Martin's Neonatal-Perinatal Medicine: Diseases of the Fetus and Infant.* 9 ed. St. Louis: Elsevier Mosby; 2011:577-595.

149. Park MK, Lee DH. Normative arm and calf blood pressure values in the newborn. *Pediatrics.* 1989;83(2):240-243.

150. Patankar N, Fernandes N, Kumar K, Manja V, Lakshminrusimha S. Does measurement of four-limb blood pressures at birth improve detection of aortic arch anomalies? *J Perinatol.* 2016;36(5):376-380.

151. Crossland DS, Furness JC, Abu-Harb M, Sadagopan SN, Wren C. Variability of four limb blood pressure in normal neonates. *Arch Dis Child Fetal Neonatal Ed.* 2004;89(4):F325-327.

152. Friedlich P, Shin C, Stein J, Istvan S. Shock in the Surgical Neonate. In: Kleinman CS, Seri I, Polin RA, eds. *Hemodynamics and Cardiology: Neonatology Questions and Controversies.* 2 ed: Elsevier Health Sciences; 2012:311-319.

153. Walker V. Newborn Evaluation. In: Gleason CA, Juul SE, eds. *Avery's Diseases of the Newborn.* 10 ed. Philadelphia PA: Elsevier; 2018:289-311.

154. Phelps C, Shivapour J. Cardiovascular Problems of the Neonate. In: Martin RJ, Fanaroff AA, Walsh MC, eds. *Fanaroff and Martin's Neonatal-Perinatal Medicine: Diseases of the Fetus and Infant.* 11 ed. Philadelphia: Elsevier; 2020:1364-1373.

155. Miscellaneous Congenital Cardiac Conditions. In: Park MK, Salamat M, eds. *Park's Pediatric Cardiology for Practitioners.* 7 ed. Philadelphia PA: Elsevier; 2021:224-236.

156. Valvular Heart Disease. In: Park MK, Salamat M, eds. *Park's Pediatric Cardiology for Practitioners.* 7 ed. Philadelphia PA: Elsevier; 2021:288-296.

157. Osborn DA, Evans N, Kluckow M. Clinical detection of low upper body blood flow in very premature infants using blood pressure, capillary refill time, and central-peripheral temperature difference. *Arch Dis Child Fetal Neonatal Ed.* 2004;89(2):F168-173.

158. Strozik KS, Pieper CH, Roller J. Capillary refilling time in newborn babies: normal values. *Archives of disease in childhood Fetal and neonatal edition.* 1997;76(3):F193-196.

159. Strozik KS, Pieper CH, Cools F. Capillary refilling time in newborns--optimal pressing time, sites of testing and normal values. *Acta Paediatr.* 1998;87(3):310-312.

160. Chameides L. Part 2: Systematic Approach to the Seriously Ill or Injured Child. In: Chameides L, Samson RA, Schexnayder SM, Hazinski MF, eds. *Pediatric Advanced Life Support Provider Manual.* Dallas: American Heart Association; 2011:7-29.

161. Raju NV, Maisels MJ, Kring E, Schwarz-Warner L. Capillary refill time in the hands and feet of normal newborn infants. *Clin Pediatr (Phila).* 1999;38(3):139-144.

162. LeFlore JL, Engle WD. Capillary refill time is an unreliable indicator of cardiovascular status in term neonates. *Adv Neonatal Care.* 2005;5(3):147-154.

163. Lobos AT, Lee S, Menon K. Capillary refill time and cardiac output in children undergoing cardiac catheterization. *Pediatr Crit Care Med.* 2012;13(2):136-140.

164. Wodey E, Pladys P, Betremieux P, Kerebel C, Ecoffey C. Capillary refilling time and hemodynamics in neonates: a Doppler echocardiographic evaluation. *Crit Care Med.* 1998;26(8):1437-1440.

165. Gale C. Question 2. Is capillary refill time a useful marker of haemodynamic status in neonates? *Arch Dis Child.* 2010;95(5):395-397.

166. Johnson WH, Moller JH. Tools to Diagnose Cardiac Conditions in Children. In: Johnson WH, Moller JH, eds. *Pediatric Cardiology: The Essential Pocket Guide.* 3 ed: Wiley Blackwell; 2014:1-72.

167. Evans W. Chapter 1. Heart Murmurs. In: Evans W, Acherman R, Luna C, eds. *Simple & Easy Pediatric Cardiology.* Las Vegas: Childrens Heart Center Nevada Press; 2013:3-14.

168. Beerman LB, Kreutzer J, Allada V. Cardiology. In: Zitelli BJ, McIntire SC, Nowalk AJ, eds. *Zitelli and Davis' Atlas of Pediatric Physical Diagnosis.* 7 ed. Philadelphia: Elsevier; 2018:137-170.

169. Krishnamurthy G, Ratner V, Levasseur S, Rubenstein SD. Congenital Heart Disease in the Newborn Period. In: Polin RA, Yoder MC, eds. *Workbook in Practical Neonatology.* 5 ed. Philadelphia: Elsevier Saunders; 2015:244-269.

170. Cyanotic Congenital Heart Defects. In: Park MK, Salamat M, eds. *Park's Pediatric Cardiology for Practitioners.* 7 ed. Philadelphia PA: Elsevier; 2021:160-223.

171. Anyane-Yeboa K, Gupta P. Genetics of Congenital Heart Disease. In: Kleinman CS, Seri I, Polin RA, eds. *Hemodynamics and Cardiology: Neonatology Questions and Controversies.* 2 ed. Philadelphia: Elsevier Saunders; 2012:363-374.

172. O'Leary PW, Qureshi MY, Hagler DJ. Cardiac Malpositions and Abnormalities of Atrial and Visceral Situs. In: Allen HD, Shaddy RE, Penny DJ, Feltes TF, Cetta F, eds. *Moss and Adams' Heart Disease in Infants, Children, and Adolescents*. 9 ed. Philadelphia: Wolters Kluwer; 2016:1237-1261.

173. Maleszewski JJ, Edwards WD. Classification and Terminology of Cardiovascular Anomalies. In: Allen HD, Shaddy RE, Penny DJ, Feltes TF, Cetta F, eds. *Moss and Adams' Heart Disease in Infants, Children, and Adolescents*. 9 ed. Philadelphia: Wolters Kluwer; 2016:213-234.

174. Bernstein D. Abnormal Positions of the Heart and Heterotaxy Syndromes (Asplenia, Polysplenia). In: Kliegman R, Stanton B, St. Geme III J, Schor N, Behrman R, eds. *Nelson Textbook of Pediatrics*. 19 ed. Philadelphia: Elsevier Saunders; 2011: 1595-1596.

175. Hill SJ, Heiss KF, Mittal R, et al. Heterotaxy syndrome and malrotation: does isomerism influence risk and decision to treat. *Jnl Pediatric Surg*. 2014;49(6):934-937.

176. Berlin S. Diagnostic Imaging of the Neonate. In: Martin RJ, Fanaroff AA, Walsh MC, eds. *Fanaroff and Martin's Neonatal-Perinatal Medicine: Diseases of the Fetus and Infant*. 11 ed. Philadelphia: Elsevier; 2020:608-633.

177. Chest Radiography. In: Park MK, Salamat M, eds. *Park's Pediatric Cardiology for Practitioners*. 7 ed. Philadelphia: Elsevier; 2021:50-55.

178. Maleszewski JJ, Edwards WD. Cardiac Anatomy and Examination of Cardiac Specimens. In: Allen HD, Shaddy RE, Penny DJ, Feltes TF, Cetta F, eds. *Moss and Adams' Heart Disease in Infants, Children, and Adolescents*. 9 ed. Philadelphia: Wolters Kluwer; 2016:181-212.

179. Noninvasive Imaging Tools. In: Park MK, Salamat M, eds. *Park's Pediatric Cardiology for Practitioners*. 7 ed. Philadelphia PA: Elsevier; 2021:58-73.

180. Clyman RI. Patent Ductus Arteriosus in the Preterm Infant. In: Gleason CA, Juul SE, eds. *Avery's Diseases of the Newborn*. 10 ed. Philadelphia PA: Elsevier; 2018:790-800.

181. Artman M, Mahony L, Teitel DF. Chapter 12. Cardiovascular Drug Therapy. *Neonatal Cardiology*. 3 ed. New York: McGraw Hill Education; 2017:235-254.

182. Artman M, Mahony L, Teitel DF. Chapter 5. Initial Evaluation of the Newborn with Suspected Cardiovascular Disease. *Neonatal Cardiology*. 3 ed. New York: McGraw Hill Education; 2017:67-80.

183. Estes K, Nowicki M, Bishop P. Cortical hyperostosis secondary to prostaglandin E1 therapy. *J Pediatr*. 2007;151(4):441, 441.e1.

184. Woo K, Emery J, Peabody J. Cortical hyperostosis: a complication of prolonged prostaglandin infusion in infants awaiting cardiac transplantation. *Pediatrics*. 1994;93(3):417-420.

185. Obstructive Lesions. In: Park MK, Salamat M, eds. *Park's Pediatric Cardiology for Practitioners*. 7 ed. Philadelphia PA: Elsevier; 2021:143-159.

186. Ashwath R, Snyder CS. Congenital Defects of the Cardiovascular System. In: Martin RJ, Fanaroff AA, Walsh MC, eds. *Fanaroff and Martin's Neonatal-Perinatal Medicine: Diseases of the Fetus and Infant*. 10 ed. Philadelphia: Elsevier Saunders; 2015:1230-1249.

187. Artman M, Mahony L, Teitel DF. Chapter 8. Approach to the Infant with Inadequate Systemic Perfusion. *Neonatal Cardiology*. 3 ed. New York: McGraw Hill Education; 2017:137-153.

188. Basu SK, Dobrolet NC. Congenital Defects of the Cardiovascular System. In: Martin RJ, Fanaroff AA, Walsh MC, eds. *Fanaroff and Martin's Neonatal-Perinatal Medicine: Diseases of the Fetus and Infant*. 11 ed. Philadelphia: Elsevier; 2020:1342-1363.

189. Ezon DS, Penny DJ. Aortic Arch and Vascular Anomalies. In: Allen HD, Shaddy RE, Penny DJ, Feltes TF, Cetta F, eds. *Moss and Adams' Heart Disease in Infants, Children, and Adolescents*. 9 ed. Philadelphia: Wolters Kluwer; 2016:833-870.

190. Tweddell JS, Hoffman, G.M., Ghanayem, N.S., Frommelt, M.A., Mussatto, K.A. & Berger, S. . Hypoplastic Left Heart Syndrome. In: Allen HD, Shaddy RE, Penny DJ, Feltes TF, Cetta F, eds. *Moss and Adams' Heart Disease in Infants, Children, and Adolescents*. 9 ed. Philadelphia: Wolters Kluwer; 2016:1125-1161.

191. Friedland-Little JM, Zampi JD, Gajarski RJ. Aortic Stenosis. In: Allen HD, Shaddy RE, Penny DJ, Feltes TF, Cetta F, eds. *Moss and Adams' Heart Disease in Infants, Children, and Adolescents*. 9 ed. Philadelphia: Wolters Kluwer; 2016:1085-1105.

192. Evans W, Acherman R. Chapter 19. Cardiovascular Malformations. In: Evans W, Acherman R, Luna C, eds. *Simple & Easy Pediatric Cardiology*. Las Vegas: Childrens Heart Center Nevada Press; 2013:241-304.

193. Dorfman AT, Marino BS, Wernovsky G, et al. Critical heart disease in the neonate: presentation and outcome at a tertiary care center. *Pediatr Crit Care Med*. 2008;9(2):193-202.

194. Bernstein D. Cyanotic Congenital Heart Disease: Lesions Associated with Decreased Pulmonary Blood Flow. In: Kliegman R, Stanton B, St. Geme III J, Schor N, Behrman R, eds. *Nelson Textbook of Pediatrics*. 19 ed. Philadelphia: Elsevier Saunders; 2011:1573-1584.

195. Johnson WH, Moller JH. Chapter 6. Congenital Heart Disease with a Right-to-Left Shunt in Children. In: Johnson WH, Moller JH, eds. *Pediatric Cardiology: The Essential Pocket Guide*. 3 ed: Wiley Blackwell; 2014:186-232.

196. Roche SL, Greenway SC, Redington AN. Tetralogy of Fallot with Pulmonary Stenosis, Pulmonary Atresia, and Absent Pulmonary Valve. In: Allen HD, Shaddy RE, Penny DJ, Feltes TF, Cetta F, eds. *Moss and Adams' Heart Disease in Infants, Children, and Adolescents*. 9 ed. Philadelphia: Wolters Kluwer; 2016: 1029-1052.

197. Tsze DS, Vitberg YM, Berezow J, Starc TJ, Dayan PS. Treatment of tetralogy of Fallot hypoxic spell with intranasal fentanyl. *Pediatrics*. 2014;134(1):e266-269.

198. Hegenbarth MA, American Academy of Pediatrics Committee on D. Preparing for pediatric emergencies: drugs to consider. *Pediatrics*. 2008;121(2):433-443.

199. Wolfe TR, Braude DA. Intranasal medication delivery for children: a brief review and update. *Pediatrics*. 2010;126(3):532-537.

200. Bocks ML, Boe BA, Galantowicz ME. Neonatal Management of Congenital Heart Disease. In: Martin RJ, Fanaroff AA, Walsh MC, eds. *Fanaroff and Martin's Neonatal-Perinatal Medicine: Diseases of the Fetus and Infant*. 11 ed. Philadelphia: Elsevier; 2020:1393-1414.

201. Rao PS. Management of Congenital Heart Disease: State of the Art-Part II-Cyanotic Heart Defects. *Children (Basel)*. 2019;6(4):54. doi: 10.3390/children6040054.

202. Montero JV, Nieto EM, Vallejo IR, Montero SV. Intranasal midazolam for the emergency management of hypercyanotic spells in tetralogy of Fallot. *Pediatr Emerg Care*. 2015;31(4):269-271.

203. Artman M, Mahony L, Teitel DF. Chapter 6. Approach to the Cyanotic Infant. *Neonatal Cardiology*. 3 ed. New York: McGraw Hill Education; 2017:81-110.

204. Wright GE, Maeda K, Silverman NH, Hanley FL, Roth SJ. Double-Outlet Right Ventricle. In: Allen HD, Shaddy RE, Penny DJ, Feltes TF, Cetta F, eds. *Moss and Adams' Heart Disease in Infants, Children, and Adolescents*. 9 ed. Philadelphia: Wolters Kluwer; 2016:1201-1215.

References

205. Walters HLI, Mavroudis C. Double-Outlet Ventricles. In: Mavroudis C, Backer CL, eds. *Pediatric Cardiac Surgery*. 4 ed. Oxford: Wiley-Blackwell; 2013:457-491.

206. Bernstein D. Double-Outlet Right Ventricle. In: Kliegman R, Stanton B, St. Geme III J, Schor N, Behrman R, eds. *Nelson Textbook of Pediatrics*. 19 ed. Philadelphia: Elsevier Saunders; 2011:1582.

207. Lopez L, Geva T. Double-Outlet Ventricle. In: Lai WW, Mertens LL, Cohen MS, Geva T, eds. *Echocardiography in Pediatric and Congenital Heart Disease: From Fetus to Adult*. 2 ed. Chichester, West Sussex, UK: John Wiley & Sons, Ltd.; 2016:466-488.

208. Cetta F, Dearani JA, O'Leary PW, Driscoll DJ. Tricuspid Valve Disorders: Atresia, Dysplasia, and Ebstein Anomaly. In: Allen HD, Shaddy RE, Penny DJ, Feltes TF, Cetta F, eds. *Moss and Adams' Heart Disease in Infants, Children, and Adolescents*. 9 ed. Philadelphia: Wolters Kluwer; 2016:949-981.

209. Sanders SP. Hearts with Functionally One Ventricle. In: Lai WW, Mertens LL, Cohen MS, Geva T, eds. *Echocardiography in Pediatric and Congenital Heart Disease: From Fetus to Adult*. 2 ed. Chichester, West Sussex, UK: John Wiley & Sons, Ltd.; 2016: 511-540.

210. Cabalka AK, Edwards WD, Dearani JA. Truncus Arteriosus. In: Allen HD, Shaddy RE, Penny DJ, Feltes TF, Cetta F, eds. *Moss and Adams' Heart Disease in Infants, Children, and Adolescents*. 9 ed. Philadelphia: Wolters Kluwer; 2016:1053-1064.

211. Mavroudis C. Chapter 10. Truncus Arteriosus. In: Mavroudis C, Backer CL, eds. *Atlas of Pediatric Cardiac Surgery*. London: Springer; 2015:131-143.

212. Slesnick TC, Sachdeva R, Kreeger JR, Border WL. Truncus Arteriosus and Aortopulmonary Window. In: Lai WW, Mertens LL, Cohen MS, Geva T, eds. *Echocardiography in Pediatric and Congenital Heart Disease: From Fetus to Adult*. 2 ed. Chichester, West Sussex, UK: John Wiley & Sons, Ltd.; 2016:433-445.

213. Brown DW, Geva T. Anomalies of the Pulmonary Veins. In: Allen HD, Shaddy RE, Penny DJ, Feltes TF, Cetta F, eds. *Moss and Adams' Heart Disease in Infants, Children, and Adolescents*. 9 ed. Philadelphia: Wolters Kluwer; 2016:881-909.

214. Epelman M. Partial and Total Anomalous Pulmonary Venous Connections. In: Yoo S-J, MacDonald C, Babyn P, eds. *Chest Radiographic Interpretation in Pediatric Cardiac Patients*. New York: Thieme Medical Publishers, Inc.; 2010:206-214.

215. Domadia S, Kumar SR, Votava-Smith JK, Pruetz JD. Neonatal Outcomes in Total Anomalous Pulmonary Venous Return: The Role of Prenatal Diagnosis and Pulmonary Venous Obstruction. *Pediatr Cardiol*. 2018;39(7):1346-1354.

216. Seale AN, Uemura H, Webber SA, et al. Total anomalous pulmonary venous connection: morphology and outcome from an international population-based study. *Circulation*. 2010;122(25):2718-2726.

217. Cetta F, Eidem BW. Ebstein Anomaly, Tricuspid Valve Dysplasia, and Right Atrial Anomalies. In: Lai WW, Mertens LL, Cohen MS, Geva T, eds. *Echocardiography in Pediatric and Congenital Heart Disease: From Fetus to Adult*. 2 ed. Chichester, West Sussex, UK: John Wiley & Sons, Ltd.; 2016:231-242.

218. Nykanen DG. Pulmonary Atresia and Intact Ventricular Septum. In: Allen HD, Shaddy RE, Penny DJ, Feltes TF, Cetta F, eds. *Moss and Adams' Heart Disease in Infants, Children, and Adolescents*. 9 ed. Philadelphia: Wolters Kluwer; 2016:1009-1028.

219. Shahanavaz S, Hijazi ZM, Hellenbrand WE, Vincent JA. Catheter-Based Therapy in the Neonate with Congenital Heart Disease. In: Kleinman CS, Seri I, Polin RA, eds. *Hemodynamics and Cardiology: Neonatology Questions and Controversies*. 2 ed. Philadelphia: Elsevier Saunders; 2012:503-520.

220. Holzer RJ, Gauvreau K, Kreutzer J, et al. Safety and efficacy of balloon pulmonary valvuloplasty: a multicenter experience. *Catheter Cardiovasc Interv*. 2012;80(4):663-672.

221. Shi-Joon Y, Caldarone CA. Glossary of Pediatric Cardiovascular Surgical Procedures. In: Yoo S-J, MacDonald C, Babyn P, eds. *Chest Radiographic Interpretation in Pediatric Cardiac Patients*. New York: Thieme Medical Publishers, Inc.; 2010:41-54.

222. Kellenberger CJ. Tetralogy of Fallot and Related Conditions. In: Yoo S-J, MacDonald C, Babyn P, eds. *Chest Radiographic Interpretation in Pediatric Cardiac Patients*. New York: Thieme Medical Publishers, Inc.; 2010:193-202.

223. Bernstein D. Tetralogy of Fallot with Pulmonary Atresia. In: Kliegman R, Stanton B, St. Geme III J, Schor N, Behrman R, eds. *Nelson Textbook of Pediatrics*. 19 ed. Philadelphia: Elsevier Saunders; 2011:1578.

224. Morris SA, Maskatia SA, Altman CA, Ayres NA. Fetal and Perinatal Cardiology. In: Allen HD, Shaddy RE, Penny DJ, Feltes TF, Cetta F, eds. *Moss and Adams' Heart Disease in Infants, Children, and Adolescents*. 9 ed. Philadelphia: Wolters Kluwer; 2016:137-180.

225. Sana MK, Ahmed Z. Pulmonary Atresia With Ventricular Septal Defect. *StatPearls*. Treasure Island (FL)2020.

226. Qureshi AM, Justino H, Heinle JS. Transposition of the Great Arteries. In: Allen HD, Shaddy RE, Penny DJ, Feltes TF, Cetta F, eds. *Moss and Adams' Heart Disease in Infants, Children, and Adolescents*. 9 ed. Philadelphia: Wolters Kluwer; 2016: 1163-1185.

227. Roman KS. Transpositions of the Great Arteries. In: Yoo S-J, MacDonald C, Babyn P, eds. *Chest Radiographic Interpretation in Pediatric Cardiac Patients*. New York: Thieme Medical Publishers, Inc.; 2010:234-240.

228. Hornung TS, Calder L. Congenitally corrected transposition of the great arteries. *Heart*. 2010;96(14):1154-1161.

229. Gessner IH, Weber HS, Windle ML, Allen HD. Ventricular Inversion. 2015; https://emedicine.medscape.com/article/892856-overview. Accessed August 3, 2020.

230. Karlsen KA. *The S.T.A.B.L.E. Program: Post-Resuscitation / Pre-Transport Stabilization Care of Sick Infants*. 6 ed. Salt Lake City: S.T.A.B.L.E., Inc.; 2013.

231. Ward Platt M, Deshpande S. Metabolic adaptation at birth. *Seminars in fetal & neonatal medicine*. 2005;10(4):341-350.

232. Cowett RM, Farrag HM. Selected principles of perinatal-neonatal glucose metabolism. *Semin Neonatol*. 2004;9(1):37-47.

233. McGowan JE, Rozance PJ, Price-Douglas W, Hay WW. Glucose Homeostasis. In: Gardner SL, Carter BS, Enzman-Hines M, Hernandez JA, eds. *Merenstein & Gardner's Handbook of Neonatal Intensive Care*. 7th ed. St. Louis: Mosby Elsevier; 2011:353-377.

234. Philipps AF. Oxygen Consumption and General Carbohydrate Metabolism of the Fetus. In: Polin RA, Fox WW, Abman SH, eds. *Fetal and Neonatal Physiology*. 4 ed. Philadelphia: Elsevier Saunders; 2011:535-549.

235. Werny D, Taplin C, Bennett JT, Pihoker C. Disorders of Carbohydrate Metabolism. In: Gleason CA, Juul SE, eds. *Avery's Diseases of the Newborn*. 10 ed. Philadelphia PA: Elsevier; 2018:1403-1416.

236. Hay Jr WW, Raju TNK, Higgins RD, Kalhan SC, Devaskar SU. Knowledge Gaps and Research Needs for Understanding and Treating Neonatal Hypoglycemia: Workshop Report from Eunice Kennedy Shriver National Institute of Child Health and Human Development. *The Journal of Pediatrics.* 2009;155(5):612-617.

237. Koh TH, Eyre JA, Aynsley-Green A. Neonatal hypoglycaemia--the controversy regarding definition. *Arch Dis Child.* 1988;63(11):1386-1388.

238. Katz LL, Stanley CA. Disorders of Glucose and Other Sugars. In: Spitzer AR, ed. *Intensive Care of the Fetus & Neonate.* 2 ed. Philiadelphia: Elsevier Mosby; 2005:1167-1178.

239. Wilker RE. Hypoglycemia and Hyperglycemia. In: Cloherty JP, Eichenwald E, C., Hansen AR, Stark AR, eds. *Manual of Neonatal Care.* 7 ed. Philadelphia: Lippincott, Williams & Wilkins; Wolters Kluwer; 2012:284-296.

240. Lilien LD, Pildes RS, Srinivasan G, Voora S, Yeh TF. Treatment of neonatal hypoglycemia with minibolus and intravenous glucose infusion. *The Journal of pediatrics.* 1980;97(2):295-298.

241. Seo S. Umbilical Vein Catheterization. In: Ramasethu J, Seo S, eds. *MacDonald's Atlas of Procedures in Neonatology.* 6 ed. Philadelphia: Wolters Kluwer; 2020:217-223.

242. Seo S. Umbilical Artery Catheterization. In: Ramasethu J, Seo S, eds. *MacDonald's Atlas of Procedures in Neonatology.* 6 ed. Philadelphia: Wolters Kluwer; 2020:199-216.

243. Stanley CA, Rozance PJ, Thornton PS, et al. Re-evaluating "transitional neonatal hypoglycemia": mechanism and implications for management. *J Pediatr.* 2015;166(6):1520-1525 e1521.

244. Thornton PS, Stanley CA, De Leon DD, et al. Recommendations from the Pediatric Endocrine Society for Evaluation and Management of Persistent Hypoglycemia in Neonates, Infants, and Children. *J Pediatr.* 2015;167(2):238-245.

245. Gomella TL. Arterial Access: Umbilical Artery Catheterization. In: Gomella TL, Cunningham MD, Eyal FG, Tuttle D, eds. *Neonatology: Management, Procedures, On-Call Problems, Diseases, and Drugs.* 6 ed. New York: McGraw Hill Medical; 2009:203-207.

246. Gomella TL. Arterial Access: Umbilical Vein Catheterization. In: Gomella TL, Cunningham MD, Eyal FG, Tuttle D, eds. *Neonatology: Management, Procedures, On-Call Problems, Diseases, and Drugs.* 6 ed. New York: McGraw Hill Medical; 2009:243-246.

247. Choi H-Y, Rivera A, Chahine AA. Central Venous Catheterization. In: Ramasethu J, Seo S, eds. *MacDonald's Atlas of Procedures in Neonatology.* 6 ed. Philadelphia: Wolters Kluwer; 2020:233-252.

248. Kaushal S, Ramasethu J. Peripheral Arterial Catheterization. In: Ramasethu J, Seo S, eds. *MacDonald's Atlas of Procedures in Neonatology.* 6 ed. Philadelphia: Wolters Kluwer; 2020:224-232.

249. Furdon SA, Horgan MJ, Bradshaw WT, Clark DA. Nurses' Guide to Early Detection of Umbilical Arterial Catheter Complications in Infants. *Advances in Neonatal Care: Official Journal of the National Association of Neonatal Nurses.* 2006(6):242-256.

250. Gupta R, Drendel AL, Hoffmann RG, Quijano CV, Uhing MR. Migration of Central Venous Catheters in Neonates: A Radiographic Assessment. *Am J Perinatol.* 2016;33(6):600-604.

251. Srinivasan HB, Tjin ATA, Galang R, Hecht A, Srinivasan G. Migration patterns of peripherally inserted central venous catheters at 24 hours postinsertion in neonates. *Am J Perinatol.* 2013;30(10):871-874.

252. Bashir RA, Callejas AM, Osiovich HC, Ting JY. Percutaneously Inserted Central Catheter-Related Pleural Effusion in a Level III Neonatal Intensive Care Unit: A 5-Year Review (2008-2012). *JPEN J Parenter Enteral Nutr.* 2017;41(7):1234-1239.

253. Sharpe EL. Neonatal peripherally inserted central catheter practices and their association with demographics, training, and radiographic monitoring: results from a national survey. *Adv Neonatal Care.* 2014;14(5):329-335.

254. Coit AK, Kamitsuka MD, Pediatrix Medical G. Peripherally inserted central catheter using the saphenous vein: importance of two-view radiographs to determine the tip location. *J Perinatol.* 2005;25(10):674-676.

255. Colacchio K, Deng Y, Northrup V, Bizzarro MJ. Complications associated with central and non-central venous catheters in a neonatal intensive care unit. *J Perinatol.* 2012;32(12):941-946.

256. Bradshaw WT, Furdon SA. A nurse's guide to early detection of umbilical venous catheter complications in infants. *Adv Neonatal Care.* 2006;6(3):127-138; quiz 139-141.

257. Schlesinger AE, Braverman RM, DiPietro MA. Pictorial essay. Neonates and umbilical venous catheters: normal appearance, anomalous positions, complications, and potential aid to diagnosis. *AJR Am J Roentgenol.* 2003;180(4):1147-1153.

258. Nash P. Umbilical catheters, placement, and complication management. *J Infus Nurs.* 2006;29(6):346-352.

259. Gorski LA, Hadaway L, Hagle ME, et al. Infusion Therapy Standards of Practice, 8th Edition. *J Infus Nurs.* 2021;44(1S Suppl 1):S1-S224.

260. AHA. Part 9: Management of Shock. In: Samson RA, Schexnayder SM, Hazinski MF, et al., eds. *Pediatric Advanced Life Support Provider Manual.* Dallas: American Heart Association; 2016:197-238.

261. Revenis ME, Soghier L. Intraosseous Infusions. In: Ramasethu J, Seo S, eds. *MacDonald's Atlas of Procedures in Neonatology.* 6 ed. Philadelphia: Wolters Kluwer; 2020:453-458.

262. Scrivens A, Reynolds PR, Emery FE, et al. Use of Intraosseous Needles in Neonates: A Systematic Review. *Neonatology.* 2019;116(4):305-314.

263. Philbeck TE. Pain Management with the Use of IO. *Journal of Emergency Medical Services.* 2010;9(35).

264. Laptook AR, Salhab W, Bhaskar B. Admission temperature of low birth weight infants: predictors and associated morbidities. *Pediatrics.* 2007;119(3):e643-649.

265. Sahni R, Schulze K. Temperature control in newborn infants. In: Polin RA, Fox WW, Abman SH, eds. *Fetal and Neonatal Physiology.* 4 ed. Philadelphia: Elsevier Saunders; 2011:624-648.

266. Durand DJ, Mickas NA. Blood Gases: Technical Aspects and Interpretation. In: Goldsmith JP, Karotkin EH, Siede BL, eds. *Assisted Ventilation of the Neonate.* 5th ed. St. Louis: Elsevier Saunders; 2011:292-305.

267. Blackburn ST. Respiratory System. In: Blackburn ST, ed. *Maternal, Fetal & Neonatal Physiology: A Clinical Perspective.* 3 ed. St. Louis: Saunders Elsevier; 2007:315-374.

268. Hall JE. Transport of Oxygen and Carbon Dioxide in Blood and Tissue Fluids. In: Hall JE, ed. *Guyton and Hall Textbook of Medical Physiology.* 12th ed. Philadelphia: Saunders Elsevier; 2011:495-504.

269. Hall JE. Respiratory Insufficiency - Pathophysiology, Diagnosis, Oxygen Therapy. In: Hall JE, ed. *Guyton and Hall Textbook of Medical Physiology.* 12 ed. Philadelphia: Saunders Elsevier; 2011:515-523.

References

270. Kulik TJ. Physiology of Congenital Heart Disease in the Neonate. In: Polin RA, Fox WW, Abman SH, eds. *Fetal and Neonatal Physiology*. 4 ed. Philadelphia: Elsevier Saunders; 2011:777-789.

271. Andropoulos DB, Shekerdemian LS, Checchia PA, Chang AC. Cardiovascular Intensive Care. In: Allen HD, Shaddy RE, Penny DJ, Feltes TF, Cetta F, eds. *Moss and Adams' Heart Disease in Infants, Children, and Adolescents*. 9 ed. Philadelphia: Wolters Kluwer; 2016:665-713.

272. Hoffman GM, Ghanayem NS, Scott JP, Tweddell JS, Mitchell ME, Mussatto KA. Postoperative Cerebral and Somatic Near-Infrared Spectroscopy Saturations and Outcome in Hypoplastic Left Heart Syndrome. *Ann Thorac Surg*. 2017;103(5):1527-1535.

273. Hoffman GM, Stuth EA, Jaquiss RD, et al. Changes in cerebral and somatic oxygenation during stage 1 palliation of hypoplastic left heart syndrome using continuous regional cerebral perfusion. *J Thorac Cardiovasc Surg*. 2004;127(1):223-233.

274. Rais-Bahrami K, Rivera O, Short BL. Validation of a noninvasive neonatal optical cerebral oximeter in veno-venous ECMO patients with a cephalad catheter. *J Perinatol*. 2006;26(10):628-635.

275. Kaufman J, Almodovar MC, Zuk J, Friesen RH. Correlation of abdominal site near-infrared spectroscopy with gastric tonometry in infants following surgery for congenital heart disease. *Pediatr Crit Care Med*. 2008;9(1):62-68.

276. Martini S, Corvaglia L. Splanchnic NIRS monitoring in neonatal care: rationale, current applications and future perspectives. *J Perinatol*. 2018;38(5):431-443.

277. Mintzer JP, Moore JE. Regional tissue oxygenation monitoring in the neonatal intensive care unit: evidence for clinical strategies and future directions. *Pediatr Res*. 2019;86(3):296-304.

278. Mahle WT, Martin GR, Beekman RH, 3rd, Morrow WR, Section on C, Cardiac Surgery Executive C. Endorsement of Health and Human Services recommendation for pulse oximetry screening for critical congenital heart disease. *Pediatrics*. 2012;129(1):190-192.

279. Kemper AR, Lam WKK, Bocchini JA, Jr. The Success of State Newborn Screening Policies for Critical Congenital Heart Disease. *Jama*. 2017;318(21):2087-2088.

280. Glidewell J, Grosse SD, Riehle-Colarusso T, et al. Actions in Support of Newborn Screening for Critical Congenital Heart Disease - United States, 2011-2018. *MMWR Morb Mortal Wkly Rep*. 2019;68(5):107-111.

281. Ewer AK, Furmston AT, Middleton LJ, et al. Pulse oximetry as a screening test for congenital heart defects in newborn infants: a test accuracy study with evaluation of acceptability and cost-effectiveness. *Health Technol Assess*. 2012;16(2):v-xiii, 1-184.

282. Manzoni P, Martin GR, Sanchez Luna M, et al. Pulse oximetry screening for critical congenital heart defects: a European consensus statement. *Lancet Child Adolesc Health*. 2017;1(2):88-90.

283. Wong KK, Fournier A, Fruitman DS, et al. Canadian Cardiovascular Society/Canadian Pediatric Cardiology Association Position Statement on Pulse Oximetry Screening in Newborns to Enhance Detection of Critical Congenital Heart Disease. *Can J Cardiol*. 2017;33(2):199-208.

284. Narayen IC, Te Pas AB, Blom NA, van den Akker-van Marle ME. Cost-effectiveness analysis of pulse oximetry screening for critical congenital heart defects following homebirth and early discharge. *Eur J Pediatr*. 2019;178(1):97-103.

285. Oster ME, Aucott SW, Glidewell J, et al. Lessons Learned From Newborn Screening for Critical Congenital Heart Defects. *Pediatrics*. 2016;137(5):e20154573.

286. Samuel TY, Bromiker R, Mimouni FB, et al. Newborn oxygen saturation at mild altitude versus sea level: implications for neonatal screening for critical congenital heart disease. *Acta Paediatr*. 2013;102(4):379-384.

287. Guo F, Tang S, Guo T, Bartell S, Detrano R. Revised threshold values for neonatal oxygen saturation at mild and moderate altitudes. *Acta Paediatr*. 2020;109(2):321-326.

288. (AAP) AAoP. Newborn Screening: Critical Congenital Heart Defects. 2020; https://www.aap.org/en-us/advocacy-and-policy/aap-health-initiatives/PEHDIC/Pages/Newborn-Screening-for-CCHD.aspx. Accessed June 10, 2020.

289. Liberman RF, Getz KD, Lin AE, et al. Delayed diagnosis of critical congenital heart defects: trends and associated factors. *Pediatrics*. 2014;134(2):e373-381.

290. Mahle WT, Newburger JW, Matherne GP, et al. Role of pulse oximetry in examining newborns for congenital heart disease: a scientific statement from the AHA and AAP. *Pediatrics*. 2009;124(2):823-836.

291. Meberg A, Brugmann-Pieper S, Due R, Jr., et al. First day of life pulse oximetry screening to detect congenital heart defects. *The Journal of pediatrics*. 2008;152(6):761-765.

292. Bhola K, Kluckow M, Evans N. Post-implementation review of pulse oximetry screening of well newborns in an Australian tertiary maternity hospital. *J Paediatr Child Health*. 2014;50(11):920-925.

293. CDC. Congenital Heart Defects Information for Healthcare Providers. 2020; https://www.cdc.gov/ncbddd/heartdefects/hcp.html. Accessed June 10, 2020.

294. Martin GR, Ewer AK, Gaviglio A, et al. Updated Strategies for Pulse Oximetry Screening for Critical Congenital Heart Disease. *Pediatrics*. 2020;146(1):e20191650.

295. O'Shea J, Dempsey EM. A comparison of blood pressure measurements in newborns. *Am J Perinatol*. 2009;26(2):113-116.

296. Troy R, Doron M, Laughon M, Tolleson-Rinehart S, Price W. Comparison of noninvasive and central arterial blood pressure measurements in ELBW infants. *J Perinatol*. 2009;29(11):744-749.

297. Lalan S, Blowey D. Comparison between oscillometric and intra-arterial blood pressure measurements in ill preterm and full-term neonates. *J Am Soc Hypertens*. 2014;8(1):36-44.

298. Nuntnarumit P, Yang W, Bada-Ellzey HS. Blood pressure measurements in the newborn. *Clinics in perinatology*. 1999;26(4):981-996.

299. Arafat M, Mattoo TK. Measurement of blood pressure in children: recommendations and perceptions on cuff selection. *Pediatrics*. 1999;104(3):e30.

300. Pejovic B, Peco-Antic A, Marinkovic-Eric J. Blood pressure in non-critically ill preterm and full-term neonates. *Pediatr Nephrol*. 2007;22(2):249-257.

301. Berger A. How does it work? Oscillatory blood pressure monitoring devices. *BMJ*. 2001;323:919.

302. DiFiore JM. Biomedical Engineering Aspects of Neonatal Cardiorespiratory Monitoring. In: Martin RJ, Fanaroff AA, Walsh MC, eds. *Fanaroff and Martin's Neonatal-Perinatal Medicine: Diseases of the Fetus and Infant*. 10 ed. Philadelphia: Elsevier Saunders; 2015:522-535.

303. Stebor AD. Basic principles of noninvasive blood pressure measurement in infants. *Adv Neonatal Care*. 2005;5(5):252-261; quiz 262-264.

304. Devinck A, Keukelier H, De Savoye I, Desmet L, Smets K. Neonatal blood pressure monitoring: visual assessment is an unreliable method for selecting cuff sizes. *Acta Paediatr.* 2013;102(10):961-964.

305. Kirk A. Pulmonology. In: Tschudy MM, Arcara KM, eds. *The Harriet Lane Handbook*. 19 ed. Philadelphia: Elsevier Mosby; 2012:584-605.

306. Nicks BA, McGinnis HD, Borron SW, et al. Acute Lactic Acidosis. 2018; https://emedicine.medscape.com/article/768159-overview. Accessed June 26, 2020.

307. Gunnerson KJ, Harvey CE, Talavera F, Pinksy MR, Franklin C. Lactic Acidosis. 2018; https://emedicine.medscape.com/article/167027-overview. Accessed June 26, 2020.

308. Wright CJ, Posencheg MA, Seri I, Evans JR. Fluid, Electrolyte, and Acid-Base Balance. In: Gleason CA, Juul SE, eds. *Avery's Diseases of the Newborn*. 10 ed. Philadelphia PA: Elsevier; 2018:368-389.

309. Askenazi D, Selewski D, Willig L, Warady BA. Acute Kidney Injury and Chronic Kidney Disease. In: Gleason CA, Juul SE, eds. *Avery's Diseases of the Newborn*. 10 ed. Philadelphia PA: Elsevier; 2018:1280-1307.

310. Workeneh BT, Agraharkar M, Gupta R, Lederer E, Batuman V. Acute Kidney Injury. 2018; https://emedicine.medscape.com/article/243492-overview. Accessed June 27, 2020.

311. Wandrup J, Kroner J, Pryds O, Kastrup KW. Age-related reference values for ionized calcium in the first week of life in premature and full-term neonates. *Scand J Clin Lab Invest.* 1988;48(3):255-260.

312. Loughead JL, Mimouni F, Tsang RC. Serum ionized calcium concentrations in normal neonates. *Am J Dis Child.* 1988;142(5):516-518.

313. Namgung Ran, Tsang RC. Neonatal Calcium, Phosphorus, and Magnesium Homeostasis. In: Polin RA, Fox WW, Abman SH, eds. *Fetal and Neonatal Physiology*. 4 ed. Philadelphia: Elsevier Saunders; 2011:384-402.

314. Abrams SA, Tiosano D. Disorders of Calcium, Phosphorus, and Magnesium Metabolism in the Neonate. In: Martin RJ, Fanaroff AA, Walsh MC, eds. *Fanaroff and Martin's Neonatal-Perinatal Medicine: Diseases of the Fetus and Infant*. 11 ed. Philadelphia: Elsevier; 2020:1611-1642.

315. AHA. Part 10 Recognition of Arrhythmias. In: Samson RA, Schexnayder SM, Hazinski MF, Meeks R, Knight LJ, eds. *Pediatric Advanced Life Support Provider Manual*. Dallas: American Heart Association; 2016:239-252.

316. Letterio J, Pateva I, Petrosiute A, Ahuja S. Hematologic and Oncologic Problems in the Fetus and Neonate. In: Martin RJ, Fanaroff AA, Walsh MC, eds. *Fanaroff and Martin's Neonatal-Perinatal Medicine: Diseases of the Fetus and Infant*. 11 ed. Philadelphia: Elsevier; 2020:1416-1475.

317. Medicine UNLo. Partial Thromboplastin Time (PTT) Test. 2020; https://medlineplus.gov/lab-tests/partial-thromboplastin-time-ptt-test/v. Accessed June 27, 2020.

318. Medicine UNLo. Prothrombin Time Test and INR (PT/INR). 2020; https://medlineplus.gov/lab-tests/prothrombin-time-test-and-inr-ptinr/. Accessed June 27, 2020.

319. Clinical Use of Coagulation Tests. UpToDate; 2020. Accessed June 27, 2020.

320. Ottolini MC, Lundgren K, Mirkinson LJ, Cason S, Ottolini MG. Utility of complete blood count and blood culture screening to diagnose neonatal sepsis in the asymptomatic at risk newborn. *Pediatr Infect Dis J.* 2003;22(5):430-434.

321. Christensen RD, Rothstein G, Hill HR, Hall RT. Fatal early onset group B streptococcal sepsis with normal leukocyte counts. *Pediatr Infect Dis.* 1985;4(3):242-245.

322. Del Vecchio A, Christensen RD. Neonatal neutropenia: what diagnostic evaluation is needed and when is treatment recommended? *Early Hum Dev.* 2012;88 Suppl 2:S19-24.

323. Schmutz N, Henry E, Jopling J, Christensen RD. Expected ranges for blood neutrophil concentrations of neonates: the Manroe and Mouzinho charts revisited. *J Perinatol.* 2008;28(4):275-281.

324. McPherson RJ, Juul S. Patterns of thrombocytosis and thrombocytopenia in hospitalized neonates. *J Perinatol.* 2005;25(3):166-172.

325. Wiedmeier SE, Henry E, Sola-Visner MC, Christensen RD. Platelet reference ranges for neonates, defined using data from over 47,000 patients in a multihospital healthcare system. *J Perinatol.* 2009;29(2):130-136.

326. Sola MC. Evaluation and treatment of severe and prolonged thrombocytopenia in neonates. *Clinics in perinatology.* 2004;31(1):1-14.

327. Sola-Visner M, Saxonhouse MA, Brown RE. Neonatal thrombocytopenia: what we do and don't know. *Early Hum Dev.* 2008;84(8):499-506.

328. Esper F. Postnatal Bacterial Infections. In: Martin RJ, Fanaroff AA, Walsh MC, eds. *Fanaroff and Martin's Neonatal-Perinatal Medicine: Diseases of the Fetus and Infant*. 11 ed. Philadelphia: Elsevier; 2020:789-808.

329. Ohls RK, Christensen RD, Kamath-Rayne BD, et al. A randomized, masked, placebo-controlled study of darbepoetin alfa in preterm infants. *Pediatrics.* 2013;132(1):e119-127.

330. Patel S, Ohls RK. Darbepoetin Administration in Term and Preterm Neonates. *Clin Perinatol.* 2015;42(3):557-566.

331. Messier AM, Ohls RK. Neuroprotective effects of erythropoiesis-stimulating agents in term and preterm neonates. *Curr Opin Pediatr.* 2014;26(2):139-145.

332. da Graca RL, Hassinger DC, Flynn PA, Sison CP, Nesin M, Auld PA. Longitudinal changes of brain-type natriuretic peptide in preterm neonates. *Pediatrics.* 2006;117(6):2183-2189.

333. El-Khuffash A, Molloy EJ. Are B-type natriuretic peptide (BNP) and N-terminal-pro-BNP useful in neonates? *Archives of disease in childhood Fetal and neonatal edition.* 2007;92(4):F320-324.

334. Farombi-Oghuvbu I, Matthews T, Mayne PD, Guerin H, Corcoran JD. N-terminal pro-B-type natriuretic peptide: a measure of significant patent ductus arteriosus. *Archives of disease in childhood Fetal and neonatal edition.* 2008;93(4):F257-260.

335. Koch A, Singer H. Normal values of B type natriuretic peptide in infants, children, and adolescents. *Heart.* 2003;89(8):875-878.

336. Davlouros PA, Karatza AA, Xanthopoulou I, et al. Diagnostic role of plasma BNP levels in neonates with signs of congenital heart disease. *Int J Cardiol.* 2011;147(1):42-46.

337. Maisel A. Updated algorithms for using B-type natriuretic peptide (BNP) levels in the diagnosis and management of congestive heart failure. *Crit Pathw Cardiol.* 2004;3(3):144-149.

338. Cantinotti M, Passino C, Storti S, Ripoli A, Zyw L, Clerico A. Clinical relevance of time course of BNP levels in neonates with congenital heart diseases. *Clin Chim Acta.* 2011;412(23-24):2300-2304.

339. Nir A, Lindinger A, Rauh M, et al. NT-pro-B-type natriuretic peptide in infants and children: reference values based on combined data from four studies. *Pediatr Cardiol.* 2009;30(1):3-8.

References

340. Kulkarni M, Gokulakrishnan G, Price J, Fernandes CJ, Leeflang M, Pammi M. Diagnosing significant PDA using natriuretic peptides in preterm neonates: a systematic review. *Pediatrics.* 2015;135(2):e510-525.

341. Ko HK, Lee JH, Choi BM, et al. Utility of the rapid B-type natriuretic peptide assay for detection of cardiovascular problems in newborn infants with respiratory difficulties. *Neonatology.* 2008;94(1):16-21.

342. Chong D, Chua YT, Chong SL, Ong GY. What Raises Troponins in the Paediatric Population? *Pediatr Cardiol.* 2018;39(8):1530-1534.

343. Zaidi AN, Daniels CJ. Myocardial Ischemia in the Pediatric Population. In: Allen HD, Shaddy RE, Penny DJ, Feltes TF, Cetta F, eds. *Moss and Adams' Heart Disease in Infants, Children, and Adolescents.* 9 ed. Philadelphia: Wolters Kluwer; 2016:1455-1463.

344. Trevisanuto D, Picco G, Golin R, et al. Cardiac troponin I in asphyxiated neonates. *Biol Neonate.* 2006;89(3):190-193.

345. Bader D, Kugelman A, Lanir A, Tamir A, Mula E, Riskin A. Cardiac troponin I serum concentrations in newborns: a study and review of the literature. *Clin Chim Acta.* 2006;371(1-2):61-65.

346. Mahajan VS, Jarolim P. How to interpret elevated cardiac troponin levels. *Circulation.* 2011;124(21):2350-2354.

347. Trevisanuto D, Picco G, Golin R, et al. Cardiac troponin I in asphyxiated neonates. *Biol Neonate.* 2006;89(3):190-193.

348. Mitchell AL. Congenital Anomalies. In: Martin RJ, Fanaroff AA, Walsh MC, eds. *Fanaroff and Martin's Neonatal-Perinatal Medicine: Diseases of the Fetus and Infant.* 11 ed. Philadelphia: Elsevier; 2020:489-511.

349. Cassidy SB, Allanson JE. Introduction. In: Cassidy SB, Allanson JE, eds. *Management of Genetic Syndromes.* 3 ed. Hoboken NJ: John Wiley & Sons; 2010:1-7.

350. Gardner RM, Sutherland GR, Shaffer LG. Chromosome Analysis. *Chromosome Abnormalities and Genetic Counseling.* 4 ed. New York, NY: Oxford University Press; 2012:21-26.

351. Treff NR, Levy B, Su J, Northrop LE, Tao X, Scott RT. SNP microarray-based 24 chromosome aneuploidy screening is significantly more consistent than FISH. *MHR: Basic science of reproductive medicine.* 2010;16(8):583-589.

352. Cheng EY. Prenatal Diagnosis. In: Gleason CA, Juul SE, eds. *Avery's Diseases of the Newborn.* 10 ed. Philadelphia PA: Elsevier; 2018:190-200.

353. American College of Obstetricians and Gynecologists' Committee on Practice Bulletins—Obstetrics, Committee on Genetics, and the Society for Maternal–Fetal Medicine. Practice Bulletin No. 162: Prenatal Diagnostic Testing for Genetic Disorders. *Obstet Gynecol.* 2016;127(5):e108-122.

354. Gregg AR, Skotko BG, Benkendorf JL, et al. Noninvasive prenatal screening for fetal aneuploidy, 2016 update: a position statement of the American College of Medical Genetics and Genomics. *Genet Med.* 2016;18(10):1056-1065.

355. Miller DT, Adam MP, Aradhya S, et al. Consensus statement: chromosomal microarray is a first-tier clinical diagnostic test for individuals with developmental disabilities or congenital anomalies. *Am J Hum Genet.* 2010;86(5):749-764.

356. Borghesi A, Mencarelli MA, Memo L, et al. Intersociety policy statement on the use of whole-exome sequencing in the critically ill newborn infant. *Ital J Pediatr.* 2017;43(1):100.

357. Belkadi A, Bolze A, Itan Y, et al. Whole-genome sequencing is more powerful than whole-exome sequencing for detecting exome variants. *Proc Natl Acad Sci U S A.* 2015;112(17):5473-5478.

358. Meienberg J, Bruggmann R, Oexle K, Matyas G. Clinical sequencing: is WGS the better WES? *Hum Genet.* 2016;135(3):359-362.

359. Friedman SH, Thomson-Salo F, Ballard AR. Support for the Family. In: Martin RJ, Fanaroff AA, Walsh MC, eds. *Fanaroff and Martin's Neonatal-Perinatal Medicine: Diseases of the Fetus and Infant.* 11 ed. Philadelphia: Elsevier; 2020:690-702.

360. Lee AY, Taghon T, McClead R, Crandall W, Davis T, Brilli RJ. Safety and Quality in the Heart Center. In: Allen HD, Shaddy RE, Penny DJ, Feltes TF, Cetta F, eds. *Moss and Adams' Heart Disease in Infants, Children, and Adolescents.* 9 ed. Philadelphia: Wolters Kluwer; 2016:1781-1793.

361. Gooding JS, Cooper LG, Blaine AI, Franck LS, Howse JL, Berns SD. Family support and family-centered care in the neonatal intensive care unit: origins, advances, impact. *Semin Perinatol.* 2011;35(1):20-28.

362. Bracht M, O'Leary L, Lee S, O'Brien K. Implementing family-integrated care in the NICU: a parent education and support program. *Adv Neonatal Care.* 2013;13(2):115-126.

Index

The letter f after a page number indicates a figure and the letter t indicates a table.

A

Acidosis, 29, 30, 43, 65
  reverse, 96
Adenosine, 36–37
  adverse reactions, 37
  dose and, 36
  drug interactions, 37
  patient monitoring and, 36
  warnings/precautions, 37
Airway module
  O_2 content and, 160
  O_2 saturation, hemoglobin, and CHD, 160
Anti-factor Xa activity, 171
Aortic run-off lesion, 18
Aortic valve, 78
  bicuspid, 78
  unicuspid, 78
Aortic valve stenosis (AS), 44, 78, 79f, 188f
  anatomic features of critical, 78f
  critical, 188f
    with a closing ductus arteriosus, 79f
Aortic valvotomy, 188f
Arteriovenous malformation (AVM), 44
Asplenia syndrome, 58, 60f, 61t
Atrial septal defect (ASD), 13, 15, 15f, 16
Atrioventricular canal defect, 13
Atrioventricular discordance, 144
Atrioventricular septal defect, 13
Atrioventricular valve (AV), 14, 14f
Auscultation of the heart, 49
Autoimmune disorders, 31

B

Balloon atrial septostomy, 143, 143f
Balloon valvuloplasty, 188f, 198f
  pulmonary atresia post, 181f
Beta blockers, 95
Bilateral left-sidedness, 58
Bilateral right-sidedness, 58
Blalock Taussig shunt, 192
  emergency placement of, 96
Blood gas, 168
Blood pressure module, 166-167
  measuring blood pressure
    arm/leg, 42
    arterial, 166
    oscillometric, 166–167, 167f
Blood sugar, 168
Blood urea nitrogen (BUN), 169
Bradycardia, 30
Bradypnea, 29
Bronchopulmonary dysplasia, 26
B-type natriuretic peptide (BNP), 173

C

Calcium, ionized, 170
Capillary refill time (CRT), 46, 47f
Cardiac decompensation, 43
Cardiac disease, features of pulmonary disease versus, 65t

Cardiac output, 32
Cardiogenic shock, 148
Cardiopulmonary bypass, 180
Central cyanosis, 25
CHARGE syndrome, 20, 20f, 175
  CHD7 gene, 20
  clinical characteristics of, 21t
  diagnosing, 20, 21t
  most common cardiac defects, 20
Chromosomal microarray analysis, 175
Chromosome analysis, 174
Coagulation tests, 171
Coaptation defect, 120
Coarctation of the aorta (COA), 74, 74f, 75f, 120, 184f
  surgical repair of the aortic arch, 184–185f
Color, skin, 25
  abnormal, 25
  normal, 25
Complete atrioventricular septal defect (AVSD), 14
  balanced, 14
  unbalanced, 14
Complete blood count with differential, 172
Complete heart block, 30, 31f
  primary causes of, 31–32
Congenital heart defects
  critical, 3
  exposures that increase risk for, 6t
Congenital heart disease (CHD)
  ductal dependency and, 68
    left-sided obstructive lesions, 68
    right-sided obstructive lesions, 68
  incidence of, 3, 3f
  infants born with, per year, 3f
  options for palliation or surgical repair of, 179–215
  stabilizing the cyanotic neonate with suspected, 86
  syndromes and chromosomal abnormalities associated with, 13
    CHARGE syndrome, 20, 20f
    monosomy X (Turner syndrome--XO chromosomes), 19, 19f
    trisomy 13 (Patau syndrome), 17, 17f, 172, 174
    trisomy 18 (Edwards syndrome), 16, 16f, 172, 174
    trisomy 21 (Down syndrome), 13, 13f, 172, 174
    22q11.2 deletion syndrome, 22–23, 23f, 175
    VACTERL association, 22, 22f
  U.S. annual rate of, 3f
Congestive heart failure (CHF)
  respiratory signs of, 29
Conotruncal area, 24, 24f
Creatinine, 169
Critical congenital heart defects (CCHD), 3
Critical congenital heart disease, 162
  pulse oximetry screening (POS) for, 162–165, 165f
  screening protocols for, 164, 164f, 165f
  timing of screening, 163, 163f
Cyanosis, 25

central, 25
  reverse differential, 28, 28f, 139, 139f
Cyanotic congenital heart disease, 86, 86f, 197f, 207f
  ductal dependent for pulmonary blood flow, 125-145, 125f
  not ductal dependent, 87-123
Cyanotic neonate
  stabilizing with ductal dependent pulmonary blood flow, 125, 125f
  stabilizing with suspected congenital heart disease, 86

D

Dextrocardia, 58, 59f
  with situs inversus totalis, 58, 59f
DiGeorge syndrome (22 q211.2 deletion syndrome), 22-23, 23f, 175
Diagnostic tests
  cardiomegaly, 62, 62f
  chest x-ray, 62
  echocardiogram, 63, 63f
  electrocardiogram (ECG), 63
  pulmonary vascular markings (PVM), 62
Differential diagnosis, 64, 65t
Diuretics, 84
Dopamine, 84
Double outlet right ventricle (DORV), 16, 98–101, 98f
  anatomic features of, 98
  with noncommitted VSD, 100
  with subaortic VSD, 99, 99f
    pulmonary stenosis and, 99
    without pulmonary stenosis, 99
  with subpulmonic VSD, 100
  surgical repair of, 100–101, 100f, 101f
  types of, 99–100
Ductus arteriosus (DA), 68, 69f
  stent for, 196f, 199f, 209

E

Ebstein anomaly, 120–124
  anatomic features of, 120f, 121f
  associated defects of, 121
  chest x-ray and
    heart size and shape, 122
    pulmonary vasculature, 122
  clinical presentation, 122, 122f
    arrhythmia and, 122
    congestive heart failure and, 122
    cyanosis, 122
    heart murmur and, 122
    initial stabilization and, 123, 123f
    surgical repair-cone repair, 206f
    underlying concepts, 124
Echocardiogram, 63, 63f
Electrocardiogram (ECG), 63
Electrolytes and renal function tests, 169
Emotional support module, 176–177, 176f, 177f
Endocardial cushion defect, 13
Eosinophils, 172
Epinephrine, 84
Erythropoiesis-stimulating agents (ESAs), 172
Esmolol, 95

Index

F

Fatty tissue necrosis, 35
Fibrinogen, 171
Fluorescence in situ hybridization (FISH)
    process, 174–175
Fontan connection, 181f
Foramen ovale, 81

G

Gasping, 29
Genetic testing, 174–175
Gestational diabetes and obesity, 10, 10f
Glenn shunt, 181f, 193f, 203f
Glucose, 148
    production rate, 148
    utilization rate, 148

H

Heart murmur, 52
    blood forced through a narrowed area
        such as a ventricular septal defect, 52
    blood forced through a stenotic valve, 52
        blood forced through stenotic
    pulmonary arteries, 52
    blood forced through stenotic systemic
        arteries, 52
    bruit, 44
    increased blood flow across normal
        structures, 52
    non pathologic murmurs
        closure of the ductus arteriosus, 55
        peripheral pulmonic stenosis, 55
        Still's murmur, 55
    pathologic, 56
    regurgitation of blood through an
        incompetent valve, 52
    systemic approach to auscultating for a,
        53, 53f
    systolic ejection, 78, 82
    thrill, 54
    timing, 54
Heart sounds, 49–51
Hemi-Fontan operation, 193f
Heterotaxy, 58
History and patient assessment
    congenital heart disease (CHD)
        exposures that increase risk for, 6t
        incidence of, 3
    history and patient presentation, 4
    maternal medical history, 5
    neonatal history, 4
    pregnancy, labor, and delivery history, 4–5
    recurrence risk, 5
Hydrops fetalis (HF), 32
Hyperactive precordium, 18, 48
Hypercyanotic/tet spells, 93–97, 93f, 94f
    causes of, 93–94
    treatment of, 95–96, 97t
Hyperkalemia, 169
Hyperpneic respirations, attempt to
    decrease, 96
Hypertrophic cardiomyopathy (HCM), 11
Hyperviscosity, signs of, 25
Hypocalcemia, 170

Hypokalemia, 169
Hypomagnesemia, 170
Hyponatremia, 169
Hypoplastic left heart syndrome (HLHS),
    80–81, 190–196f
    anatomic features of, 80f
    case study of 1-day old infant with, 85
    with a closing ductus arteriosus, 81f
    dependent upon a right-to-left shunt at
        the ductus arteriosus for systemic
        perfusion, 69f
    hybrid approach, 196f
    Norwood procedure for, 180
    post Fontan procedure, 181f
    procedural steps--Hemi-Fontan
        procedure, 194f
    stage 1 Norwood operation, 191–192f
    stage 2 operation, 193f
    stage 3 Fontan operation, 195f
Hypothalamus, 158
Hypothermia, 158
Hypoxemia, 30, 159
Hypoxia, 159
    tissue, 159

I

"Icing" vagal maneuver, performing, 34–35
Infant of the diabetic mother (IDM), 10
    congenital heart disease (CHD), 11
    hypertrophic cardiomyopathy (HCM), 11
Inotropes, 84
International normalized ratio (INR), 171
Interrupted aortic arch (IAA), 76–77, 76f,
    186–187f
    anatomic features of, 76f
    surgical repair of, 184–187f
    with a closing ductus arteriosus, 77f
Intracardiac defect (ASD), 124
Ionized calcium, 170

K

Karyotype, 174

L

Lab work module, 168–173
    blood gas, 168
    blood sugar, 168
    electrolytes and renal function tests,
        169–170
        blood urea nitrogen (BUN) and
            creatinine, 169
        cardiac enzymes: B- type natriuretic
            peptide (BNP) and troponin, 173
        complete blood count with
            differential, 172
        ionized calcium, 170
        liver function tests (LFTs), 171
        magnesium, 170–171
        sodium and potassium, 169
    lactic acid/lactate, 168–169
Lactic acid, 168–169
Large for gestational age (LGA), 9, 9f
Left isomerism, 58
Left-sided obstructive lesions, 73-85, 73f,
    183f

clinical presentation, 82, 83f
    chest x-ray and, 82, 83f
    cyanosis and, 82
    heart sounds and, 82
    murmur and, 82
initial stabilization and, 84
    blood pressure support and, 84
    NICU management and, 84
    O₂ saturation goal and, 84
    PGE infusion and, 84
    respiratory support and, 84
Left-sided organs, 58
Left-to-right shunt, 68, 69f, 124
Levocardia, 58
Liver enzymes, 171
Liver function tests (LFTs), 171
Liver size and location, 57, 57f
L-transposition, 145, 145f
Lung parenchymal disease, 26
Lymphocytes, 172

M

Magnesium, 170–171
Maternal autoimmune disease, 32
Maternal medical history, 5
Meconium aspiration syndrome, 26
Milrinone, 84
Monocytes, 172

N

Near Infrared Reflective Spectroscopy (NIRS)
    Monitoring, 161
Necrosis, fatty tissue, 35
Neonatal history, 4
Neurologic status, 8
Neutrophils, 172
Next generation sequencing (NGS), 175

O

Obstructive shock, 148
Oscillometric measurement, 166–167, 167f

P

Partial thromboplastin time (PTT), 171
Patent ductus arteriosus (PDA), 13, 16
    as hemodynamically significant, 18
    persistent, 18
Patient assessment, 8–64
Peripheral arterial line (PAL), 152
Persistent patent ductus arteriosus (PDA), 18
Pharmacology prostaglandin E1, 70–72, 70f
    actions, 70
    dose, 70
    indications, 70
    infusion rules, 71
    side effects, 71
    treatment goals, 70
Platelets, 172
Pneumonia, 26
Point of maximal impulse (PMI), 48
Polysplenia syndrome, 58, 60t, 61t
Polyvalvular disease, 16
Potassium, 169
Precordial activity, 48
Preductal and postductal O₂ saturation, 26
    monitoring, 27

Pregnancy, labor, and delivery history, 4–5
Prenatal cell-free DNA (cfDNA) testing, 174
Preterm infant, respiratory distress in, 4
Propranol, 95
Prostaglandin E2 (PGE2), 18
Prothrombin time (PT), 171
Pulmonary atresia
    dependent upon a left-to-right shunt
        at the ductus atteriosus for pulmonary
        perfusion, 69f
    with intact ventricular septum (PA-IVS),
        125f, 126–130
        anatomic features of, 126f, 127f
        clinical presentation, 128–129, 129f
        initial stabilization, 128
        surgical and palliative options,
            208–211f
        ventriculocoronary connections and,
            130, 131f
    with ventricular septal defect (PA-VSD),
        125f, 132–135, 132f, 133f, 212f
        chest x-ray, 135
            heart shape, 135
            heart size, 135
            pulmonary vasculature, 135
        clinical presentation, 134–135, 134f,
            135f
            cyanosis, 134
            heart sounds, 134
            murmur, 134
        initial stabilization, 135
        and major aortopulmonary collateral
            arteries, (MAPCAs) 213f
        Pulmonary atresia post balloon
            valvuloplasty, 181f
Pulmonary disease, features of cardiac
    disease versus, 65t
Pulmonary hypertension of the newborn
    (PPHN), 4
Pulmonary stenosis (PS), 16
    subvalvar, 98
    valvar, 98
Pulmonary vascular markings (PVM), 62
Pulmonary vascular resistance (PVR), 93
Pulse
    abnormal, 45
    bounding, 45
    brachial, 44, 45, 104
    classification of, 44
    difficult to feel, 45
    femoral, 44, 45, 104
    normal, 44
    pedal, 44
    posterior tibialis, 44
Pulse oximetry, 161
    screening for critical congenital heart
        disease (CCHD), 162–165, 162f
        CCHD screen protocols, 164, 164f,
            165f
        purpose of POS, 162
        timing of CCHD screening, 163, 163f
Pulse pressure, 40
    causes of narrow or wide, 41f

R
Recommended universal newborn screening
    panel (RUSP), 162
Recurrence risk, 5
Regional oximetry monitoring–near infrared
    reflective spectroscopy (NIRS)monitoring,
    161
Respiratory distress syndrome, 26
Respiratory signs of CHF, 29
Reverse acidosis, 96
Reverse differential cyanosis, 28, 28f, 136,
    139, 139f
Right isomerism, 58
Right-sided organs, 58
Right-to-left shunt, 68, 69f
Right ventricular outflow tract (RVOT) stent,
    199f
Ross procedure, 189f

S
Sano shunt, 192
Secundum ASD, 15
Sepsis, risk factors for, 4–5
Shock, 43
    septic/distributive, 45
Single nucleotide polymorphism (SNP), 175
Single ventricle palliation, 181f
Sinus bradycardia, 30
Sinus tachycardia, 32
    versus supraventricular tachycardia, 32
Situs inversus, 13, 16
Situs solitus, 58
Sjögren syndrome, 31
Skin perfusion and appearance, 46
Small for gestational age (SGA) infants, 12, 12f
Sodium, 169
S.T.A.B.L.E. Program, 1
Subvalvar pulmonary stenosis, 98
Sugar and safe care module, 147–157
    glucose production and utilization rate,
        148
    initial IV fluid rate and target glucose
        levels, 147–148
    IV access and central lines, 149, 149f
    peripherally inserted central catheter
        (PICC), 155–156, 156f, 157f
    umbilical artery catheter (UAC) and
        peripheral arterial line (PAL), 152,
        152f, 153f
    umbilical catheter safety, 154
    umbilical vein catheter, 150, 151f
Supraventricular tachycardia (SVT), 33, 33f
    adenosine in treating, 36–37
    Ebstein anomaly and, 121
    sinus tachycardia versus, 32
    termination of, 34, 36, 37
    treatment of, 34
Systematic vascular resistance (SVR), 93
Systemic lupus erythematosus, 31

T
Tachycardia, 32
    supraventricular, 33, 33f
Tachypnea, 29
Targeted gene panel (TGP), 175
Temperature module, 158, 158f
Tetralogy of Fallot (TOF), 13, 16, 87f, 88–92
    clinical presentation
        anatomic features of, 88f
        chest x-ray, 91, 91f
        cyanosis
            acyanotic ("pink tet"), 90
            cyanotic ("blue tet"), 90
        heart shape, 91
        heart sounds, 90
        initial stabilization, 92, 92f
        murmur, 90
        with severe PS, 89f
    Surgical repair of, 201f
    palliative options for, 198–200f
Thermoregulation, 158
Third-degree atrioventricular block, 30
Thrombocytes, 172
Tissue hypoxia, 159
Torsades de Pointes, 171
Total anomalous pulmonary venous
    connection (TAPVC), 87f, 112–121
    cardiac, 116, 116f
    chest x-ray
        with obstruction, 118
        without obstruction, 118
    clinical presentation
        with obstruction, 118
        without obstruction, 118
    infracardiac, 117, 117f
    initial stabilization
        without obstruction, 119
        with obstruction, 119
    supracardiac, 114, 114f, 115f
    total anomalous pulmonary venous,
        118–119, 119f
    types of, 112–113, 112f, 113f
Transposition of the great arteries (TGA),
    124, 125f, 136–143, 136f, 137f
    arterial switch operation, 214–215f
    chest x-ray, 140, 140f
        heart size and pulmonary vasculature,
            140, 140f
    clinical presentation, 138–139, 138f
        cyanosis, 138
        reverse differential cyanosis, 139
    D-TGA, difference between L-TGA and,
        144–145
    initial stabilization--TGA with IVS, 141–
        142
Tricuspid atresia, 87f, 102–107, 202–203f
    anatomic features of, 102f
    chest x-ray
        heart size, 106
        pulmonary vasculature, 106
    clinical presentation, 104
        cyanosis, 104, 105f
    clinical presentation of
        heart sounds, 104
        murmur, 104
        pulses, 104

Index

T (continued)

thrill, 104
with congenitally corrected transposition of the great arteries, 102
with D-TGA, 106f
initial stabilization, 108
with normally related great arteries, 102, 102f, 106f
with transposition of the great arteries, 102, 103, 103f, 107f
Trisomy 13 (Patau syndome), 17, 17f, 172, 174
Trisomy 18 (Edwards syndrome), 16, 16f, 172, 174
Trisomy 21 (Down syndrome), 13, 13f, 172, 174
Troponin, 173
Truncus arteriosus, 87f, 108–111, 204–205f
anatomic features of, 108, 108f
clinical presentation of, 110f
chest x-ray, 110, 111f
congestive heart failure, 110
cyanosis, 110
heart sounds, 110
murmur, 110
initial stabilization, 111, 111f
post surgical repair, 181f
truncal valve, 108
types of, 109, 109f

U

Umbilical artery catheter (UAC), 152
Umbilical catheter safety, 154
Umbilical vein catheter (UVC), 150
Urea, 169

V

VACTERL association, 22, 22f
Vagal maneuvers, 35f
Valvar stenosis, 98
Velo-cardio-facial syndrome, 22
Velopharyngeal incompetence, 23
Ventricle palliation, single, 181f
Ventricular inversion, 144
Ventricular septal defect (VSD), 13, 16, 76
incidence and location, 15, 15f
Vital signs
blood pressure (BP), 38, 39f, 40
heart rate and rhythm, 30
respiratory rate and effort, 29

W

White blood cells, 172
types of, 173
Whole exome sequencing (WES), 175
Whole genome sequencing (WGS), 175
William's syndrome, 175
Wolff-Parkinson-White syndrome, 122